Bone Marrow

abbreviation	expansion
AS-PCR	allele-specific
CBC	complete blood count
CEP	centromere enumeration probes
CMA	chromosomal microarray
CT	computed tomography
DNA	deoxyribonucleic acid
EDTA	ethylenediaminetetraacetic acid
FFPE	formalin-fixed paraffin embedded
FISH	fluorescence in situ hybridization
HCT	hematocrit
HGB	hemoglobin
Ig	immunoglobulin
IHC	immunohistochemistry
LOH	loss of heterozygosity
MCV	mean corpuscular volume
MRD	minimal residual disease
NCCN	National Comprehensive Cancer Network
NGS	next generation sequencing
PCR	polymerase chain reaction
PET	positron emission tomography
qPCR	quantitative PCR
qRT-PCR	quantitative RT-PCR
RBC	red blood cell
RNA	ribonucleic acid
RT-PCR	reverse transcriptase PCR
SNP	single nucleotide polymorphism
VAF	variant allele frequency
WBC	white blood cell
WHO	World Health Organization

Rose C Beck & Erika M Moore

MOLECULAR HEMATOPATHOLOGY
An Integrated Case-Based Approach

Publishing Team

Jeffrey Carlson (design)
Erik N Tanck & Annabelle Ulalulae (production)
Joshua Weikersheimer (publishing direction)

Notice

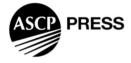

ISBN 978-089189-6814

Printed in the United States of America

25 24 23 22 21

MOLECULAR
HEMATOPATHOLOGY
An Integrated Case-Based Approach

Rose C Beck, MD, PhD
Associate Professor, Department of Pathology
Director, Hematopathology Fellowship
Director, Hematology Laboratory
University Hospitals of Cleveland, Case Western Reserve University School of Medicine
Cleveland, Ohio

Erika M Moore, MD
Assistant Professor of Pathology, Division of Hematopathology
Director, Hematology Laboratory
University of Pittsburgh School of Medicine
Pittsburgh, Pennsylvania

Contributors
(by last name)

Rose C Beck, MD, PhD
Associate Professor, Department of Pathology
Director, Hematopathology Fellowship
Director, Hematology Laboratory
University Hospitals of Cleveland,
Case Western Reserve University School of Medicine
Cleveland, Ohio

Ramya Gadde, MBBS
Assistant Professor, Department of Pathology
University Hospitals of Cleveland,
Case Western Reserve University School of Medicine
Cleveland, Ohio

Catherine Gestrich, DO
Resident in Pathology, Department of Pathology
University Hospitals of Cleveland,
Case Western Reserve University School of Medicine
Cleveland, Ohio

Nathaniel Havens, DO
Resident in Pathology, Department of Pathology
University Hospitals of Cleveland, Case Western
Reserve University School of Medicine
Cleveland, Ohio

Annette S Kim, MD, PhD
Associate Professor, Department of Pathology
Brigham & Women's Hospital, Harvard Medical School
Boston, Massachusetts

Jingwei Li, MD, PhD
Resident in Pathology, Department of Pathology
Brigham & Women's Hospital, Harvard Medical School
Boston, Massachusetts

Howard J Meyerson, MD
Professor, Department of Pathology
Section Head of Hematopathology
Director, Flow Cytometry Laboratory
University Hospitals of Cleveland,
Case Western Reserve University School of Medicine
Cleveland, Ohio

Erika M Moore, MD
Assistant Professor of Pathology,
Division of Hematopathology
Director, Hematology Laboratory
University of Pittsburgh School of Medicine
Pittsburgh, Pennsylvania

Amelia Nakanishi, MD
Fellow in Forensic Pathology
Miami Dade Medical Examiner Department
Miami, Florida

Megan O Nakashima, MD
Assistant Professor, Pathology & Laboratory Medicine
Institute
Director, Hematopathology Fellowship
Cleveland Clinic Lerner College of Medicine
Staff Hematopathologist, Cleveland Clinic
Cleveland, Ohio

Valentina Nardi, MD
Assistant Professor, Department of Pathology
Massachusetts General Hospital,
Harvard Medical School
Boston, Massachusetts

Priyatharsini Nirmalanantham
Resident in Pathology, Department of Pathology
University Hospitals of Cleveland,
Case Western Reserve University School of Medicine
Cleveland, Ohio

Kwadwo Oduro, MD, PhD
Assistant Professor, Department of Pathology
University Hospitals of Cleveland,
Case Western Reserve University School of Medicine
Cleveland, Ohio

Sarah Ondrejka, DO
Assistant Professor, Pathology & Laboratory Medicine
Institute
Cleveland Clinic Lerner College of Medicine
Medical Director, Manual Hematology Laboratory
Staff Hematopathologist, Cleveland Clinic
Cleveland, Ohio

Herleen Rai, MD
Clinical Fellow in Transfusion Medicine, Department of
Transfusion Medicine
National Institutes of Health (NIH)
Bethesda, Maryland

Bryan Rea, MD
Assistant Professor of Pathology
Department of Pathology, Division of Hematopathology
University of Pittsburgh School of Medicine
Pittsburgh, Pennsylvania

Christopher B Ryder, MD, PhD
Assistant Professor, Department of Pathology
University Hospitals of Cleveland,
Case Western Reserve University School of Medicine
Cleveland, Ohio

Shashirekha Shetty, PhD
Associate Professor, Department of Pathology
Director, Cytogenetics Laboratory,
Center for Human Genetics
Associate Director, Laboratory Genetics & Genomics
Fellowship Program
University Hospitals of Cleveland,
Case Western Reserve University School of Medicine
Cleveland, Ohio

Theresa Spivey, MD
Resident in Pathology, Department of Pathology
University Hospitals of Cleveland,
Case Western Reserve University School of Medicine
Cleveland, Ohio

Olga Weinberg, MD
Associate Professor, Harvard Medical School
Director of Hematopathology & Flow Cytometry
Boston Children's Hospital
Boston, Massachusetts

John Van Arnam, MD, MS
Houston, Texas

David Zemmour, MD, PhD
Fellow in Hematopathology, Department of Pathology
Brigham & Women's Hospital, Harvard Medical School
Boston, Massachusetts

*Special thanks to Navid Sadri, MD, PhD, and Jennifer
Yoest, MD, from the University Hospitals of Cleveland
Division of Genomic & Molecular Pathology, for their
valued expertise.*

Contents

ISBN 978-089189-6814

Part 2: Lymphoid & histiocytic neoplasms

 ISBN 978-089189-6814

Self-Study & Reference

                                              ISBN 978-089189-6814

Rose C Beck & Erika M Moore

P

Preface

In the last 30 years, the field of hematopathology has undergone several revolutionary periods, including the development of a classification system defining distinct, "real" entities (later evolved to the current WHO classification of hematologic neoplasms), advances in sophisticated immunophenotyping such as flow cytometry, and most recently, an explosion in molecular/genetic testing that greatly expands how we understand the pathophysiology of hematologic disease.

The aim of this book is to provide readers a practical learning experience through actual hematopathology cases where a combination of morphologic analysis, flow cytometry, and genetic testing (cytogenetics, FISH, PCR, and/or NGS) was used at diagnostic evaluation. Although genetic testing is also used in benign hematology, the focus of this book is on neoplastic hematopoietic disorders and related conditions. The goal was not simply to include an example of every hematologic neoplasm having a defined cytogenetic or molecular abnormality, but to include cases whose evaluations illustrate how specific chromosomal and molecular findings are used for diagnosis, prognostication, and/or consideration for targeted therapy. Entities are named according to the 2017 WHO Classification of Tumours of Haematopoietic and Lymphoid Tissues.

Many of the individual case chapters include summary tables which compare the described malignancy with similar entities, so that even if a specific hematologic neoplasm is not represented as a chapter, it will likely be included in one of these summary tables. Two sets of quiz questions are also provided for aiding in self-study. The Appendices briefly review basic cytogenetic and molecular techniques and standard nomenclature, with a guide to reading the NGS figures presented in some chapters.

The reaches, applications, and ramifications of the genomic revolution are still being developed and explored, and we as pathologists have much to anticipate in the years to come. We hope this book inspires and excites the reader by demonstrating how novel advances in molecular and cellular biology translate to modern pathology practice.

Rose C Beck, MD, PhD
Associate Professor of Pathology
University Hospitals of Cleveland, Case Western Reserve University
Cleveland, Ohio

Erika M Moore, MD
Assistant Professor of Pathology
University of Pittsburgh Medical School
Pittsburgh, Pennsylvania

Howard Meyerson

1

Chronic myeloid leukemia presenting with t(9;22)(q34.1;q11.2) *BCR-ABL1* & trisomy 8

History A 57-year-old woman with a past medical history of obesity, hypertension and diabetes was noted to have leukocytosis on a routine CBC at her primary care physician's office. She demonstrated no specific symptoms other than mild shortness of breath. The patient had an "intentional" weight loss of 60 lb over the last year. The spleen was not palpable due to body habitus. The CBC is shown in the table to the right.

The patient was sent to the emergency department and admitted for further evaluation. A bone marrow biopsy was performed with flow cytometry and genetic studies.

Morphology & flow cytometry The peripheral blood smear revealed a marked granulocytic left shift with predominance of myelocytes and without toxic changes **f1.1**. Blasts were increased but <10% of WBCs, and basophils were detected at 3%. No dysplasia was noted. The bone marrow aspirate smear was hypercellular, with increased myeloid:erythroid ratio of 12:1 and a myelocyte "bulge" in the differential. Blasts were enumerated at 1.5% in the aspirate. The clot section and trephine core biopsy were markedly hypercellular (~100% cellularity) and demonstrated granulocyte predominance, small hypolobate megakaryocytes, and scattered foamy histiocytes **f1.2**. Blast clusters were not seen. Flow cytometry revealed a granulocyte predominance and 1% blasts without a phenotypic abnormality, although monocytes showed partial expression of CD56.

Genetics/molecular results Chromosome analysis revealed 47,XX,+8,t(9;22)(q34;q11.2) in all 20 metaphases **f1.3**. FISH was positive for *BCR-ABL1* rearrangement in 97% of cells **f1.4**. The normalized copy number (NCN) of *BCR-ABL* fusion transcripts (*BCR-ABL/ABL*) as determined by qRT-PCR

WBC	327.9 × 10⁹/L
Differential	
Polymorphonuclear leukocytes	32%
Bands	19%
Lymphocytes	1%
Monocytes	2%
Eosinophils	2%
Basophils	3%
Metamyelocytes	9%
Myelocytes	20%
Promyelocytes	9%
Blasts	3%
RBC	2.81 × 10¹²/L
HGB	9.9 g/dL
HCT	29.0%
MCV	103 fL
RDW	21.4%
Platelets	169 × 10⁹/L

was 78.122% for the major breakpoint using the international scale (IS) and 0.13% NCN for the minor breakpoint fusion. A diagnosis of **chronic myeloid leukemia with trisomy 8** was rendered.

Discussion Chronic myeloid leukemia (CML) is characterized by the presence of the Philadelphia (Ph) chromosome, t(9;22)(q34;q11.2), which results from translocation of *ABL1* on chromosome 9 to *BCR* on chromosome 22 in a pluripotent hematopoietic stem cell. The resulting fusion leads to a constitutively active ABL1 kinase that drives multiple molecular

ISBN 978-0891896-6814

1 *Chronic myeloid leukemia presenting with t(9;22)(q34.1;q11.2) BCR-ABL1 & trisomy 8*

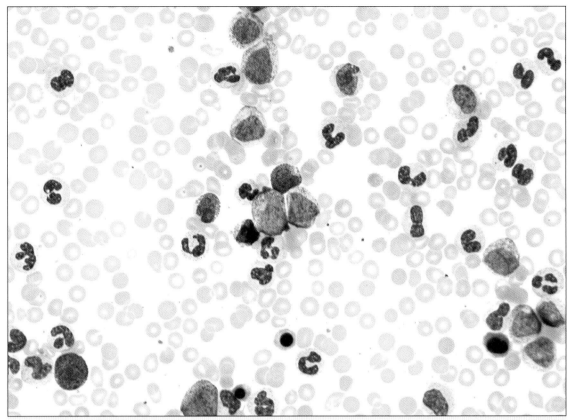

f1.1 Peripheral blood smear demonstrating left-shifted myeloid series with predominance of myelocytes

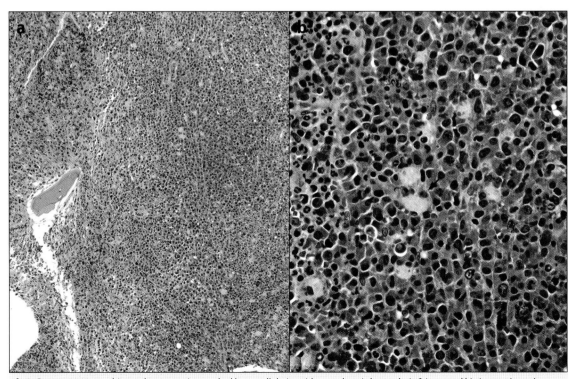

f1.2 Bone marrow core biopsy demonstrating marked hypercellularity with granulocytic hyperplasia & increased histiocytes (arrow)

1 *Chronic myeloid leukemia presenting with t(9;22)(q34.1;q11.2) BCR-ABL1 & trisomy 8*

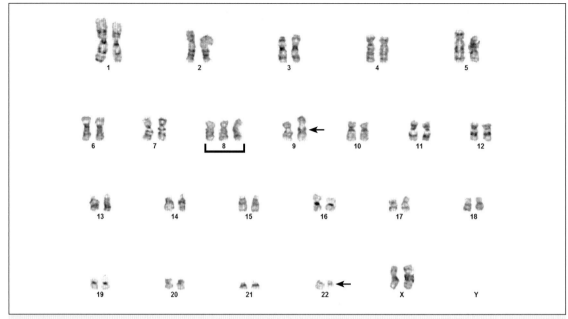

f1.3 Karyotype demonstrating reciprocal translocation (arrows) resulting in t(9;22)(q34;q11.2) as well as trisomy 8 (bracket)

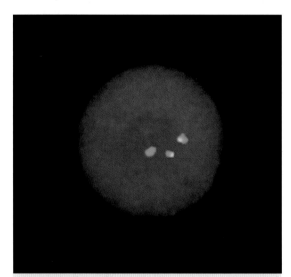

f1.4 Dual fusion FISH probes for *BCR* (green) & *ABL1* (orange) show 1 green signal, 1 orange signal, and 2 yellow fusion signals, indicative of *BCR-ABL1* translocation

pathways leading to cell proliferation, growth-factor independence, and decreased apoptosis of granulocytic progenitors. The end result is an overabundance of granulocytes in the blood, marrow, and spleen, with an increase in immature forms. At presentation in the chronic phase (CP), blasts are usually seen in blood but do not exceed 10%, with fewer blasts in the bone marrow (typically <2%). Basophils and eosinophils are virtually always increased in blood, and ~1/2 of individuals present with elevated platelet counts, with

1/3 having platelet counts exceeding $1,000 \times 10^9/L$. In the bone marrow, the granulocytes are normal but have a predominance of myelocytes ("myelocyte bulge"), whereas megakaryocytes are small and hypolobate ("dwarf" megakaryocytes), albeit usually lacking separated nuclear lobes (a finding that may be present in myelodysplastic syndromes [MDSs]). Pseudo-Gaucher cells are common in the bone marrow and reflect the exuberant cell turnover in CML which overwhelms the normal lipid metabolism machinery of marrow histiocytes. Erythroid precursors display normal morphology but are decreased.

Presenting symptoms relate to the underlying pathophysiology and include fatigue and malaise caused by anemia, as well as early satiety, weight loss, and left upper quadrant fullness owing to an enlarged spleen. Symptoms from leukostasis such as confusion, headache, and/or hypoxia are uncommon even when the WBC is quite elevated, although visual disturbances may be present because of sludging of white cells in retinal veins. Approximately 50% of patients are asymptomatic at diagnosis, however, as in this case.

Before the advent of tyrosine kinase inhibitor (TKI) therapy, classically CML progressed through 3 distinct phases: CP, the most common phase at presentation, with the features described in this case and typically lasting 3-5 years; an accelerated phase (AP) with disease progression lasting 6-9 months; and a blast phase (BP), morphologically equivalent to acute

ISBN 978-089189-6814

t1.1 Comparison of CML accelerated phase criteria published by the NCCN & the WHO

Criteria	Guideline	
	NCCN 2020	**WHO 2017**
PB or BM myeloblasts	≥15% & <30%	10%-19%
PB myeloblasts and promyelocytes combined	≥30%	N/A
Persistent or increasing WBC, unresponsive to therapy	N/A	>10 × 10⁹/L
PB basophilia	≥20%	≥20%
Thrombocytopenia, unrelated to therapy	≤100 × 10⁹/L	≤100 × 10⁹/L
Thrombocytosis, unresponsive to therapy	N/A	>1000 × 10⁹/L
ACA in Ph+ cells	Any	major route [+8, i(17q), +Ph, +19] or complex or 3q26 abnormalities at diagnosis or any new ACA on therapy

ACA, additional chromosomal abnormality; BM, bone marrow; CML, chronic myeloid leukemia; N/A, not available; NCCN, National Comprehensive Cancer Network; PB, peripheral blood; WHO, World Health Organization

leukemia and carrying a poor prognosis. The blasts in BP have a myeloid phenotype in 80% of cases, with most of the remaining cases having a B-lymphoblast phenotype (extremely rare cases of BP having T-lymphoblast phenotype have been reported). The current universal use of TKIs in CML, however, has changed the behavior of the disease dramatically, with very few patients progressing and terminating in BP. Nonetheless, in some patients, the condition still progresses and rare individuals may unpredictably and suddenly develop BP, usually B-lymphoblastic disease, while receiving TKI therapy. Progression through the phases is frequently related to the acquisition of additional genetic abnormalities. Clinical, genetic, and laboratory criteria have been proposed for the designation of AP, with the exact criteria being debatable. Distinct criteria for AP suggested by the World Health Organization (WHO) and National Comprehensive Cancer Network (NCCN) are compared in **t1.1**. Patients presenting in AP may require additional treatment, including consideration for hematopoietic stem cell transplantation; BP presentation is treated as acute myeloid leukemia with the addition of TKIs.

The differential diagnosis for CML includes leukemoid reaction, non-CML myeloproliferative neoplasms (MPNs), MDS/myeloproliferative neoplasms (MDS/MPN), and myeloid/lymphoid neoplasms with eosinophilia (MLNEos) and gene rearrangement. By definition, the WBC is elevated in leukemoid reaction, but the blood counts are generally not as high as seen in CML and rarely more than 100 × 10⁹/L. In addition, neutrophils in leukemoid reaction often demonstrate reactive changes such as toxic granulation and Döhle bodies,

which are lacking in CML. Basophilia is usually absent in leukemoid reaction but is invariably present in CML. Although MPNs, MDS/MPNs, and MLNEos may manifest with leukocytosis with left shift, basophilia, and splenomegaly, the absence of the Ph chromosome allows for distinguishing these disorders from CML. CML rarely shows monocytosis and almost never displays >10% monocytes, helping to morphologically distinguish it from the MDS / MPN overlap neoplasm, chronic myelomonocytic leukemia (CMML). The presence of granulocyte dysplasia excludes CP CML and should point toward an MDS / MPN neoplasm such as atypical CML or CMML. Rarely, patients with CML may present with isolated thrombocytosis mimicking a non-CML MPN. Genetic studies in these individuals will identify the *BCR-ABL1* rearrangement, however.

The sine qua non of CML is the presence of the *BCR-ABL1* fusion gene resulting from a reciprocal translocation of chromosomes 9 and 22, t(9;22) (q34;q11). The derivative chromosome 22, which is abnormally small on karyotype, is referred to as the Philadelphia (Ph) chromosome (named after its place of discovery). The Ph chromosome can be seen by karyotype in 90%-95% of patients with CML and is also found in ~25% of adults with de novo B-lymphoblastic leukemia/lymphoma (B-ALL; see **Case 51**). However, in 5%-10% of CML cases, the *BCR-ABL1* fusion is cryptic on karyotype but is detected by FISH; thus, FISH should be performed at diagnosis in all suspect cases. Variant 3-way chromosomal translocations are known to occur (~5% of cases) and may cause an abnormal FISH pattern, but these appear to have little clinical impact.

1 *Chronic myeloid leukemia presenting with t(9;22)(q34.1;q11.2) BCR-ABL1 & trisomy 8*

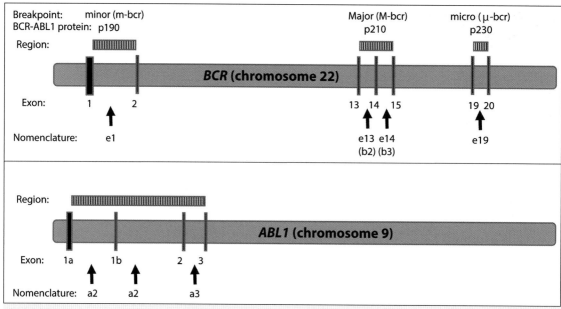

f1.5 Schematic of the various *BCR* & *ABL1* breakpoints leading to different BCR-ABL1 fusion protein products in CML

The majority of breakpoints in *BCR* are clustered within a 5.8-kb region spanning exons 12-16, called the "major" breakpoint cluster region (M-bcr; **f1.5**). The usual breakpoint in *ABL1* is between exons 1 and 2. Two types of fusion transcripts are generated based on these breakpoints: *BCR* exon 13 with *ABL1* exon 2 (referred to as e13a2 or b2a2), present in ~40% of CML patients, and *BCR* exon 14 with *ABL1* exon 2 (e14a2 or b3a2), occurring in ~50% of CML patients. The protein created from either of these M-bcr fusions (p210) has a molecular weight of 210 kd. Only minor differences in responses to TKIs have been noted between patients expressing e13a2 or e14a2 M-bcr fusion transcripts and some patients (~12%) express both because of alternative splicing **f1.5**.

Occasionally *BCR-ABL1* fusions occur outside of the M-bcr , most commonly within a 55-kb sequence of intron 1 called the "minor" bcr (m-bcr), which produces the e1a2 fusion and a smaller molecular weight protein (p190). Only ~1% of CML cases have an m-bcr fusion. Notably, because of alternative splicing, a small amount of m-bcr transcripts is detected in most patients with CML who have an M-bcr fusion, as seen in this case. The m-bcr fusion also occurs in most cases of Ph-positive de novo B-ALL. Importantly, CML patients having predominantly p190 protein appear to have an inferior response to TKI therapy, with fewer and usually short-lived responses. Less common *BCR* breaks occur in intron 19 at the "micro" bcr (μ-bcr), producing the e19a2 fusion and a larger protein of 230 kd (p230).

Disease in these individuals is associated with thrombocytosis and leukocytosis composed of mostly mature neutrophils. Other, very rare *BCR* breaks outside the aforementioned regions or after exon 2 of *ABL1* do occur, and these may not be detected with standard RT-PCR assays (as described later in this discussion).

Quantitation of *BCR-ABL1* transcripts using RT-PCR is important for monitoring disease. Primers are typically designed to detect the major and minor breakpoints but usually do not distinguish between different M-bcr transcripts. In practice, it is important to understand the limitations of a particular assay, because most do not detect breaks outside the major and minor regions. As a result, a negative RT-PCR result for *BCR-ABL1* does NOT exclude CML at diagnosis, depending on the assay used. In addition, the rare patient with a *BCR-ABL1* translocation undetectable by a particular PCR assay cannot be followed with that assay. Quantitation is normalized via use of an internal control gene, most typically *ABL1*, *BCR*, or *GUSB*, and interlaboratory correlation is possible by determining the percentage of *BCR-ABL1* relative to an internationally accepted standardized baseline (IS). It is important to note that *BCR-ABL1* transcripts can be detected with qRT-PCR in ~30% of normal individuals at low levels (eg, <0.1% IS), and these individuals should not be diagnosed as having CML.

Response to TKI therapy can be assessed based on morphologic absence of disease with normalization

ISBN 978-089189-6814 ©2021 ASCP

t1.2 Frequency & clinical significance of ACAs detected at CML diagnosis

Abnormality	Frequency, of cases having ACA at diagnosis (%)	Prognosis
>1 ACA	19	Poor
–Y	39	No effect
Trisomy 8	14	Mildly adverse to no effect
Additional Ph	8	Mildly adverse to no effect
3q26 abnormality	1.5	Poor
i(17q)	2.5	Poor
–7/del(7q)	2.5	Poor
Trisomy 19	4	Unclear
Others including del(9q34)	27	Likely no effect

ACA, additional chromosomal abnormalities; CML, chronic myeloid leukemia

of blood counts (hematologic response), using karyotyping and FISH (cytogenetic response), or quantitation of *BCR-ABL1* transcripts using molecular methods (molecular response), with molecular response being the most sensitive indicator of the presence of residual disease. Thus, therapy response can be semiquantitated based on whether a complete hematologic, cytogenetic, or a molecular response has been reached. In patients undergoing TKI therapy, the degree of the reduction of *BCR-ABL1* transcripts in peripheral blood correlates with these milestones and is predictive of disease behavior; therefore, repeat marrow studies are generally not necessary. It is recommended that *BCR-ABL1* levels be <10% IS at 3-6 months and <1% IS at 12 months after therapy. *BCR-ABL1* levels at 0.1% IS at 12 months are associated with low probability of subsequent disease progression. The inability to reach these minimal levels at the specified time points indicates therapy failure and should prompt both a medication change and sequencing of *BCR-ABL1* to identify drug resistance mutations that occur in the kinase domain. Such mutations are detectable in ~50% of patients with treatment failure and/or progression; >80 amino acid substitutions have been associated with resistance to TKIs. The T315I mutation is particularly problematic and is known to confer resistance to all known TKIs except ponatinib.

Chromosomal abnormalities in addition to the Ph chromosome (additional chromosome abnormalities, or ACAs) may develop during the course of disease or less commonly, may be present at diagnosis. ACAs occur in ~5% of cases that would otherwise be considered in CP, but as the disease progresses, ACAs become more frequent, with ~30% of patients in AP and 50%-80% of cases in BP demonstrating ACAs. The accumulation of chromosomal abnormalities and genetic defects is

a hallmark of disease progression in CML and these abnormalities are often associated with other indicators of AP **t1.1**. Early studies identified trisomy 8, a second Ph chromosome, isochromosome 17q (i17q), and trisomy 19 as the most common secondary genetic events. These ACAs have therefore been referred to as the "major route" abnormalities and all other secondary genetic events considered minor pathway aberrations. Studies differ on the significance of various aberrations, especially in relation to the timing of acquisition and type of the additional abnormality. Nonetheless, ACAs developing during the course of CML are generally considered a feature of acceleration, although not all ACAs appear to be equally detrimental for patient outcomes **t1.2**. The major route ACAs account for 10%-50% of CML cases having clonal evolution and have been shown to impart an inferior outcome in CML compared to other ACAs in some studies. As a result, some guidelines accept only the major route ACAs as indicators of AP (European LeukemiaNet) whereas others (WHO and NCCN) suggest that any ACA occurring during therapy is indicative of AP. More recent analysis in patients treated with TKIs has shed some doubt that all major route ACAs impart a poor prognosis. Parsing out the effects of isolated abnormalities is difficult because of the co-occurrence of many of the major route ACAs. For example, when trisomy 8 is identified, it occurs as an isolated ACA in only 20% of these cases, as observed in the current case. Isolated trisomy 8 occurring in CML otherwise classifiable as CP, in particular, does not appear to be associated with a worse outcome, and it has been suggested that other accelerated features contribute to the adverse prognosis formerly associated with this abnormality. Similar findings have been seen with the acquisition of a second Ph chromosome. Thus, trisomy 8 and an additional Ph chromosome appear not as deleterious as the other major route abnormalities such as i(17q).

Similar differences in prognostic significance exist for the minor route abnormalities. The loss of chromosome Y in men, the most common ACA in CML across all cases, has been shown to have no prognostic significance, mirroring its presence in the general population. Clonal cytogenetic abnormalities in Ph-negative cells may occur in 5%-10% of patients during TKI therapy and do not seem to adversely affect outcome except for abnormalities of chromosome 7, which carries an increased risk for myelodysplasia and acute leukemia (likely unrelated to the underlying CML). In contrast, abnormalities involving chromosome region 3q26 and complex chromosomal abnormalities (>1 ACA) have been shown to impart a poor prognosis. Other isolated minor route abnormalities seem to fall somewhere in between.

The impact of ACAs when detected at diagnosis has been difficult to assess because of the rarity of these occurrences (<5%) and the aforementioned co-occurrence of different abnormalities. There is agreement that loss of the derivative chromosome 9 (reciprocal translocation of the Ph chromosome) detected at diagnosis does not affect patient outcome in the TKI era. Discrepant results have been reported for other ACAs, however. In actual practice, patients presenting with >1 ACA, the major route ACAs, particularly i(17q), and the minor route 3q26 aberration may be considered "high risk" but usually do not lead to alteration of the initial therapy. It remains controversial whether to consider patients with major route ACA at diagnosis as being in AP if no other feature of acceleration is present. Finally, the significance of somatic mutations in CML, including those present in other myeloid neoplasms, is unclear at present and is a current area of study.

This patient presented in CP disease based on blood counts and histology, but with an isolated trisomy 8 as an ACA at diagnosis. Although technically considered AP by some criteria, standard CML therapy with imatinib was initiated, given more recent data suggesting minimally adverse effects of trisomy 8 in CML otherwise classifiable as CP. Ten months after the initiation of therapy, her blood *BCR-ABL1* level was at 0.385% (<1%) IS, indicating a good response.

Diagnostic pearls/pitfalls

- Cases of chronic myeloid leukemia (CML), by definition, must have the Philadelphia (Ph) chromosome, t(9;22)(q34;q11.2), resulting from the translocation of *ABL1* on chromosome 9 to *BCR* on chromosome 22.

- The typical *BCR-ABL1* fusion transcript encodes for the p210 protein as the result of fusion of *ABL1* exon 2 with the major breakpoint region (M-bcr) of *BCR* involving exons 13 or 14. These transcripts are referred to as e13a2 and e14a2, respectively.

- FISH should be used to detect the Ph chromosome in all new suspect cases, because the t(9;22)(q34;q11.2) translocation is cryptic (not detectable) on karyotyping in 5%-10% of patients and quantitative reverse transcriptase polymerase chain reaction (qRT-PCR) for *BCR-ABL1* may be negative if the *BCR-ABL1* fusion occurs outside the major and minor breakpoint regions typically assessed with most assays.

- Low-level (<1%) *BCR-ABL1* transcripts may be found on qRT-PCR in normal individuals and should not lead to a diagnosis of CML.

- Failure to reach tyrosine kinase inhibitor (TKI) therapy milestones indicates drug failure and should trigger a medication change and sequencing of *BCR-ABL1* to identify drug resistance mutations.

- There is a lack of concordance between various organizations regarding the criteria used to define the accelerated phase (AP) and blast phase (BP) of CML.

- Additional chromosomal abnormalities (ACAs) are found in ~5% of CML patients in the chronic phase (CP) and at diagnosis, 30% of patients in AP, and 50%-80% of patients in BP. The major route ACAs are the most commonly encountered ACAs except for loss of chromosome Y, and include trisomy 8, an additional Ph chromosome, i(17q), and trisomy 19. Major route ACAs frequently occur together.

- Isolated ACAs appear to differ in prognostic significance, with trisomy 8 and an additional Ph chromosome having less of an impact compared to i(17q), complex abnormalities (>1 ACA), and abnormalities of chromosome 3q26. Trisomy 8 and an additional Ph chromosome may not affect prognosis when detected in a patient without other evidence of AP.

Readings

Akard LP, Cortes JE, Albitar M, et al. Correlations between cytogenetic and molecular monitoring among patients with newly diagnosed chronic myeloid leukemia in chronic phase: post hoc analyses of the Rationale and Insight for Gleevec High-Dose Therapy study. Arch Pathol Lab Med. 2014;138(9):1186-92. **DOI: 10.5858/arpa.2013-0584-OA**

Alhuraiji A, Kantarjian H, Boddu P, et al. Prognostic significance of additional chromosomal abnormalities at the time of diagnosis in patients with chronic myeloid leukemia treated with frontline tyrosine kinase inhibitors. Am J Hematol. 2018;93(1):84-90. **DOI: 10.1002/ajh.24943**

Baccarani M, Castagnetti F, Gugliotta G, et al; International *BCR-ABL* Study Group. The proportion of different *BCR-ABL1* transcript types in chronic myeloid leukemia: an international overview. Leukemia. 2019;33(5):1173-83. **DOI: 10.1038/s41375-018-0341-4**

Baccarani M, Deininger MW, Rosti G, et al. European LeukemiaNet recommendations for the management of chronic myeloid leukemia: 2013. Blood. 2013;122(6):872-84. **DOI: 10.1182/blood-2013-05-501569**

Branford S, Kim DDH, Apperley JF, et al; International CML Foundation Genomics Alliance. Laying the foundation for genomically-based risk assessment in chronic myeloid leukemia. Leukemia. 2019;33(8):1835-50. **DOI: 10.1038/s41375-019-0512-y**

Castagnetti F, Gugliotta G, Breccia M, et al; GIMEMA CML Working Party. The *BCR-ABL1* transcript type influences response and outcome in Philadelphia chromosome-positive chronic myeloid leukemia patients treated frontline with imatinib. Am J Hematol. 2017;92(8):797-805. **DOI: 10.1002/ajh.24774**

Castagnetti F, Testoni N, Luatti S, et al. Deletions of the derivative chromosome 9 do not influence the response and the outcome of chronic myeloid leukemia in early chronic phase treated with imatinib mesylate: GIMEMA CML Working Party analysis. J Clin Oncol. 2010;28(16):2748-54. **DOI: 10.1200/JCO.2009.26.7963**

Cortes JE, Talpaz M, Giles F, et al. Prognostic significance of cytogenetic clonal evolution in patients with chronic myelogenous leukemia on imatinib mesylate therapy. Blood. 2003;101(10):3794-800. **DOI: 10.1182/blood-2002-09-2790**

Cross NCP, White HE, Evans PAS, et al. Consensus on *BCR-ABL1* reporting in chronic myeloid leukaemia in the UK. Br J Haematol. 2018;182(6):777-88. **DOI: 10.1111/bjh.15542**

Fabarius A, Leitner A, Hochhaus A, et al; Schweizerische Arbeitsgemeinschaft für Klinische Krebsforschung (SAKK) and the German CML Study Group. Impact of additional cytogenetic aberrations at diagnosis on prognosis of CML: long-term observation of 1151 patients from the randomized CML Study IV. Blood. 2011;118(26):6760-8. **DOI: 10.1182/blood-2011-08-373902**

Flis S, Chojnacki T. Chronic myelogenous leukemia, a still unsolved problem: pitfalls and new therapeutic possibilities. Drug Des Devel Ther. 2019;13:825-43. **DOI: 10.2147/DDDT.S191303**

Foroni L, Wilson G, Gerrard G, et al. Guidelines for the measurement of *BCR-ABL1* transcripts in chronic myeloid leukaemia. Br J Haematol. 2011;153(2):179-90. **DOI: 10.1111/j.1365-2141.2011.08603.x**

Hanfstein B, Lauseker M, Hehlmann R, et al; SAKK and the German CML Study Group. Distinct characteristics of e13a2 versus e14a2 *BCR-ABL1* driven chronic myeloid leukemia under first-line therapy with imatinib. Haematologica. 2014;99(9):1441-7. **DOI: 10.3324/haematol.2013.096537**

Issa GC, Kantarjian HM, Gonzalez GN, et al. Clonal chromosomal abnormalities appearing in Philadelphia chromosome-negative metaphases during CML treatment. Blood. 2017;130(19):2084-91. **DOI: 10.1182/blood-2017-07-792143**

Lauseker M, Bachl K, Turkina A, et al. Prognosis of patients with chronic myeloid leukemia presenting in advanced phase is defined mainly by blast count, but also by age, chromosomal aberrations and hemoglobin. Am J Hematol. 2019;94(11):1236-1243. **DOI: 10.1002/ajh.25628**

Jabbour E, Kantarjian H. Chronic myeloid leukemia: 2018 update on diagnosis, therapy and monitoring. Am J Hematol. 2018;93(3):442-59. **DOI: 10.1002/ajh.25011**

Jain P, Kantarjian H, Patel KP, et al. Impact of *BCR-ABL* transcript type on outcome in patients with chronic-phase CML treated with tyrosine kinase inhibitors. Blood. 2016;127(10):1269-75. **DOI: 10.1182/blood-2015-10-674242**

Luatti S, Castagnetti F, Marzocchi G, et al; Gruppo Italiano Malattie Ematologiche dell'Adulto (GIMEMA) Working Party on CML. Additional chromosomal abnormalities in Philadelphia-positive clone: adverse prognostic influence on frontline imatinib therapy: a GIMEMA Working Party on CML analysis. Blood. 2012;120(4):761-7. **DOI: 10.1182/blood-2011-10-384651**

Majlis A, Smith TL, Talpaz M, O'Brien S, Rios MB, Kantarjian HM. Significance of cytogenetic clonal evolution in chronic myelogenous leukemia. J Clin Oncol. 1996;14(1):196-203. **DOI: 10.1200/JCO.1996.14.1.196**

Marzocchi G, Castagnetti F, Luatti S, et al; Gruppo Italiano Malattie EMatologiche dell'Adulto (GIMEMA) Working Party on Chronic Myeloid Leukemia. Variant Philadelphia translocations: molecular-cytogenetic characterization and prognostic influence on frontline imatinib therapy, a GIMEMA Working Party on CML analysis. Blood. 2011;117(25):6793-800. **DOI: 10.1182/blood-2011-01-328294**

Mitelman F, Levan G, Nilsson PG, et al. Non-random karyotypic evolution in chronic myeloid leukemia. Int J Cancer. 1976;18(1):24-30. **DOI: 10.1002/ijc.2910180105**

Primo D, Tabernero MD, Rasillo A, et al. Patterns of BCR/ABL gene rearrangements by interphase fluorescence in situ hybridization (FISH) in *BCR/ABL*+ leukemias: incidence and underlying genetic abnormalities. Leukemia. 2013;17(6):1124-9. **DOI: 10.1038/sj.leu.2402963**

Quintás-Cardama A, Kantarjian H, Shan J, et al. Prognostic impact of deletions of derivative chromosome 9 in patients with chronic myelogenous leukemia treated with nilotinib or dasatinib. Cancer. 2011;117(22):5085-93. **DOI: 10.1002/cncr.26147**

Rea D, Etienne G, Nicolini F, et al. First-line imatinib mesylate in patients with newly diagnosed accelerated phase-chronic myeloid leukemia. Leukemia. 2012;26(10):2254-9. **DOI: 10.1038/leu.2012.92**

Verma D, Kantarjian HM, Jones D, et al. Chronic myeloid leukemia (CML) with P190 *BCR-ABL*: analysis of characteristics, outcomes, and prognostic significance. Blood. 2009;114(11):2232-5. **DOI: 10.1182/blood-2009-02-204693**

Wang W, Cortes JE, Tang G, et al. Risk stratification of chromosomal abnormalities in chronic myelogenous leukemia in the era of tyrosine kinase inhibitor therapy. Blood. 2016;127(22):2742-50. **DOI: 10.1182/blood-2016-01-690230**

Wang W, Cortes JE, Lin P, et al. Impact of trisomy 8 on treatment response and survival of patients with chronic myelogenous leukemia in the era of tyrosine kinase inhibitors. Leukemia. 2015;29(11):2263-6. **DOI: 10.1038/leu.2015.96**

Wang W, Cortes JE, Lin P, et al. Clinical and prognostic significance of 3q26.2 and other chromosome 3 abnormalities in CML in the era of tyrosine kinase inhibitors. Blood. 2015;126(14):1699-706. **DOI: 10.1182/blood-2015-05-646489**

Wasilewska EM, Panasiuk B, Gniot M, et al. Clonal chromosomal aberrations in Philadelphia negative cells such as monosomy 7 and trisomy 8 may persist for years with no impact on the long term outcome in patients with chronic myeloid leukemia. Cancer Genet. 2017;216-217:1-9. **DOI: 10.1016/j.cancergen.2017.04.066**

Zaccaria A, Testoni N, Valenti AM, et al; GIMEMA Working Party on CML. Chromosome abnormalities additional to the Philadelphia chromosome at the diagnosis of chronic myelogenous leukemia: pathogenetic and prognostic implications. Cancer Genet Cytogenet. 2010;199(2):76-80. **DOI: 10.1016/j.cancergencyto.2010.02.003**

2

Erika M Moore & Rose C Beck

Polycythemia vera with *JAK2* V617F & *ASXL1* mutation

History A 68-year-old female with a history of breast cancer treated with chemotherapy developed polycythemia 1 year later, with routine CBC showing a HGB of 17.2 g/dL (177 g/L) and HCT of 53.4%. Her serum erythropoietin level was 1.3 mIU/mL (1.3 IU/L; normal 2.6-18.5 mIU/mL [2.6-18.5 IU/L]). A bone marrow biopsy with genetic studies was performed. CBC at the time of the biopsy is shown to the right.

WBC	$13.8 \times 10^9 / L$
RBC	$6.72 \times 10^{12} / L$
HGB	17.7 g / dL
HCT	55.2%
MCV	94 fL
RDW	19.5%
Platelets	$456 \times 10^9 / L$

Morphology & flow cytometry The peripheral blood smear showed no morphologic abnormalities, and the bone marrow aspirate showed normal erythropoiesis and granulopoiesis, with a normal myeloid:erythroid ratio of 1.7:1, though few megakaryocytes with cloudlike nuclei were noted **f2.1**. The bone marrow core biopsy demonstrated hypercellularity for age (70%) because of pan-hyperplasia, including increased megakaryocytes forming occasional small clusters. Some of the megakaryocytes exhibited enlarged, hyperlobated nuclei, whereas others had condensed, cloudlike nuclei. A reticulin stain did not show an increase in reticulin fibrosis, and flow cytometry revealed no definite abnormalities.

Genetics/molecular results Chromosome analysis revealed a normal female karyotype; FISH was not performed. A targeted myeloid NGS panel was positive for *JAK2* p.V617F (c.1849G>T) with 73% variant allele frequency (VAF) **f2.2** and *ASXL1* p.Q768* (c.2302C>T) with 46% VAF.

Based on the laboratory, morphologic, and genetic findings including *JAK2* V617F mutation, a final diagnosis of **polycythemia vera** (PV) was rendered.

Discussion PV is a chronic myeloproliferative neoplasm which results in unchecked RBC production. Virtually all patients harbor a somatic *JAK2* gain-of-function mutation at the stem cell level, leading to cytokine-independent proliferation of erythroid cells, granulocytes, and megakaryocytes. This results in pan myelosis in the blood and bone marrow, but patients typically present with symptoms related specifically to increased RBC mass; the 2017 WHO diagnostic criteria for PV are listed in **t2.1**. Thrombosis is a well-known complication and any patient with Budd-Chiari syndrome or mesenteric, portal, or splenic vein thrombosis should undergo evaluation for PV. Microvascular thrombi also occur, resulting in parasthesias, headaches, and visual disturbances. Many patients will have plethora and/or splenomegaly on physical examination. Most patients are treated with phlebotomy to decrease red cell mass, along with aspirin, but if adverse prognostic factors are present, cytoreductive therapy such as hydroxyurea may also be used.

The disease has 2 main phases : the polycythemic (proliferative) phase and post-polycythemic myelofibrosis. In the polycythemic phase, hemoglobin and hematocrit are increased in the peripheral blood and patients may also have neutrophilia and

ISBN 978-089189-6814

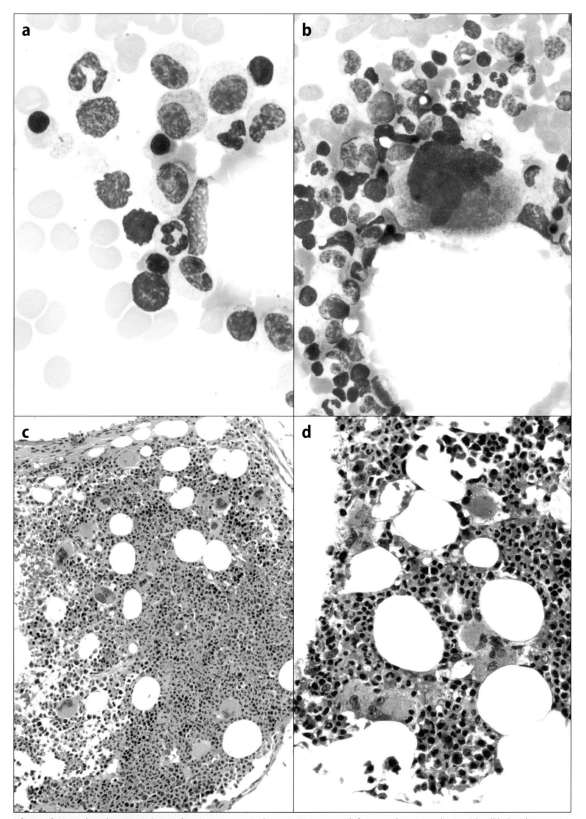

f2.1 a, b Normal erythropoiesis & granulopoiesis present in the aspirate smear, with few megakaryocytes having "cloudlike" nuclei;
c, d sections of the core biopsy show pan-hyperplasia with increased, enlarged megakaryocytes, which form small clusters

2 Polycythemia vera with JAK2 V617F & ASXL1 mutation

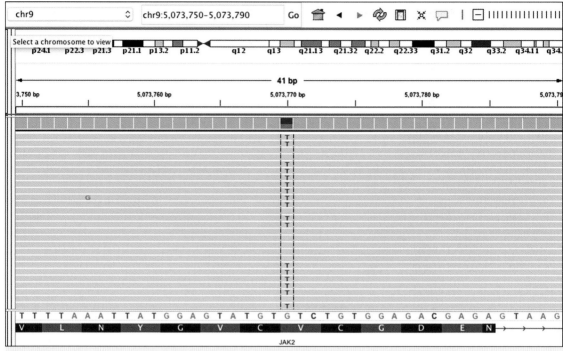

f2.2 Somatic variant analysis using a targeted myeloid NGS panel. Annotated reads mapped to the *JAK2* locus demonstrate p.V617F (c.1849G>T), highlighted in red (hg19, IGV browser) [see **fA.8**, p312]

t2.1 World Health Organization 2017 diagnostic criteria for polycythemia vera

Diagnosis requires all 3 major criteria or the first 2 major criteria plus the minor criterion*

Major criteria

1. Elevated hemoglobin or hematocrit (men: >16.5 g/dL [>165 g/L], >49%; women: >16.0 g/dL [>160 g/L], >48%) or increased red blood cell mass >25% above mean normal predicted value

2. Age-adjusted hypercellular bone marrow with pan-myelosis including megakaryocytic proliferation with pleomorphic, mature megakaryocytes

3. *JAK2* V617F or JAK2 exon 12 mutation

Minor criterion

1. Subnormal serum erythropoietin level

A bone marrow biopsy may not be required in patients with sustained absolute erythrocytosis & hemoglobin levels >18.5 g/dL (>185 g/L) in men (hematocrit >55.5%) or >16.5 g/dL (>165 g/L) in women (hematocrit >49.5%) if major criterion 3 & the minor criterion are present

thrombocytosis. The bone marrow is hypercellular for age, with panmyelosis. Erythropoiesis is normoblastic, granulocytes may be slightly left-shifted, and megakaryocytes are generally pleomorphic. The megakaryocytes may form loose clusters but typically do not exhibit markedly abnormal morphology or very tight clusters, as can be seen in primary myelofibrosis

(PMF). No significant dysplasia should be evident. Most patients will lack stainable iron because of increased erythrocyte production. Fibrosis is not a characteristic feature, but a small subset of patients may have a mild increase in reticulin fibers at diagnosis. Approximately 15%-25% of patients may eventually progress to the post-polycythemic myelofibrosis phase. These patients will have findings that are essentially identical to those of PMF, with anemia and a leukoerythoblastic picture in the peripheral blood, marked reticulin, and collagen fibrosis in the bone marrow, with decreased erythropoiesis and granulopoiesis, and increased, hyperchromatic, and bizarre-appearing megakaryocytes, often forming tight clusters **t2.2**. Therefore, a diagnosis of post-polycythemic myelofibrosis can only be made when there is a well-documented prior diagnosis of PV **t2.2**. Rarely, patients with PV may also progress to a myelodysplastic-like phase or even acute myeloid leukemia.

Most PV patients (>95%) have the *JAK2* V617F mutation, while <5% harbor an alternative gain-of-function *JAK2* mutation, usually within exon 12. *JAK2* is a tyrosine kinase that mediates downstream signaling via phosphorylation of cytokine receptors and recruitment and phosphorylation of effector proteins, including the STAT transcription factors and those in the RAS/MAPK and PI3K/AKT pathways. The V617F is a gain-of-function mutation that results in constitutive activation

ISBN 978-089189-6814   ©2021 ASCP

t2.2 WHO 2017 diagnostic criteria for post-polycythemia vera myelofibrosis

Required criteria

1. Documentation of a previous diagnosis of WHO-defined PV

2. Bone marrow fibrosis of grade 2-3 (on 0-3 scale) or 3-4 (on 0-4 scale)

Additional criteria (2 are required)

Anemia below the reference range for age, gender, and altitude or sustained loss of need for phlebotomy or cytoreductive therapy for erythrocytosis

Leukoerythroblastosis

Increasing splenomegaly (newly palpable or >5 cm from baseline [distance from left costal margin])

Development of at least 2 of the following: >10% weight loss in 6 months, night sweats, unexplained fever (>37.5°C)

of *JAK2*, leading to cytokine-independent hematopoietic cell growth through activation of the erythropoietin, thrombopoietin, and granulocyte colony-stimulating factor receptors, resulting in panmyelosis.

JAK2 V617F is not specific to PV and is also seen in approximately half of essential thrombocythemia (ET) and PMF cases, and more rarely in other myeloid malignancies such as myelodysplastic syndrome (MDS), as well as in clonal hematopoiesis of indeterminate potential (CHIP; see **Case 17**). A subset of PV cases has a very high *JAK2* V617F allelic frequency (>50%), resulting from a homozygous mutant clone acquired via uniparental disomy of the 9q24 locus (which encompasses the *JAK2* gene). These PV patients with V617F homozygosity tend to have higher hemoglobin and white blood cell counts but lower platelet counts. Similarly, *JAK2* V617F-mutated ET cases usually have higher hemoglobin and lower platelet counts than non-*JAK2* mutated ET cases. As mentioned, <5% of patients with PV have a different gain-of-function *JAK2* mutation in exon 12. Among myeloproliferative neoplasms, *JAK2* exon 12 mutations are unique to PV and are typically associated with isolated erythrocytosis. A subset of PV patients will also have concurrent cytogenetic abnormalities, commonly gains of chromosomes 8 and 9; patients with disease progression also have a much higher incidence of cytogenetic aberrancies.

Although abnormalities in *JAK2* are the driver mutation in PV, a portion of cases have secondary mutations. Although the data on the implications of these mutations are not extensive, recent studies have shown that some mutations have an independent poor prognostic impact, particularly *ASXL1* mutations (as seen in this case). Other gene mutations that appear to have prognostic impact include mutations in *IDH2*, *RUNX1*, *SRSF2*, and other spliceosome genes.

Diagnostic pearls/pitfalls

– Essentially all patients with polycythemia vera (PV) have a *JAK2* V617 mutation or *JAK2* exon 12 gain-of-function mutation.

– Thrombosis is a common complication of PV and all patients presenting with a major vein thrombosis should be evaluated for PV.

– Although elevated hemoglobin and hematocrit levels are major criteria for PV, many patients will also have neutrophilia and/or thrombocytosis.

– Although the megakaryocytes in PV are pleomorphic and can be atypical, tight clusters and overtly bizarre morphology are not characteristic in the polycythemic phase and should point to the possibility of another myeloproliferative neoplasm or progression to post-PV myelofibrosis .

– The findings in post-polycythemia myelofibrosis look identical to those of primary myelofibrosis and therefore, a patient must have a well-documented history of PV to receive a diagnosis of post-PV myelofibrosis.

Readings

Andréasson B, Pettersson H, Wasslavik C, et al. *ASXL1* mutations, previous vascular complications and age at diagnosis predict survival in 85 WHO-defined polycythaemia vera patients. Br J Haematol. 2020;189(5):913-9. doi: 10.1111/bjh.16450

Levine R, Pardanani A, Tefferi A, Gilliland DG. Role of *JAK2* in the pathogenesis and therapy of myeloproliferative disorders. Nat Rev Cancer. 2007;7(9):673-83. **DOI: 10.1038/nrc2210**

Skoda R, Duek A, Grisouard J. Pathogenesis of myeloproliferative neoplasms. Exp Hematol. 2015;43(8):599-608. **DOI: 10.1016/j. exphem.2015.06.007**

Swerdlow SH, Campo E, Harris NL, et al. World Health Organization Classification of Tumours of Haematopoietic and Lymphoid Tissues. 4th ed. Lyon, France: IARC Press, 2017. ISBN-13: 9789283244943

Tefferi A, Guglielmelli P, Lasho TL, et al. Mutation-enhanced international prognostic systems for essential thrombocythaemia and polycythaemia vera. Br J Haematol. 2020 Apr;189(2):291-302. Epub 2020 Jan 16. **DOI: 10.1111/bjh.16380**

Tefferi A, Lasho TL, Guglielmelli P, et al. Targeted deep sequencing in polycythemia vera and essential thrombocythemia. Blood Adv. 2016;1(1):21-30. **DOI: 10.1182/bloodadvances.2016000216**

Tefferi A, Lavu S, Mudireddy M, et al. *JAK2* exon 12 mutated polycythemia vera: Mayo-Careggi MPN Alliance study of 33 consecutive cases and comparison with *JAK2* V617F mutated disease. Am J Hematol. 2018;93:E93-6. **DOI: 10.1002/ajh.25017**

Vainchenker W, Kralovics R. Genetic basis and molecular pathophysiology of classical myeloproliferative neoplasms. Blood. 2017;129(6):667-79. **DOI: 10.1182/blood-2016-10-695940**

3

Nathaniel P Havens & Rose C Beck

Essential thrombocytosis with *CALR* type 1 mutation

History A 77-year-old female with past medical history of chronic fatigue, hypothyroidism, peripheral neuropathy, ataxia, and arthritis was referred to hematology for evaluation of macrocytic anemia. CBC at the time of the biopsy is shown to the right. Vitamin B_{12} and folate levels were within normal ranges. A bone marrow biopsy with peripheral smear review was performed for further evaluation.

Morphology & flow cytometry The main finding in the peripheral blood smear was thrombocytosis with many small platelets **f3.1**. The WBCs appeared normal. The bone marrow aspirate smear was hemodilute and suboptimal for evaluation, but examination of the touch preparation showed complete, maturing erythropoiesis and granulopoiesis without evidence of dysplasia. The megakaryocytes, however, were atypically enlarged and hyperlobate. Increased atypical megakaryocytes were also present in the core biopsy, some in loose clusters, and many with hyperlobate, "staghorn" nuclei **f3.2**. A reticulin stain showed no definite increase in reticulin fibrosis. Flow cytometry revealed no definite abnormalities.

Genetics/molecular results Chromosome analysis showed a normal female karyotype, and FISH studies were negative for del(5q), monosomy 5, del(7q), monosomy 7, trisomy 8, del(17p), and del(20q). A targeted myeloid NGS panel was positive for *CALR* p.L367fs*46 (c.1099_1150del) with 43% variant allele frequency (VAF).

Based on the findings of a *CALR* mutation and absence of *BCR-ABL1* translocation (by karyotype) in conjunction with the laboratory and morphologic findings, a diagnosis of **essential thrombocytosis** (ET) was rendered.

WBC	$6.8 \times 10^9 / L$
RBC	$3.69 \times 10^{12} / L$
HGB	11.5 g/dL
HCT	38.2%
MCV	104 fL
RDW	13.4%
Platelets	$641 \times 10^9 / L$

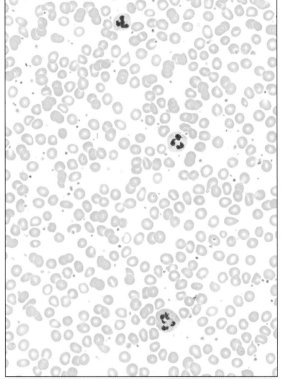

f3.1 Peripheral blood demonstrating thrombocytosis with normal-appearing platelets & normal white blood cells

ISBN 978-089189-6814   ©2021 ASCP

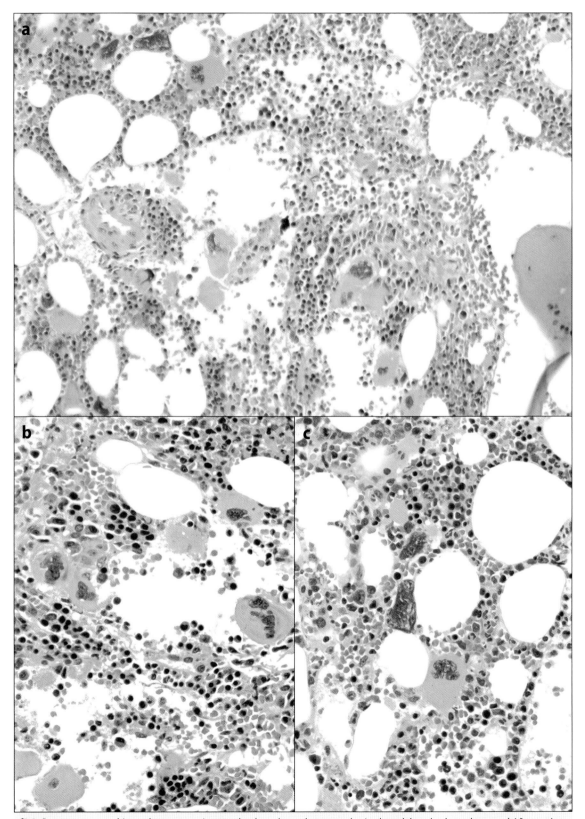

f3.2 Bone marrow core biopsy demonstrates increased, enlarged megakaryocytes having hyperlobated or hyperdense nuclei & occurring in clusters

t3.1 World Health Organization (WHO) 2017 diagnostic criteria for essential thrombocytosis (ET)

All of the following major criteria
or
the first 3 major criteria in addition to both the minor criteria must be satisfied to render a diagnosis of ET

Major criteria

1. Thrombocytosis with platelet count ≥450 × 10⁹/L

2. Bone marrow biopsy with megakaryocyte proliferation, including increased mature, enlarged megakaryocytes, many with hyperlobate nuclei, and almost no left shift or increase in erythropoiesis or granulopoiesis; very infrequently, minor increase in reticulin fibrosis (grade 1)

3. Must not fulfill WHO criteria for primary myelofibrosis, polycythemia vera, *BCR-ABL1*-positive chronic myeloid leukemia (CML), or other myeloid neoplasm

4. Presence of *JAK2, CALR,* or *MPL* mutation

Minor criteria

Identification of clonal marker
or
Exclusion of causes of reactive thrombocytosis

A bone marrow biopsy may not be required in patients with sustained absolute erythrocytosis & hemoglobin levels >18.5 g/dL (>185 g/L) in men (hematocrit >55.5%) or >16.5 g/dL (>165 g/L) in women (hematocrit >49.5%) if major criterion 3 & the minor criterion are present

Discussion ET is a myeloproliferative neoplasm (MPN) characterized by marked thrombocytosis in the peripheral blood and the absence of other accompanying cytoses or cytopenias. The 2017 World Health Organization (WHO) diagnostic criteria **t3.1** require a thrombocytosis with platelet count of ≥450 × 10⁹/L and bone marrow biopsy with evidence of megakaryocyte proliferation, including mature, enlarged megakaryocytes with hyperlobate nuclei. Almost no left shift or increase in erythropoiesis or neutrophil granulopoiesis should be present. A minor increase in reticulin fibrosis (grade 1) may seldom be seen. If WHO criteria can be fulfilled for primary myelofibrosis, polycythemia vera, or *BCR-ABL1*-positive chronic myeloid leukemia (CML), then a diagnosis of ET must not be rendered. Finally, if the presence of a *JAK2, CALR,* or *MPL* mutation cannot be confirmed, then a clonal marker must be identified or causes of reactive thrombocytosis must be excluded.

ET is often discovered incidentally after routine laboratory studies in asymptomatic individuals (>50% of cases). Other patients may present with hemorrhage, most commonly at mucosal surfaces, or with sequelae of vascular occlusion. Severe cases may have thrombosis of major arteries and veins. In ~15%-20% of patients, the physical examination may be significant for mild palpable splenomegaly. Although ET generally follows an indolent course,

infrequent complications of severe hemorrhage or thrombosis may occur. Leukemic transformation or progression to myelofibrosis is rare.

The bone marrow of most cases of ET will demonstrate a normal karyotype, though nonspecific abnormalities such as trisomy 8 or del(20q) are rarely present. The main genetic findings in ET are observed at the molecular level, with driver mutations in 3 signaling genes, *JAK2, CALR,* and *MPL,* found in most cases. None of these mutations is specific to ET and they are frequently found in other myeloid neoplasms, especially PV and PMF. About 12% of cases of ET lack mutations in any of these 3 genes and are designated as "triple-negative." The *JAK2* V617F mutation in exon 14 is present in 50%-60% of cases and confers an increased risk of thrombosis compared to *CALR*-mutated or triple-negative ET cases. Mutations in *CALR* are present in ~30% of ET cases and are associated with a higher platelet count, lower hemoglobin level, and lower WBC count than cases with *JAK2* V617F . The presence of *MPL* mutation is rare (3% of cases) and may increase the risk of progression to myelofibrosis. No significant difference in the risk of leukemic transformation is evident among these 3 driver mutations, however, and overall survival when adjusted for age and sex is similar among ET patients with *JAK2, CALR,* and *MPL* gene mutations and those with triple-negative status.

ISBN 978-089189-6814

Pathogenic *CALR* variants induce a frameshift in exon 9; the most common of these are type 1, a 52-bp deletion (p.L367fs*46) seen in this patient, and type 2, a 5-bp insertion (p.K385fs*47). These two variants comprise more than 80% of pathogenic *CALR* mutations, which cause abnormal binding of calreticulin to the thrombopoietin receptor (MPL) due to loss of a KDEL motif that normally causes retention of calreticulin in the endoplasmic reticulin. Mutant calreticulin bound to MPL results in excessive platelet production and megakaryocyte proliferation through the JAK-STAT pathway. Type 1 and type 2 *CALR* mutations are both characterized by higher platelet counts than the *JAK2* p.V617F mutation in patients with ET; however, the difference is more pronounced with type 2 *CALR* mutation. Despite this, type 2 *CALR* mutation is associated with a lower rate of thrombotic events than type 1 mutation and especially *JAK2* p.V617F. Despite these differences, however, there is no significant difference in overall or thrombosis-free survival between patients having type 1 and type 2 *CALR* mutations.

Mutations in myeloid-associated genes other than *JAK2*, *CALR*, or *MPL* are found in approximately half of ET cases, and in particular, at least one mutation in *SH2B3*, *IDH2*, *U2AF1*, *SF3B1*, *EZH2*, or *TP53* has adverse prognostic significance, being associated with decreased overall survival independent of age and karyotype. The presence of *TP53* mutation, in particular, is associated with an increased risk of leukemic transformation.

Diagnostic pearls/pitfalls
– Essential thrombocytosis (ET) is marked by thrombocytosis without significant dysplasia or abnormal cell counts. Therefore, it is especially important to rule out reactive causes for the elevated platelet count.
– The prefibrotic phase of primary myelofibrosis (PMF) may resemble ET, although in PMF, hypercellularity, granulocytic hyperplasia, and distinct atypia of megakaryocytes, including forms with "bulbous" or "cloudlike" nuclei, are usually more evident. Distinction between the 2 entities may be difficult based on histologic evaluation alone, especially in suboptimal biopsy samples.
– *CALR* exon 9 mutation is the second most common mutation found in ET, with most exon 9 variants being type 1 or type 2. Although both type 1 and type 2 variants are characterized by higher platelet counts than those seen with *JAK2* mutations, the

risk of thrombosis remains lower. Although type 1 is associated with increased risk of progression to myelofibrosis, overall and thrombosis-free survival rates are similar between patients having either variant.
– The presence of thrombocytosis with dysplasia or abnormal cell counts should prompt investigation for a different myeloproliferative neoplasm (MPN) or myelodysplastic syndrome (MDS)/MPN overlap neoplasm. In particular, MDS/MPN with ring sideroblasts and thrombocytosis (see **Case 15**) may have similar findings to ET including enlarged, hyperlobated megakaryocytes and a *JAK2* mutation. Thus, careful evaluation for the presence of erythroid dysplasia and ring sideroblasts is necessary to help distinguish between the two entities.

Readings
Elala YC, Lasho TL, Gangat N, et al. Calreticulin variant stratified driver mutational status and prognosis in essential thrombocythemia. Am Hematol. 2016;91(5):503-6. **DOI: 10.1002/ajh.24338**

Klampfl T, Gisslinger H, Harutyunyan AS, et al. Somatic mutations of calreticulin in myeloproliferative neoplasms. N Engl J Med. 2013;369(25):2379-90. **DOI: 10.1056/NEJMoa1311347**

National Comprehensive Cancer Network (NCCN) Guidelines for Myeloproliferative Neoplasms, version 1.2020. **https://www.nccn.org/professionals/physician_gls/pdf/mpn.pdf**

Pietra D, Rumi E, Ferretti VV, Di Buduo CA, et al. Differential clinical effects of different mutation subtypes in *CALR*-mutant myeloproliferative neoplasms. Leukemia. 2016;30(2):431 **DOI: 10.1038/leu.2015.277**

Spivak J. Myeloproliferative neoplasms. N Engl J Med. 2017;(376):2168-81. **DOI: 10.1056/NEJMra1406186**

Swerdlow SH, Campo E, Harris NL, et al. World Health Organization Classification of Tumours of Haematopoietic and Lymphoid Tissues. 4th ed. Lyon, France: IARC Press; 2017. **ISBN: 978-9283224310**

Tefferi A, Lasho TL, Guglielmelli P, et al. Targeted deep sequencing in polycythemia vera and essential thrombocythemia. Blood Adv. 2016;1(1):21-30. **DOI: 10.1182/bloodadvances.2016000216**

Tefferi A, Wassie EA, Guglielmelli P, et al. Type 1 versus Type 2 calreticulin mutations in essential thrombocythemia: a collaborative study of 1027 patients. Am J Hematol. 2014;89(8):E121-4. **DOI: 10.1002/ajh.23743**

Vainchenker W, Kralovics R. Genetic basis and molecular pathophysiology of classical myeloproliferative neoplasms. Blood. 2017;129(6):667-79. **DOI: 10.1182/blood-2016-10-695940**

Rose C Beck

4

Chronic neutrophilic leukemia with *CSF3R* T618I

History A 63-year-old female with no significant past medical history was found to have leukocytosis after evaluation for knee pain and was referred to an oncologist. CBC results are shown to the right. Review of the medical record indicated the patient had an elevated WBC ($18\text{-}40 \times 10^9/\text{L}$) over the preceding 2 years. A bone marrow biopsy with peripheral blood smear review was then performed.

WBC	$44.5 \times 10^9/\text{L}$
HGB	14.2 g / dL
HCT	43.8%
MCV	89 fL
Platelets	$163 \times 10^9/\text{L}$

Morphology & flow cytometry The peripheral smear demonstrated leukocytosis composed of mostly mature neutrophils with toxic granulation, with 2% metamyelocytes and myelocytes and no blasts **f4.1**. The bone marrow aspirate showed a granulocytic predominance (myeloid:erythroid ratio 8:1) with occasional toxic changes but no dysplastic features. Blasts were not increased and dysplasia of the erythroid and megakaryocytic lineages was also not seen **f4.2a**. The core biopsy and clot section demonstrated similar findings as the aspirate, with 100% cellularity **f4.2b**. There was no morphologic evidence for a plasma cell neoplasm and flow cytometry did not show any significant abnormalities.

Based on the morphologic findings and extended history of unexplained leukocytosis, a descriptive diagnosis was initially rendered, but with concern for a **myeloproliferative neoplasm** (MPN), specifically **chronic neutrophilic leukemia** (CNL).

Genetics/molecular results The karyotype was normal and FISH was negative for *BCR-ABL1*, del(5q), monosomy 5, del(7q), monosomy 7, trisomy 8, del(17p), and del(20q). A targeted myeloid NGS panel was positive for the presence of several pathogenic variants: *CSF3R* p.T618I (c.1853C>T) at 45% variant allele frequency (VAF) and *CSF3R* p.Y787* (c.2361T>A) at 50% VAF **f4.3**.

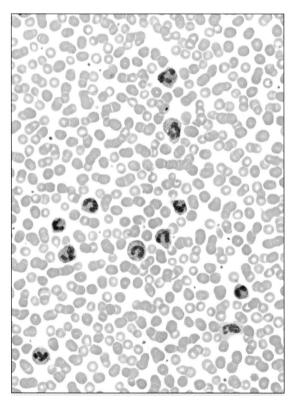

f4.1 Blood smear showing neutrophilia with mostly mature forms & toxic granulation

ISBN 978-089189-6814

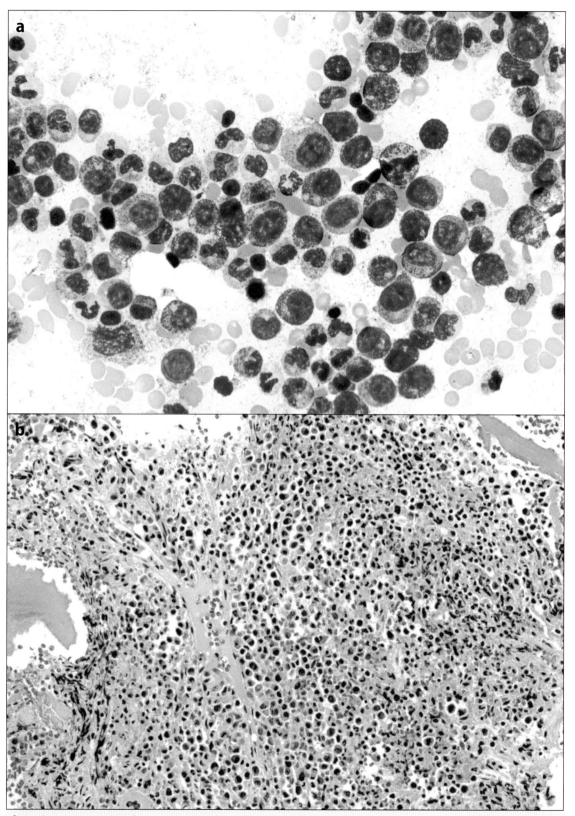

f4.2 a Bone marrow aspirate demonstrating granulocytic hyperplasia without significant dysplasia in any of the 3 hematopoietic lineages; **b** core biopsy section demonstrating hypercellularity with granulocyte predominance

4 Chronic neutrophilic leukemia with CSF3R T618I

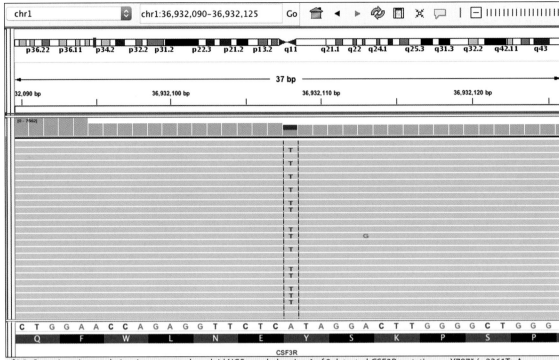

f4.3 Somatic variant analysis using a targeted myeloid NGS panel, showing 1 of 2 detected *CSF3R* mutations, p.Y787* (c.2361T>A; highlighted in red); this mutation results in a premature stop codon, TAA (hg19, Integrative Genomics Viewer [IGV] browser, showing the reverse strand) [see **fA.8**, p312]

t4.1 World Health Organization (WHO) 2017 diagnostic criteria for CNL

1. Blood leukocytosis ≥25,000/µL (≥25 × 10⁹/L), with segmented and band neutrophils ≥80% of white cells & without dysgranulopoiesis; immature granulocytes (promyelocytes, myelocytes & metamyelocytes) are <10% of white cells; only rare myeloblasts present; monocytes are <1,000/µL (<1 ×10⁹/L)
2. Hypercellular bone marrow with increased neutrophils with normal-appearing maturation & <5% blasts
3. Not meeting WHO criteria for CML or any other myeloproliferative neoplasm
4. No evidence of rearrangement of *PDGFRA*, *PDGFRB*, or *FGFR1*, or *PCM1-JAK2* fusion
5. Presence of *CSF3R* p.T618I or other activating *CFS3R* mutation **or** persistent, unexplained neutrophilia (3 months) with splenomegaly. If a plasma cell neoplasm is present, demonstration of clonality of myeloid cells on genetic or molecular studies because of a frequent association of plasma cell neoplasm with reactive neutrophilia)

CML, chronic myeloid leukemia; CNL, chonic neutophylic leukemia

With the addition of the molecular findings, a final diagnosis of **chronic neutrophilic leukemia** was rendered.

Discussion CNL is a rare MPN characterized by sustained peripheral blood neutrophilic leukocytosis without significant left shift (<10% immature granulocytes) and lack of dysplastic morphology. Patients are often older, with a median age of 66.5 years at diagnosis, and may be asymptomatic or have symptoms associated with hepatosplenic involvement, with splenomegaly occurring in ~1/3 of affected individuals. The course of the disease is usually aggressive, with median survival of 2-3 years. Disease progression is often accompanied by increasing WBC, worsening cytopenia and organomegaly, and transformation to acute myeloid leukemia (AML) in 10%-20% of cases.

Histologically, CNL most closely resembles benign leukemoid reaction, but it can also mimic *BCR-ABL1*-positive chronic myeloid leukemia (CML) or atypical CML (see **t14.2** of **Case 14** for a comparison of these entities); therefore, CNL cannot be diagnosed by morphology alone. Based on World Health Organization (WHO) 2017 criteria **t4.1**, the diagnosis of CNL requires leukocytosis ≥25,000/µL (≥25 × 10⁹/L), with ≥80% neutrophils that are predominantly mature (<10% immature forms) and no dysplasia.

ISBN 978-089189-6814   ©2021 ASCP

Often there is toxic granulation in the neutrophils, as seen in this case. Genetic and molecular testing must be performed to exclude other chronic myeloid neoplasms that have recurrent genetic abnormalities, such as *BCR-ABL1*-positive CML and *JAK2*-associated MPN. A rare neutrophilic variant of CML, CML-N, is characterized by prominent neutrophilia and may be confused with CNL. CML-N is associated with the e19/a2 breakpoints for *BCR-ABL1*, resulting in a larger, p230 BCR-ABL fusion protein that is detectable with FISH (see **Case 1**).

Depending on the strictness of diagnostic criteria applied, 80%-100% of CNL cases have activating mutations in *CSF3R* (*colony stimulating factor 3 receptor*), which encodes for the transmembrane granulocyte colony-stimulating factor (G-CSF) receptor, important for neutrophil maturation, proliferation, and survival. The most common *CSF3R* mutation detected in CNL is p.T618I in exon 14. This and other activating mutations of *CSF3R* result in constitutive signaling through the JAK/STAT pathway. Approximately 25% of CNL cases have both a membrane-proximal mutation such as *CSF3R* p.T618I and a truncation mutation in the cytoplasmic tail region, as demonstrated by the *CSF3R* p.Y787* mutation in this patient. Truncation mutations disrupt normal receptor trafficking and turnover, resulting in increased expression of the G-CSF receptor at the cell surface. Clinically, the presence of the p.T618I mutation in particular is associated with more aggressive disease including a higher WBC and lower hemoglobin and platelet counts. Mutations in *CSF3R* are not specific to CNL and are found in severe congenital neutropenia and hereditary neutrophilia, as well as infrequently in other myeloid neoplasms such as atypical CML and AML.

Mutations in other genes besides *CSF3R* are also found in most CNL cases, with the median burden of myeloid-associated mutations identified at 3.6 using whole exome sequencing. *SETBP1* mutations, which also occur in atypical CML and chronic myelomonocytic leukemia (CMML), have been reported in 14%-56% of CNL cases. Other frequently mutated genes in CNL include *ASXL1*, *TET2*, *CBL*, and spliceosome genes such as *SRSF2* and *U2AF1*. Rarely, mutations in *JAK2* and *CALR* have been reported in CNL; the presence of these mutations should prompt investigation for a different MPN.

Chromosome analysis detects a normal karyotype in most CNL cases. If present, chromosomal aberrations include those typically associated with myeloid neoplasm, such as trisomy 8, del(11q), and del(20q).

There is no standard therapy for CNL, and treatment regimens include supportive care, cytoreductive agents, and targeted therapy with the JAK2 inhibitor ruxolitinib, which has shown variable effectiveness.

Diagnostic pearls/pitfalls

– The neutrophilic leukocytosis of chronic neutrophilic leukemia (CNL) closely resembles a benign leukemoid reaction and is composed of mostly segmented neutrophils and bands, without dysplasia and sometimes with toxic granulation.

– CNL may be confused with other myeloproliferative neoplasms (MPNs) having a prominent granulocytic component, such as *BCR-ABL*-positive chronic myeloid leukemia (CML), the neutrophilic variant of *BCR-ABL*-positive CML, and atypical CML.

– Molecular and genetic testing are both critical for evaluating suspected cases of CNL, to assess for *CSF3R* mutations and to exclude alterations found in other MPNs, especially *BCR-ABL1*.

– Over 80% of CNL cases have at least 1 mutation in *CSF3R*, which helps to confirm the diagnosis in the appropriate clinicopathologic context.

Readings

Maxson JE, Gotlib J, Pollyea DA, et al. Oncogenic *CSF3R* mutations in chronic neutrophilic leukemia and atypical CML. N Engl J Med. 2013;368(19):1781-90. **DOI: 10.1056/NEJMoa1214514**

Maxson JE, Tyner JW. Genomics of chronic neutrophilic leukemia. Blood. 2017;129(6):715-22. **DOI: 10.1182/blood-2016-10-695981.**

McClure RF, Ewalt MD, Crow J, et al. Clinical significance of DNA variants in chronic myeloid neoplasms: a report of the Association for Molecular Pathology. J Mol Diagn. 2018;20(6):717-37. **DOI: 10.1016/j.jmoldx.2018.07.002**

Meggendorfer M, Haferlach T, Alpermann T, et al. Specific molecular mutation patterns delineate chronic neutrophilic leukemia, atypical chronic myeloid leukemia, and chronic myelomonocytic leukemia. Haematologica. 2014;99(12):e244-6. **DOI: 10.3324/haematol.2014.113159**

Pardanani A, Lasho TL, Laborde RR, et al. *CSF3R* T618I is a highly prevalent and specific mutation in chronic neutrophilic leukemia. Leukemia. 2013;27(9):1870-3. **DOI: 10.1038/leu.2013.122**

Swerdlow SH, Campo E, Harris NL, et al. World Health Organization Classification of Tumours of Haematopoietic and Lymphoid Tissues. 4th ed. Lyon, France: IARC Press; 2017.

Szuber N, Elliott M, Tefferi A. Chronic neutrophilic leukemia: 2020 update on diagnosis, molecular genetics, prognosis, and management. Am J Hematol. 2020;95(2):212-24. **DOI: 10.1002/ajh.25688**

Zhang H, Wilmot B, Bottomly D, et al. Genomic landscape of neutrophilic leukemias of ambiguous diagnosis. Blood. 2019;134(11):867-79. **DOI: 10.1182/blood.2019000611**

5

Erika M Moore

Chronic eosinophilic leukemia with clonal abnormalities

History An 87-year-old female was referred to an oncologist because of a 1-year history of persistent, unexplained peripheral blood eosinophilia (absolute eosinophil count of 6.7×10^9/L) and thrombocytopenia. CBC results are shown at right. A bone marrow biopsy with peripheral blood smear review was performed for further evaluation.

Morphology & flow cytometry The peripheral smear demonstrated eosinophilia composed predominantly of mature eosinophils including some atypical forms with cytoplasmic vacuolation and abnormal localization of cytoplasmic granules **f5.1a**, **b**. The bone marrow aspirate smear showed normal trilineage hematopoiesis with increased eosinophils and eosinophil precursors, totaling 22% by differential count. Blasts were not increased and there was no overt dysplasia. The core biopsy was hypercellular with granulocytic hyperplasia and increased eosinophils **f5.1c**, **d**.

Flow cytometric studies demonstrated an increase in eosinophils, which normally have more uniformly high side scatter characteristics, slightly brighter CD45, and brighter HLA-DR than neutrophils **f5.2**. No phenotypic abnormalities were identified on flow cytometry.

Genetics/molecular results Initial FISH studies were negative for a *BCR-ABL1* translocation and for rearrangements of *PDGFRA*, *PDGFRB*, *FGFR1*, and *JAK2*. Karyotype analysis demonstrated trisomy 8 and loss of Y in 10 cells and additional FISH confirmed trisomy 8 in 90% of nuclei examined **f5.3**. A targeted NGS panel demonstrated *TET2* p.R1452* (c.4354C>T) with 21% variant allele frequency (VAF) **f5.4**.

WBC	13.8×10^9/L
Differential	
Polymorphonuclear leukocytes	33%
Bands	3%
Lymphocytes	10%
Monocytes	5%
Eosinophils	49%
RBC	5.21×10^{12}/L
HGB	14.9 g/dL
HCT	44.7%
MCV	86 fL
RDW	14%
Platelets	17×10^9/L

Based on these genetic and molecular findings, which indicated the presence of clonal hematopoiesis, a final diagnosis of **chronic eosinophilic leukemia** (CEL), not otherwise specified, was rendered.

Discussion CEL, not otherwise specified, is a myeloproliferative neoplasm characterized by an unexplained persistent elevation in eosinophils accompanied by organ involvement and dysfunction. Tissue damage is mediated by both infiltration of the eosinophils and cytokine-induced damage from contents of eosinophilic granules, and most often involves the heart but can also affect the lungs, skin, gastrointestinal tract, and central nervous system. The peripheral smear demonstrates predominantly mature eosinophils that may have normal morphology or may be atypical, with nuclear irregularities,

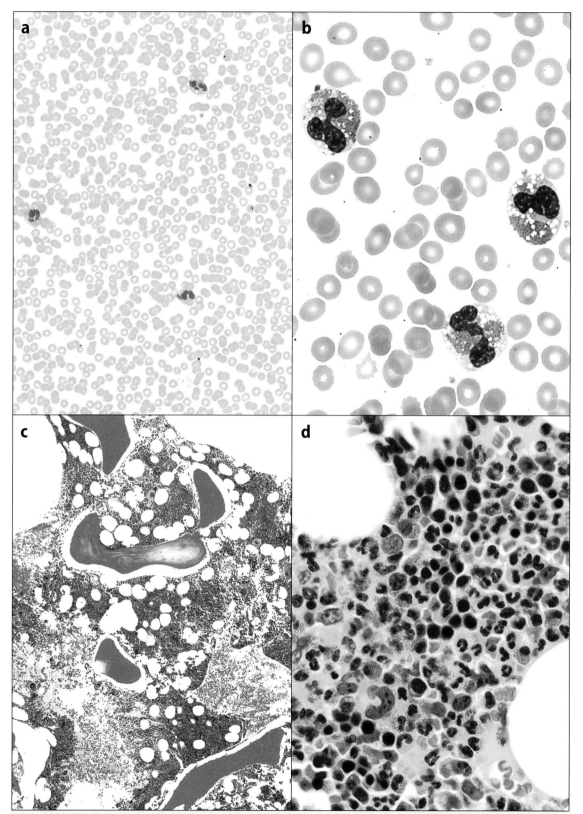

f5.1 The peripheral blood smear reveals **a** eosinophilia, including atypical forms, with cytoplasmic vacuolation & **b** abnormal localization of granules; **c, d** bone marrow core biopsy reveals hypercellular bone marrow with increased eosinophils

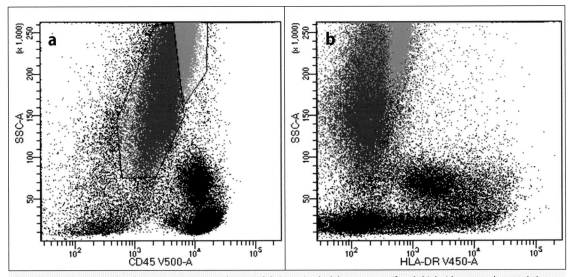

f5.2 Flow cytometric studies demonstrating increased eosinophils (green), which have more uniformly high side scatter characteristics and **a** brighter CD45 and **b** HLA-DR than neutrophils & neutrophil precursors (red)

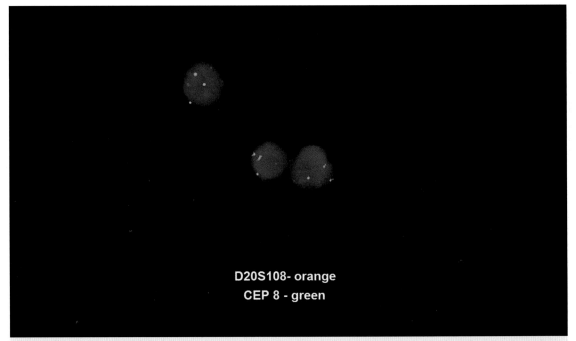

f5.2 Single color FISH probes D20S108 (20q, orange) & CEP 8 (8 centromere, green) showing a third green signal indicative of trisomy 8

cytoplasmic vacuoles, or abnormal localization of cytoplasmic granules. It is important to note, however, that eosinophilic atypia is not specific to neoplastic conditions. A concurrent neutrophilia is often present in CEL, and the bone marrow is typically hypercellular with increased eosinophils. Granulocytic dysplasia may be present. Charcot-Leyden crystals, although not common, may be seen in involved tissue; these crystals are formed from lysophospholipase present in

eosinophilic granules. They are slender and pointed on both ends and can be highlighted by a trichrome stain. Charcot-Leyden crystals are not specific to CEL and can be present in any condition with eosinophilia and tissue infiltration.

CEL is a diagnosis of exclusion and all possible reactive causes of eosinophilia must be ruled out, including allergies, autoimmune disorders, parasitic infection,

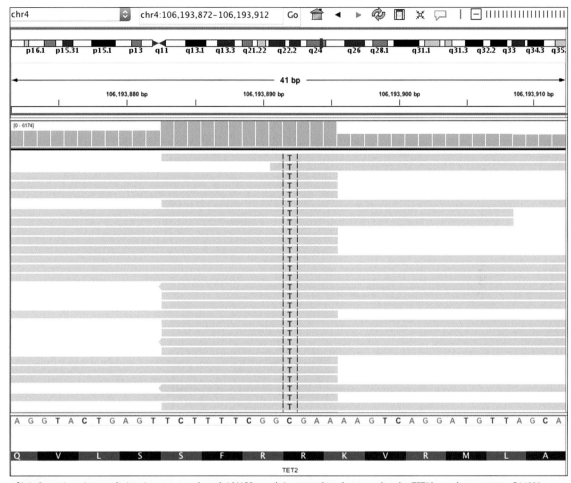

f5.4 Somatic variant analysis using a targeted myeloid NGS panel. Annotated reads mapped to the *TET2* locus demonstrate p.R1452* (c.4354C>T), highlighted in red (hg19, Integrative Genomics Viewer [IGV] browser) [see **fA.8**, p312]

and pulmonary syndromes, among other etiologies. Once reactive conditions have been excluded, a thorough investigation must be undertaken to evaluate for other hematopoietic neoplasms that may present with eosinophilia, including chronic myeloid leukemia, acute myeloid leukemia, systemic mastocytosis, and myeloid/lymphoid neoplasms with eosinophilia with specific gene rearrangements of *PDGFRA*, *PDGFRB*, *FGFR1*, or *PCM1-JAK2*. In addition to these disorders in which the eosinophils originate from the neoplastic clone, other hematopoietic neoplasms such as T-cell lymphomas and Hodgkin lymphoma can be associated with a secondary eosinophilia in which the eosinophils are not clonal. Rarely, eosinophilia can result from cytokine release from a phenotypically abnormal, clonal T-cell population that is not overt lymphoma; this disorder is categorized as "lymphocytic variant of hypereosinophilic syndrome" and responds to anti-interleukin 5 monoclonal antibody therapy. Thus, because of the occurrence of clonal or secondary

eosinophilia in different types of hematopoietic neoplasms, a comprehensive analysis of the clinical history, laboratory findings, bone marrow morphology with flow cytometry, and cytogenetic and molecular findings is critical. If another neoplastic process is excluded, a diagnosis of CEL requires either increased blasts (>2% in the peripheral blood or >5% in the bone marrow) or evidence of clonality **t5.1**. In the absence of these features, cases of unexplained persistent eosinophilia with organ involvement must be classified as idiopathic hypereosinophilic syndrome (HES). Patients who lack organ involvement are categorized as having idiopathic hypereosinophilia **t5.2**.

Defining a clonal abnormality in CEL can be challenging because there are no CEL-specific cytogenetic or molecular abnormalities. In general, cytogenetic abnormalities usually associated with myeloid neoplasms such as trisomy 8, deletion 7, or abnormalities of 17p, are supportive of a diagnosis of

t5.1 World Health Organization (WHO) 2017 diagnostic criteria for chronic eosinophilic leukemia, not otherwise specified

1. Eosinophilia (eosinophil count >1.5 × 10⁹/L)
2. WHO criteria for *BCR-ABL1*-positive chronic myeloid leukemia, polycythemia vera, essential thrombocythemia, primary myelofibrosis, chronic neutrophilic leukemia, chronic myelomonocytic leukemia, and *BCR-ABL1*-negative atypical chronic myeloid leukemia are not met
3. No rearrangement of *PDGFRA*, *PDGFRB*, or *FGFR1*, and no *PCM1-JAK2*, *ETV6-JAK2*, or *BCR-JAK2* fusion
4. Blast cells constitute <20% of the cells in the peripheral blood and bone marrow, and inv(16)(p13.1q22), t(16;16)(p13.1;q22), t(8;21)(q22;q22.1), and other diagnostic features of acute myeloid leukemia are absent
5. A clonal cytogenetic or molecular abnormality or blast cells account for ≥2% of cells in the peripheral blood or ≥5% in the bone marrow

t5.2 Comparison of possible diagnoses in patients with persistent, unexplained blood eosinophilia*

	IE	HES	CEL
tissue damage from eosinophilic infiltrate	no	yes	may be present
evidence of non-CEL hematopoietic neoplasm	no	no	no
increased blasts	no	no	may be present
clonal genetic abnormality†	no	no	may be present

Reactive, allergic, infectious, and inflammatory causes must first be excluded

†*In cases having mutations associated with clonal hematopoiesis of indeterminate potential as the sole abnormality, these findings should be interpreted with caution*

CEL, chronic eosinophilic leukemia; HES, hypereosinophilic syndrome; IE, idiopathic eosinophilia

CEL but with the caveat that other myeloid neoplasms that may have similar cytogenetic findings must be excluded first. In the past, evidence of clonality in CEL was largely based on cytogenetic abnormalities but with the advent of targeted NGS panels, it is now standard practice to incorporate molecular data into the assessment for clonality in CEL. This is supported by a study examining somatic mutations detected in HES patients (defined by absence of increased blasts or clonal cytogenetic abnormalities). This study demonstrated that while survival of CEL was significantly worse than survival in HES cases without somatic mutations, cases of HES with mutations had survival outcomes similar to cases of CEL. Commonly identified mutations include *ASXL1*, *TET2*, *EZH2*, *SETBP1*, *JAK2*, and *DNMT3A*. A subset of these mutations, however, has also been documented in elderly individuals without hematologic disease (clonal hematopoiesis of indeterminate potential, CHIP; see **Case 17**). Therefore, caution is suggested before making a diagnosis of CEL based solely on identification of a known CHIP-related mutation. The presence of >1 mutation and/or higher variant allele frequencies may favor a neoplastic process over CHIP; however, currently, there are no specific criteria to guide interpretation of mutational data when evaluating patients with hypereosinophilia.

The prognosis for patients with CEL is generally poor and no standard treatment exists. Some patients can be managed with hydroxyurea, and case reports have described patients responding to interferon α and imatinib; however, median reported survival times are approximately 22 months, and in some patients, the condition will transform to acute myeloid leukemia.

In this patient, the presence of both trisomy 8 and a *TET2* mutation indicated clonal hematopoiesis and supported a diagnosis of CEL, in the absence of an identifiable cause for the eosinophilia. Because of her advanced age, no treatment was initiated.

Diagnostic pearls/pitfalls

– There are many causes of reactive and secondary eosinophilia, all of which need to be excluded before making a diagnosis of chronic eosinophilic leukemia, which requires evidence of clonality or an increase in blasts.

– Persistent eosinophilia with organ damage in the absence of a clonal abnormality or increase in blasts is considered idiopathic hypereosinophilic syndrome.

– Eosinophilic dysplasia can be seen in reactive eosinophilia and is not a definitive indication of a hematopoietic neoplasm.

– Low-level mutations in certain genes such as *ASXL1*, *DNMT3A*, *TET2*, and *JAK2* may be an incidental finding in elderly patients rather than evidence of a clonal neoplasm and should be evaluated with caution in the context of other clinicopathologic factors.

Readings

Helbig G, Soja A, Bartkowska-Chrobok A, et al. Chronic eosinophilic leukemia–not otherwise specified has a poor prognosis with unresponsiveness to conventional treatment and high risk of acute transformation. Am J Hematol. 2012;87(6):643-5. **DOI: 10.1002/ajh.23193**

Helbig G, Stella-Holowiecka B, Majewski M, et al. Interferon alpha induces a good molecular response in a patient with chronic eosinophilic leukemia (CEL) carrying the JAK2V617F point mutation. Haematologica. 2007;92(11):e118-9. **DOI: 10.3324/haematol.11841**

Hu Z, Boddu PC, Loghavi S, et al. A multimodality work-up of patients with hypereosinophilia. Am J Hematol. 2018;93(11):1337-46. **DOI: 10.1002/ajh.25247**

Reiter A, Gotlib J. Myeloid neoplasms with eosinophilia. Blood. 2017;129(6):704-14. **DOI: 10.1182/blood-2016-10-695973**

Shomali W, Gotlib J. World Health Organization-defined eosinophilic disorders: 2019 update on diagnosis, risk stratification, and management. Am J Hematol. 2019;94(10):1149-67. **DOI: 10.1002/ajh.25617**

Swerdlow SH, Campo E, Harris NL, et al. World Health Organization Classification of Tumours of Haematopoietic and Lymphoid Tissues. 4th ed. Lyon, France: IARC Press; 2017. **ISBN: 978-9283224310**

Wang S, Tam W, Tsai A, et al. Targeted next-generation sequencing identifies a subset of idiopathic hypereosinophilic syndrome with features similar to chronic eosinophilic leukemia, not otherwise specified. Mod Pathol. 2016;29:854-64. **DOI: 10.1038/modpathol.2016.75**

Yamada O, Kitahara K, Imamura K, et al. Clinical and cytogenetic remission induced by interferon-α in a patient with chronic eosinophilic leukemia associated with a unique t(3;9;5) translocation. Am J Hematol. 1998;58(2):137-41. **DOI: 10.1002/(sici)1096-8652(199806)58:2<137::aid-ajh 9>3.0.co;2-t**

Christopher Ryder

6

Systemic mastocytosis with an associated hematopoietic neoplasm

History An 83-year-old male with an unremarkable past medical history presented to his primary care physician with fatigue and was found to be pancytopenic. CBC results are shown at right. A bone marrow biopsy with peripheral blood smear review was performed for further evaluation of his cytopenias.

WBC	1.3×10^9/L
RBC	2.91×10^{12}/L
HGB	8.9 g/dL
HCT	26.8%
MCV	92.2 fL
RDW	19.3%
Platelets	46×10^9/L

Morphology & flow cytometry The peripheral blood smear showed normocytic anemia with anisopoikilocytosis, neutropenia with few dysplastic neutrophils and basophils, rare blasts, and thrombocytopenia **f6.1**. The aspirate smears and core biopsy demonstrated granulocytic dysplasia as well as atypical megakaryocytes, including small, hypolobate forms as well as forms having discrete, separated nuclear lobes **f6.2a**. Blasts were increased, enumerated at 15% of marrow cells in the aspirate smear, and a CD34 IHC stain highlighted ~10%-15% blasts **f6.2b**. Flow cytometric studies likewise identified an increased population of myeloblasts (10% of events) **f6.3**. Overall, the biopsy findings were consistent with a diagnosis of myelodysplastic syndrome (MDS) with excess blasts 2.

In addition to the aforementioned findings, the aspirate smears contained atypical spindle-shaped, hypogranular mast cells (consistent with type I atypical mast cells, versus type II atypical mast cells which are round and hypogranular), which accounted for 40%-50% of all mast cells **f6.4a**. A single well-formed mast cell aggregate was apparent in the clot section **f6.4b**.

IHC for CD117 and tryptase highlighted increased mast cells, including frequent spindle-shaped forms and several small aggregates in the core biopsy specimen **f6.5**. Aberrant CD25 expression by mast cells was demonstrated by IHC **f6.5**. A discrete mast cell population was not identified by flow cytometry. These findings indicated the presence of a concurrent mast cell neoplasm, and a final diagnosis of **systemic mastocytosis with an associated hematopoietic neoplasm** (SM-AHN) was rendered.

Genetics/molecular results Cytogenetic analysis revealed a normal male karyotype and FISH studies did not identify any AML or MDS-associated recurrent genetic alterations. A myeloid NGS panel revealed 3 high-frequency pathogenic variants: *ASXL1* I919Nfs*5 (variant allele frequency [VAF] 47%), *RUNX1* splice site (c.532+1G>T; VAF 44%), and *SRSF2* P95H (VAF 42%), as well as a low frequency *KIT* D816V mutation (c.2447A>T; VAF 2%).

ISBN 978-089189-6814 ©2021 ASCP

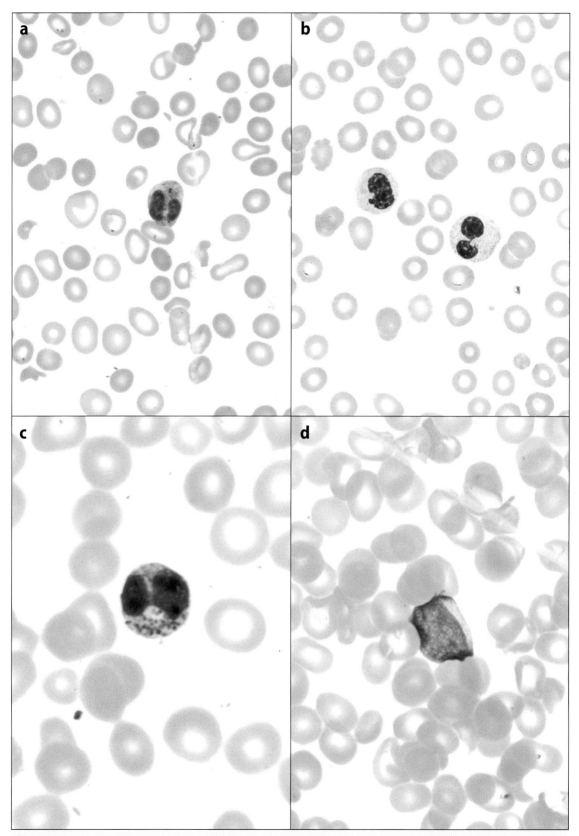

f6.1 Peripheral blood showing **a** red cell anisopoikilocytosis, **a**, **b** dysplastic neutrophils, **c** hypogranular basophil, and **d** a circulating blast

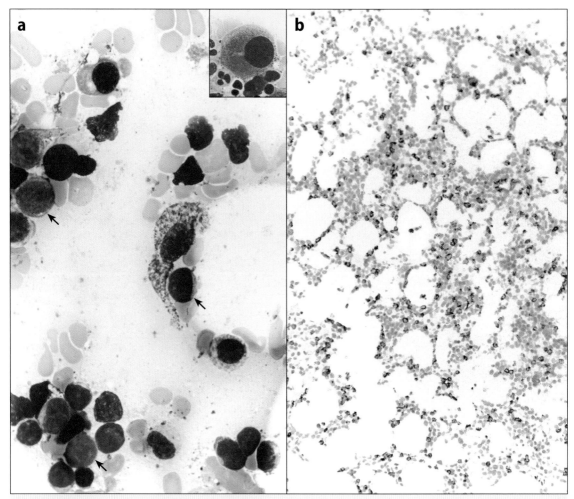

f6.2 **a** Bone marrow aspirate smear highlighting increased blasts (arrows) & dysplastic hypolobated megakaryocyte (inset); **b** CD34 stain on bone marrow clot section demonstrating increased blasts

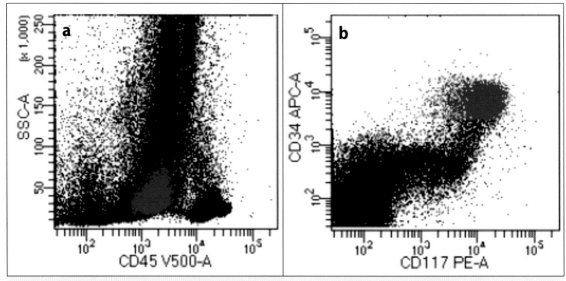

f6.3 Flow cytometry demonstrates an increase in **b** CD34-positive CD117-positive myeloblasts (10% of events)

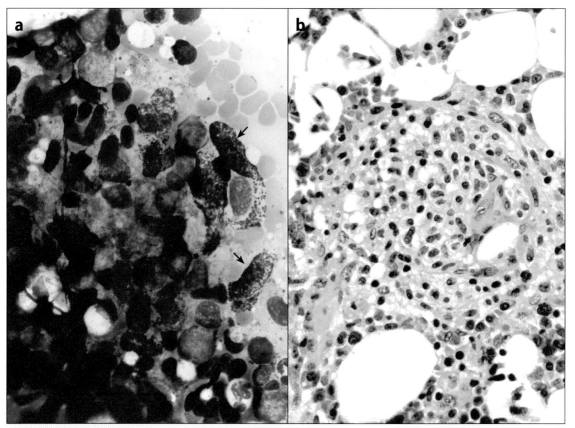

f6.4 a Bone marrow aspirate smear containing increased & atypical spindle-shaped mast cells (arrows); **b** bone marrow clot section demonstrating a mast cell aggregate

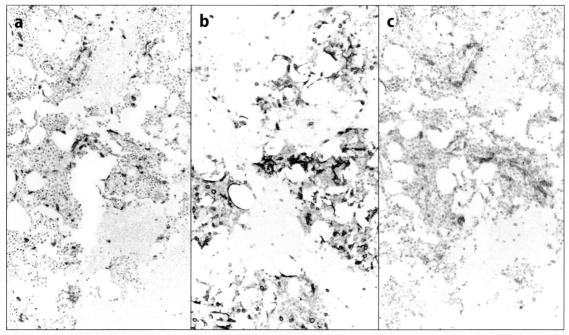

f6.5 a Tryptase & **b** CD117 immunostains performed on the bone marrow clot section highlight spindled mast cells, which have **c** atypical expression of CD25

t6.1 World Health Organization (WHO) 2017 classification of mastocytoses

Cutaneous mastocytosis (CM)

Urticaria pigmentosa/saculopapular CM
Diffuse CM
Mastocytoma of skin

Systemic mastocytosis (SM)

Indolent SM
Smoldering SM
Aggressive SM
SM with an associated clonal hematopoietic neoplasm
Mast cell leukemia

Mast cell sarcoma

t6.2 World Health Organization (WHO) 2017 diagnostic criteria for systemic mastocytosis (SM)

Major criterion

Dense, multifocal aggregates of mast cells detected in bone marrow and/or other extracutaneous organs

Minor criteria

In biopsy sections, >25% of mast cells show atypical morphology or, in aspirate smears, >25% of mast cells are immature or atypical
Mast cells aberrantly express CD2 and/or CD25 (by flow cytometry or immunohistochemistry)
KIT point mutation at codon 816 detected in bone marrow, blood, or other extracutaneous organs
Serum total tryptase persistently elevated >20 ng/mL (not valid in cases of SM with an associated hematopoietic neoplasm)

Diagnosis of SM is made if the major criterion plus 1 minor criterion or at least 3 minor criteria are met

Discussion Mastocytosis is a neoplastic, clonal proliferation of mast cells, with systemic mastocytosis (SM) and cutaneous mastocytosis (CM) being the most common variants **t6.1**. CM most commonly occurs in pediatric patients, whereas SM is generally an adult disease associated with multiorgan involvement, often including bone marrow, with accompanying organ dysfunction and overall shortened survival. When SM occurs in the context of a distinct other hematopoietic neoplasm, this process is termed "SM with an associated hematopoietic neoplasm" (SM-AHN); in most cases of SM-AHN, the non-mast cell neoplasm is of myeloid lineage and has been shown in some cases to be clonally related to the neoplastic mast cells. The diagnostic criteria for SM are summarized in **t6.2**.

In this case, only 1 single convincing mast cell aggregate was observed on H&E sections; however, a diagnosis of SM could still be made based on the presence of 3 minor criteria: >25% atypical mast cells in the aspirate smears, aberrant CD25 expression, and the presence of *KIT* D816V mutation. In addition, the presence of coexisting high-grade MDS indicated

a complete final diagnosis of SM-AHN. Because as many as 20% of cases of indolent SM may lack dense mast cell aggregates, investigation of minor criteria, including careful morphologic evaluation, immunohistochemistry, and molecular testing, is essential to the diagnosis. In the evaluation of aberrant antigen expression, several reports have demonstrated that CD25 is a more sensitive marker of atypical mast cells than CD2. SM is not associated with specific chromosomal abnormalities.

A pathogenic, activating variant in *KIT* (which encodes the receptor tyrosine kinase mast/stem cell growth factor receptor [SCFR], also known as c-kit or CD117) is identified in >90% of SM cases, with the vast majority of variants being D816V. Currently, it is not standard practice to test for mutations outside of codon 816, though other, rare variants with demonstrated receptor activating activity have been identified. Recommended treatment for aggressive SM, SM-AHN, or mast cell leukemia includes midostaurin, a kinase inhibitor with activity against both wild-type and D816V mutant c-kit. On the other hand, the D816V mutation confers resistance to imatinib, which has activity against wild-type c-kit.

In SM-AHN, the rate of detection of *KIT* D816V in the associated hematopoietic neoplasm (as determined using laser capture microdissection studies) varies based on the type of neoplasm, with significantly more occurrence in chronic myelomonocytic leukemia (CMML) than myeloproliferative neoplasm (MPN) and AML; co-mutation is rare in associated lymphoid neoplasms. The low VAF for the *KIT* mutation in this case suggests that it was isolated to the mast cell clone.

In SM-AHN, the prognosis is generally related to the associated neoplasm. In this case, the accompanying high-grade MDS portends a poor prognosis. Interestingly, each of the non-*KIT* mutations identified in this patient (*ASXL1, RUNX1, SRSF2*) have been independently associated with a worse overall survival in SM, including lower response rates to midostaurin. Some data suggest that these additional mutations may precede the acquisition of *KIT* mutation in SM-AHN. Still, given the low VAF of the *KIT* mutation, it remains uncertain whether the mast cell clone harbored the additional mutations in this case.

Diagnostic pearls/pitfalls

– *KIT* D816V mutation is also seen in acute myeloid leukemia (AML) and other myeloid neoplasms; therefore, the presence of a *KIT* D816V mutation alone is not diagnostic of a mast cell neoplasm.
– Aggregates of reactive mast cells may occur in the bone marrow of patients with myeloid neoplasms, and these cases should not be confused with SM-AHN. Evaluation for CD2 and/or CD25 expression can help elucidate neoplastic mast cells.
– In cases with eosinophilia, additional testing should be considered to rule out a myeloid/lymphoid neoplasm with eosinophilia and abnormalities of *PDGFRA, PDGFRB,* or *FGFR1,* as these conditions may have abnormal mast cells as a component of the disease.
– *KIT* D816V mutation occurs in a codon on exon 17; recurrent *KIT* mutations found in other neoplastic conditions (including AML and gastrointestinal stromal tumor) include mutations in exons 8 and 11. Therefore, genetic testing to aid in the diagnosis of SM must include sequencing of exon 17 or a specific assay for the D816V variant.

– Neoplastic mast cells occasionally express CD30, especially in aggressive mastocytoses. Thus, consideration of mast cell disease should be given to atypical CD30+ aggregates in bone marrow. Additionally, CD30 positivity should not dissuade from the diagnosis of mastocytosis.

Readings

Garcia-Montero AC, Jara-Acevedo M, Teodosio C, et al. KIT mutation in mast cells and other bone marrow hematopoietic cell lineages in systemic mast cell disorders: a prospective study of the Spanish Network on Mastocytosis (REMA) in a series of 113 patients. Blood. 2006;108:2366-72. **DOI: 10.1182/blood-2006-04-015545**

Jawhar M, Schwaab J, Naumann N, et al. Response and progression on midostaurin in advanced systemic mastocytosis: KIT D816V and other molecular markers. Blood. 2017;130:137-45. **DOI: 10.1182/blood-2017-01-764423**

Jawhar M, Schwaab J, Schnittger S, et al. Additional mutations in SRSF2, ASXL1 and/or RUNX1 identify a high-risk group of patients with KIT D816V(+) advanced systemic mastocytosis. Leukemia. 2016;30:136-43. **DOI: 10.1038/leu.2015.284**

Jawhar M, Schwaab J, Schnittger S, et al. Molecular profiling of myeloid progenitor cells in multi-mutated advanced systemic mastocytosis identifies KIT D816V as a distinct and late event. Leukemia. 2015;29:1115-22. **DOI: 10.1038/leu.2015.4**

Ma Y, Zeng S, Metcalfe DD, et al. The c-KIT mutation causing human mastocytosis is resistant to STI571 and other KIT kinase inhibitors; kinases with enzymatic site mutations show different inhibitor sensitivity profiles than wild-type kinases and those with regulatory-type mutations. Blood. 2002;99:1741-4. **DOI: 10.1182/blood.v99.5.1741**

Morgado JM, Sanchez-Munoz L, Teodosio CG, et al. Immunophenotyping in systemic mastocytosis diagnosis: 'CD25 positive' alone is more informative than the 'CD25 and/or CD2' WHO criterion. Mod Pathol. 2012;25:516-21. **DOI: 10.1038/modpathol.2011.192**

Pardanani A. Systemic mastocytosis in adults: 2017 update on diagnosis, risk stratification and management. Am J Hematol. 2016;91:1146-1159. **DOI: 10.1002/ajh.24553**

Sotlar K, Cerny-Reiterer S, Petat-Dutter K, et al. Aberrant expression of CD30 in neoplastic mast cells in high-grade mastocytosis. Mod Pathol. 2011;24:585-95. **DOI: 10.1038/modpathol.2010.224**

Sotlar K, Colak S, Bache A, et al. Variable presence of KIT D816V in clonal haematological non-mast cell lineage diseases associated with systemic mastocytosis (SM-AHNMD). J Pathol. 2010;220:586-95. **DOI: 10.1002/path.2677**

Sotlar K, Horny HP, Simonitsch I, et al. CD25 indicates the neoplastic phenotype of mast cells: a novel immunohistochemical marker for the diagnosis of systemic mastocytosis (SM) in routinely processed bone marrow biopsy specimens. Am J Surg Pathol. 2004;28:1319-25. **DOI: 10.1097/01.pas.0000138181.89743.7b**

Swerdlow SH, Campo E, Harris NL, Jaffe ES, Pileri SA, Stein H, Thiele J, et al. World Health Organization Classification of Tumours of Haematopoietic and Lymphoid Tissues. 4th ed. Lyon, France: IARC Press; 2017. ISBN-13: 978-9283224310

7

Rose C Beck

Clonal cytopenia of undetermined significance with *U2AF1* mutation

History A 67-year-old male with past medical history of diabetes was referred by his primary care physician to an oncologist for evaluation of thrombocytopenia. An initial presumptive diagnosis of immune-mediated thrombocytopenia was made and the patient was given a trial of steroid therapy. However, the platelet count continued to decrease, and a bone marrow biopsy with peripheral blood smear review was then performed. CBC at the time of biopsy is shown at right.

WBC	5.9×10^9/L
RBC	4.64×10^{12}/L
HGB	15.0 g/dL
HCT	41.4%
MCV	88.6 fL
RDW	12.7%
Platelets	52×10^9/L

Morphology & flow cytometry The peripheral smear showed thrombocytopenia with rare giant platelets but otherwise no morphologic abnormalities **f7.1**. The bone marrow aspirate demonstrated normal-appearing trilineage hematopoiesis, although rare hypolobate megakaryocytes were noted **f7.2a**. The core biopsy was slightly hypercellular for age (40%-50%) but with otherwise normal morphology and adequate megakaryocytes **f7.2b**. Flow cytometry did not demonstrate any abnormalities.

Genetics/molecular results Cytogenetics showed a normal karyotype; FISH studies were negative for monosomy 5, del(5q), monosomy 7, del(7q), trisomy 8, del(17p), and del(20q). A targeted myeloid NGS panel revealed *U2AF1* p.S34F(c.101C>T) with 23% variant allele frequency (VAF) **f7.3**.

Based on the morphologic, genetic, and molecular findings, a final diagnosis of **clonal cytopenia of undetermined significance** was rendered.

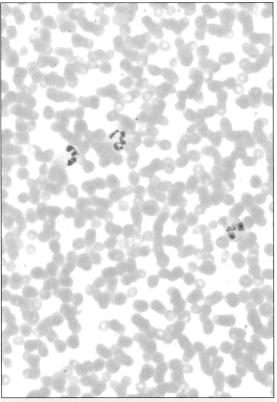

f7.1 Blood smear showing thrombocytopenia but no evidence for dysplasia

ISBN 978-089189-6814 ©2021 ASCP

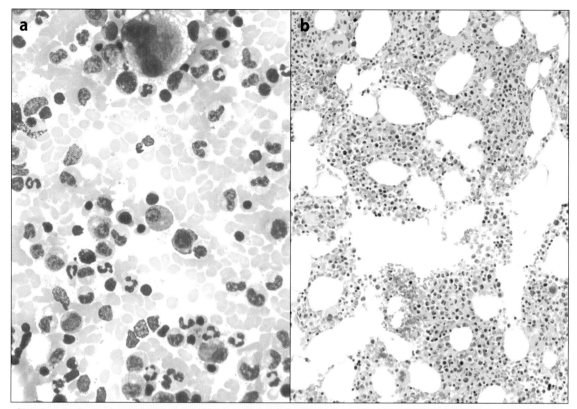

f7.2 Normal trilineage hematopoiesis present in **a** the aspirate & **b** the clot section, with mild hypercellularity for age

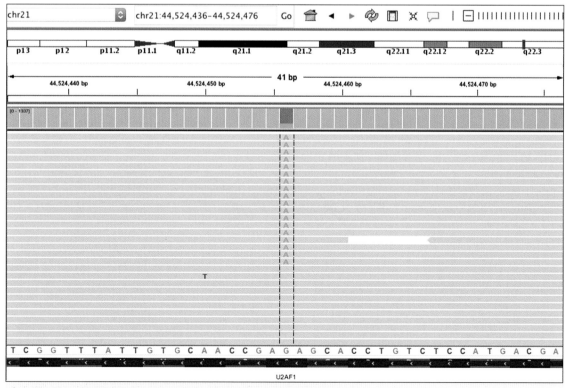

f7.3 Somatic variant analysis using a targeted myeloid NGS panel. Annotated reads mapped to the *U2AF1* locus demonstrate p.S34F(c.101C>T), highlighted in green (hg19, IGV browser, showing the reverse strand) [see **fA.8**, p312]

t7.1 Features of indolent clonal hematopoietic stem cell disorders & their comparison to myelodysplastic syndrome (MDS)

Disorder	Cytopenias	Diagnostic dysplasia	Clonal hematopoiesis*
Clonal hematopoiesis of indeterminate potential	–	–	+
Idiopathic cytopenia of undetermined significance	+	–	–
Clonal cytopenia of undetermined significance	+	–	+
MDS	+	+	±[†]

–, absence of a feature; +, presence of a feature
*As detected by mutational or cytogenetic analysis
[†]Note that ~50% of MDS cases will show a cytogenetic abnormality, while 80%-90% will show a pathogenic gene mutation depending on the size of gene panel used

Discussion The existence of persistent clonal lymphoid populations in older individuals has been well established, exemplified by monoclonal gammopathy of undetermined significance (MGUS) and monoclonal B lymphocytosis (a precursor lesion to chronic lymphocytic leukemia). In more recent years, extensive genomics analysis has shown that clonal hematopoiesis in the form of specific somatic mutations or chromosome abnormalities is detectable in the blood of individuals without evidence of hematopoietic disease and having normal CBC values. The incidence of clonal hematopoiesis increases with age, appearing in ~10% of individuals by the age of 70 years and over 15% by age 90 years, when using a detected variant allele frequency (VAF) threshold of ≥2%. The terms "age-related clonal hematopoiesis" (ARCH) or "clonal hematopoiesis of indeterminate potential" (CHIP, used hereafter) have been used to describe this phenomenon.

The somatic mutations found in CHIP are the same pathogenic mutations found in hematopoietic neoplasms. It is hypothesized that CHIP-mutated clones have a survival advantage, with neoplastic disease developing after additional genetic events occur. In fact, CHIP carries an increased risk of developing hematopoietic neoplasm, as well as an increased risk of cardiovascular disease (the latter may be from dysregulation of inflammation by cells carrying mutations). Analogous to the rate of conversion of MGUS to multiple myeloma, 0.5%-1% of individuals with CHIP will develop a hematopoietic neoplasm per year, with a higher rate occurring in those having a mutation with VAF of at least 10% or having >1 mutation. In one study, having a CHIP mutation with a VAF ≥10% in blood increased the lifetime risk of developing a hematopoietic neoplasm by 50-fold. Among individuals with CHIP who progress to hematopoietic disease, chronic myeloid neoplasms such as myelodysplastic syndrome (MDS) predominate,

although lymphoid neoplasms are also seen. The presence of CHIP before chemotherapy confers increased risk for the development of a therapy-related myeloid neoplasm in patients having tumors of either hematopoietic or nonhematopoietic origin.

The most common types of mutations found in CHIP are those occurring in genes associated with epigenetic regulation or methylation of DNA, specifically *DNMT3A* (~40%-50% of individuals with CHIP), *TET2* (~7%-10%), and *ASXL1* (~7%-10%). Not surprisingly then, these same mutations are frequently found in hematopoietic neoplasms in co-occurrence with other mutations, corroborating the hypothesis that CHIP mutations are early events in disease pathogenesis. Less common CHIP genes include *JAK2, SF3B1, SRSF2, CBL,* and even *TP53*. CHIP may also be present in the form of a chromosomal abnormality such as trisomy 8 or del(20q). Therefore, the presence of a clonal abnormality detected in blood or bone marrow, even in a gene typically associated with overt or aggressive disease, is not by itself diagnostic for malignancy.

When a patient develops unexplained cytopenia, the term "idiopathic cytopenia of undetermined significance" (ICUS) may be used, and if that patient is shown to also have clonal hematopoiesis by cytogenetic or molecular evaluation, but does not meet diagnostic criteria for myelodysplastic syndrome (MDS) or other myeloid neoplasms, the designation becomes "clonal cytopenia of undetermined significance" (CCUS). Thus, CCUS is a more immediate precursor to myeloid neoplasm than CHIP **t7.1**. Patients with CCUS have both cytopenia and evidence of clonal hematopoiesis but by definition do not meet morphologic or genetic criteria for MDS (see **Case 8**), although the bone marrow may show minimal, nondiagnostic dysplasia, as in this case. Recent studies have begun to elucidate specific risk factors in CCUS patients that predict progression to myeloid neoplasm, and both the quality and quantity of mutations play a role. CCUS patients having >1 mutation or a mutation with VAF ≥10% have significantly higher rates of progression. In addition, the presence of mutations in spliceosome genes (such as *SF3B1, SRSF2,* and *U2AF1*) or comutation of *DNMT3A, TET2,* or *ASXL1* with another gene carry a positive predictive value of >80% for the development of myeloid neoplasm. In one study, the overall 5-10 year survival rate of CCUS patients with these "high-risk" mutation patterns approximated that of patients with low-grade MDS. Thus, the detection of clonal hematopoiesis in patients with unexplained cytopenia has prognostic significance, even in the absence of diagnostic morphologic dysplasia.

Routine molecular testing performed on blood or bone marrow of patients having unexplained cytopenia but without morphologic criteria for myeloid neoplasm is, however, a matter of debate. In ICUS patients undergoing a bone marrow biopsy, the present standard for genetic testing includes karyotype with or without FISH studies to exclude MDS-defining genetic abnormalities such as del(5q), abnormalities of chromosome 7, del(17p), or recurrent translocations; however, the incidence of these types of chromosomal abnormalities in the absence of morphologic dysplasia is rare. The fact that certain high-risk mutational profiles have been delineated suggests that molecular testing in ICUS patients, especially those with a high clinical suspicion of MDS, may be warranted in routine practice. These patients will likely benefit from close monitoring for disease progression.

In this case, the presence of a mutation in the spliceosome gene *U2AF1* with a 23% VAF is highly predictive of progression to an overt myeloid neoplasm within 5-10 years. A follow-up CBC performed 2 years after the bone marrow biopsy showed the patient's thrombocytopenia to be stable at 53 × 10⁹/L, with no new cytopenias.

Diagnostic pearls/pitfalls

– The term "clonal hematopoiesis of indeterminate potential" (CHIP) is used to describe individuals having mutations or chromosomal abnormalities detected in blood, but without evidence of hematologic disease. The term "clonal cytopenia of undetermined significance" (CCUS) is used when a patient has at least one cytopenia in addition to evidence of clonal hematopoiesis.

– The somatic mutations found in CHIP are the same as pathogenic mutations found in myeloid neoplasms and include mutations in genes typically associated with overt malignancy such as *JAK2* and *TP53*. Therefore, the presence of such mutations in an otherwise normal-appearing bone marrow is not sufficient for a diagnosis of a myeloid neoplasm.

– "High risk" mutational profiles in CCUS patients include co-mutation of *DNMT3A, TET2,* or *ASXL1* with another gene or mutations in spliceosome genes (eg, *SF3B1, SRSF2, U2AF1*), as well as a mutation with VAF ≥10% or the presence of >1 mutation.

Readings

Bejar R. CHIP, ICUS, CCUS and other four-letter words. Leukemia. 2017;31(9):1869-71. **DOI: 10.1038/leu.2017.181**

Genovese G, Kähler AK, Handsaker RE, et al. Clonal hematopoiesis and blood-cancer risk inferred from blood DNA sequence. N Engl J Med. 2014;371(26):2477-87. **DOI: 10.1056/NEJMoa1409405**

Gibson CJ, Lindsley RC, Tchekmedyian V, et al. Clonal hematopoiesis associated with adverse outcomes after autologous stem-cell transplantation for lymphoma. J Clin Oncol. 2017;35(14):1598-605. **DOI: 10.1200/JCO.2016.71.6712**

Gillis NK, Ball M, Zhang Q, et al. Clonal haemopoiesis and therapy-related myeloid malignancies in elderly patients: a proof-of-concept, case-control study. Lancet Oncol. 2017;18(1):112-21. **DOI: 10.1016/S1470-2045(16)30627-1**

Gondek LP, DeZern AE. Assessing clonal haematopoiesis: clinical burdens and benefits of diagnosing myelodysplastic syndrome precursor states. Lancet Haematol. 2020 Jan;7(1):e73-e81. Epub 2019 Dec 3. **DOI: 10.1016/S2352-3026(19)30211-X**

Jaiswal S, Fontanillas P, Flannick J, et al. Age-related clonal hematopoiesis associated with adverse outcomes. N Engl J Med. 2014;371(26):2488-98. **DOI: 10.1056/NEJMoa1408617**

Jajosky AN, Sadri N, Meyerson HJ, et al. Clonal cytopenia of undetermined significance (CCUS) with dysplasia is enriched for MDS-type molecular findings compared to CCUS without dysplasia. Eur J Haematol. 2021 Jan 1. **DOI: 10.1111/ejh.13574**

Kwok B, Hall JM, Witte JS, et al. MDS-associated somatic mutations and clonal hematopoiesis are common in idiopathic cytopenias of undetermined significance. Blood. 2015;126(21):2355-61. **DOI: 10.1182/blood-2015-08-667063**

Malcovati L, Galli A, Travaglino E, et al. Clinical significance of somatic mutation in unexplained blood cytopenia. Blood. 2017;129(25):3371-8. **DOI: 10.1182/blood-2017-01-763425**

Shanmugam V, Parnes A, Kalyanaraman R, Morgan EA, Kim AS. Clinical utility of targeted next-generation sequencing-based screening of peripheral blood in the evaluation of cytopenias. Blood. 2019;134(24):2222-5. **DOI: 10.1182/blood.2019001610**

Shlush LI. Age-related clonal hematopoiesis. Blood. 2018;131(5):496-504. **DOI: 10.1182/blood-2017-07-746453**

Steensma DP. Clinical consequences of clonal hematopoiesis of indeterminate potential. Blood Adv. 2018;2(22):3404-10. **DOI: 10.1182/bloodadvances.2018020222**

Steensma DP, Bejar R, Jaiswal S, et al. Clonal hematopoiesis of indeterminate potential and its distinction from myelodysplastic syndromes. Blood. 2015;126(1):9-16. **DOI: 10.1182/blood-2015-03-631747**

Zheng G, Chen P, Pallavajjalla A, et al. The diagnostic utility of targeted gene panel sequencing in discriminating etiologies of cytopenia. Am J Hematol. 2019 Oct;94(10):1141-1148. Epub 2019 Aug 7. **DOI: 10.1002/ajh.25592**

Rose C Beck

8

Myelodysplastic syndrome with excess blasts-1 with iso(17q) & mutations in *SRSF2* & *SETBP1*

History An 85-year-old male with medical history significant for coronary artery disease presented to the emergency department (ED) due to dizziness and syncope. In the ED, testing revealed a HGB level of 7.5 g/dL and the patient was admitted and received several blood transfusions. A bone marrow biopsy with peripheral blood smear review was performed during his admission and a concurrent CBC is shown at right.

Morphology & flow cytometry The peripheral blood smear showed dysplastic granulocytes with hypolobation as well as occasional blasts, enumerated at 2% by manual differential count **f8.1**. The bone marrow aspirate demonstrated trilineage dysplasia, including erythroid cells with nuclear irregularities and pronounced basophilic stippling, hypolobated granulocytes, and many small, hypolobated megakaryocytes **f8.2a,b**. Blasts were enumerated at 8% in the aspirate smear. Many ring sideroblasts were also noted on examination of an iron stain of the clot section **f8.2c**. The core biopsy specimen was significantly hypercellular for age (90%) and contained many small, monolobated megakaryocytes **f8.3a,b**. Flow cytometry showed 6% myeloblasts without atypical antigen expression **f8.4**. Based on the morphologic findings, a diagnosis of **myelodysplastic syndrome (MDS) with excess blasts-1** was rendered.

Genetics/molecular results The karyotype showed 46,XY,i(17)(q10)[18]/46,XY[2] **f8.5a**. A FISH panel for MDS-related abnormalities was positive for del(17p) but negative for monosomy 5, del(5q), monosomy 7, del(7q), trisomy 8, and del(20q) **f8.5b**. A targeted myeloid NGS panel was also performed and showed *SRSF2* p.P95_R102delPPDSHHSR (c.284_307del24) with variant allele frequency (VAF) of 79% and *SETBP1* p.G870S (c.2608G>A) with VAF of 49% **f8.6**.

WBC	8.1×10^9/L
RBC	2.99×10^{12}/L
HGB	9.3 g/dL
HCT	27.9%
MCV	93 fL
RDW	18.7%
Platelets	100×10^9/L

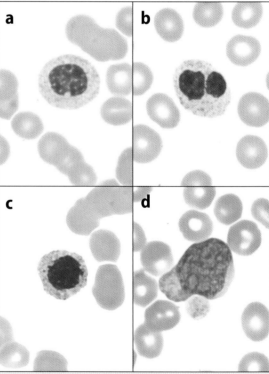

f8.1 Various atypical cells present in the peripheral blood: **a** monolobated & **b** pelgeroid neutrophils as well as **c** monolobated eosinophils & **d** 2% blasts

ISBN 978-089189-6814

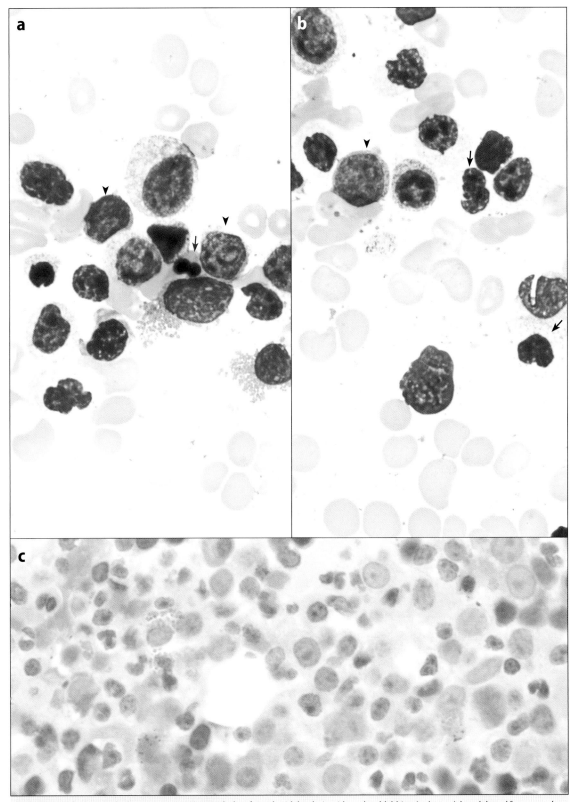

f8.2 Atypical findings in the bone marrow aspirate include **a**, **b** erythroid dysplasia with nuclear blebbing (red arrow), hypolobated/hypogranular neutrophils & granulocytic precursors (black arrows), increased blasts (arrowheads) & **c** many ring sideroblasts visible on an iron stain performed on the clot section

8 *Myelodysplastic syndrome with excess blasts-1 with iso(17q) & mutations in SRSF2 & SETBP1*

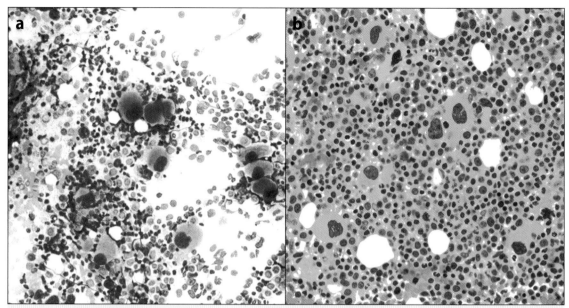

f8.3 Many hypolobated megakaryocytes can be seen in the **a** aspirate & **b** hypercellular clot section

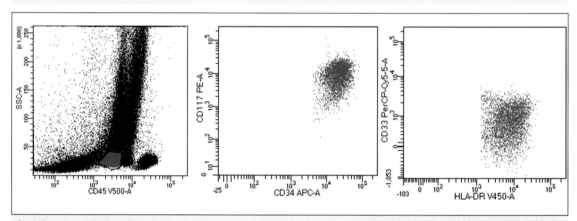

f8.4 Flow cytometry demonstrating 6% myeloblasts expressing CD34, CD117, CD33 & HLA-DR

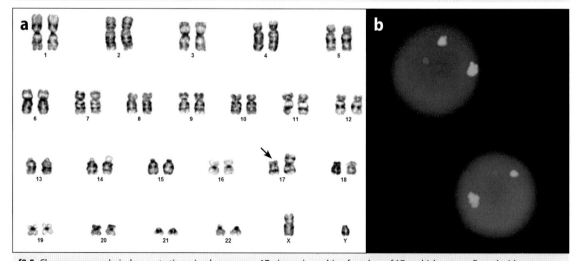

f8.5 Chromosome analysis demonstrating **a** isochromosome 17q (arrow), resulting from loss of 17p, which was confirmed with **b** FISH analysis, using single color probes for 17p (red) & 17 centromere (green)

ISBN 978-089189-6814 ©2021 ASCP

8 *Myelodysplastic syndrome with excess blasts-1 with iso(17q) & mutations in SRSF2 & SETBP1*

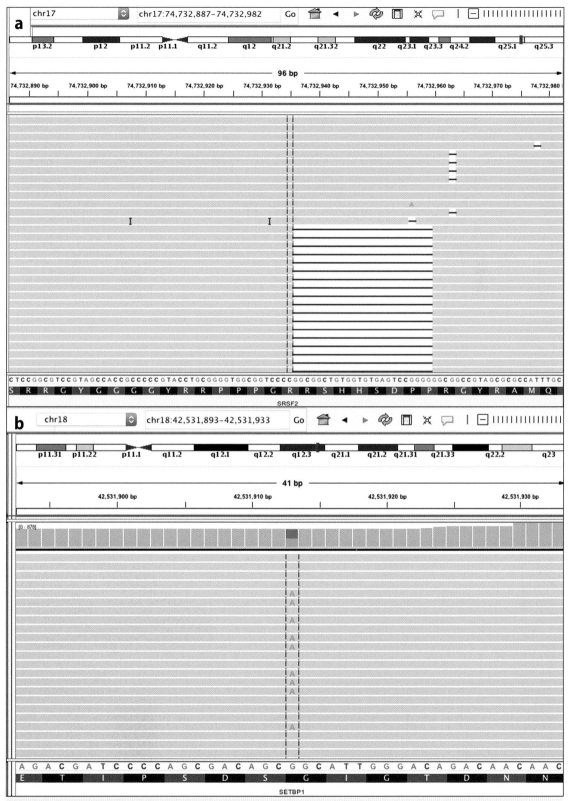

f8.6 Somatic variant analysis using a targeted myeloid NGS panel: **a** Annotated reads mapped to the *SRSF2* locus demonstrate a 24-base pair deletion (solid white with bars) resulting in p.P95_R102delPPDSHHSR; **b** At the *SETBP1* locus a p.G870S (c.2608G>A) mutation is highlighted in green (hg19, IGV browser) [see **fA.8**, p312]

t8.1 WHO 2017 classification of myelodysplastic syndromes & their diagnostic criteria

Entity	RS*	Blast %	Genetic findings
MDS-SLD	<15%/<5%[†]	BM <5%, PB <1% No Auer rods	Variable; should not fulfill criteria for MDS with isolated del(5q)
MDS-MLD	<15%/<5%[†]	BM <5%, PB <1% No Auer rods	Variable; should not fulfill criteria for MDS with isolated del(5q)
MDS with RS with SLD or MLD	≥15%/≥5%[†]	BM <5%, PB <1% No Auer rods	Variable; should not fulfill criteria for MDS with isolated del(5q)
MDS with isolated del(5q)	Any	BM <5%, PB <1% No Auer rods	del(5q) with or without 1 other chromosomal abnormality except −7 or del(7q)
MDS-EB-1	Any	BM 5%-9% or PB 2%-4% No Auer rods	Any
MDS-EB-2	Any	BM 10%-19% or PB 5%-19% Or Auer rods but BM & PB <20%	Any
MDS-U with 1% blood blasts	Any	BM <5%, PB 1% No Auer rods	Any
MDS-U with SLD & pancytopenia	Any	BM <5%, PB <1% No Auer rods	Any
MDS-U based on defining cytogenetic abnormality	<15%	BM <5%, PB <1% No Auer rods	MDS-defining abnormality (see **t8.2**)

BM, bone marrow; EB, excess blasts; PB, peripheral blood; MLD, multilineage dysplasia; MDS, myelodysplastic syndrome;
MDS-U, myelodysplastic syndrome, unclassifiable; RS, ring sideroblasts; SLD, single-lineage dysplasia; WHO, World Health Organization
*As percentage of erythroid cells in bone marrow
[†]If SF3B1 mutation is present, only 5% RS are necessary to diagnosis MDS with RS

Discussion Myelodysplastic syndrome (MDS) is a clonal hematopoietic stem cell disorder characterized by peripheral blood cytopenias in addition to morphologic dysplasia and/or characteristic genetic findings in blood or bone marrow. In the 2017 World Health Classification classification of hematopoietic neoplasms, MDS is categorized by single or multilineage dysplasia, presence of del(5q) or ring sideroblasts, and enumeration of blasts **t8.1**. The older term "refractory anemia" is now replaced by MDS as anemia may not be the presenting cytopenia in all patients. Diagnosis of MDS requires morphologic dysplasia in at least 10% of cells in a single hematopoietic lineage, unless disease-defining chromosomal abnormalities are present **t8.2**. Therefore, adequate preparation of Wright-stained aspirate smears is essential for the evaluation of morphology as well as blast count. Patients with an increasing blast count have a higher risk for transformation to acute myeloid leukemia (AML).

There is a wide range of clinical behavior among MDS patients, and the International Prognostic Scoring System (IPSS) is commonly used by oncologists for risk stratification. The IPSS score incorporates the following clinical and laboratory factors: karyotype, bone marrow blast percentage, and peripheral cell counts (hemoglobin, platelets, absolute neutrophil count) at presentation. Higher blast percentage and lower cell counts result in a higher IPSS score, as do more unfavorable karyotypic abnormalities such as monosomy 7, del(7q), del(17p), inv(3), and a complex karyotype (having at least 3 chromosomal abnormalities).

In aggregate, chromosomal abnormalities are found in only ~50% of MDS cases, whereas a myeloid-associated somatic mutation is found in up to 90% of cases depending on the number of genes examined. Despite the frequent presence of somatic mutations in MDS, at present, the only mutated gene incorporated into MDS classification is *SF3B1*, seen in MDS with ring sideroblasts **t8.1** (see also **Case 10**). There are no cytogenetic or molecular abnormalities entirely specific to MDS, and many of the abnormalities listed in **t8.2** & **t8.3** are frequently found in other myeloid neoplasms or even individuals without evidence of hematologic disease (see **Cases 7 & 17** for a discussion of clonal hematopoiesis of indeterminate potential [CHIP]).

ISBN 978-089189-6814   ©2021 ASCP

t8.2 Recurrent cytogenetic abnormalities that may be disease-defining for MDS*

Chromosomal gains/losses	Frequency in MDS (%)	Balanced translocations	Frequency in MDS (%)
del(5q)	10	t(11;16)(q23.3;p13.3)	<3
loss of 7 or del(7q)	10	t(3;21)(q26.2;q22.1)	<3
gain of 8*	10	t(1;3)(p36.3;q21.2)	1
del(20q)*	5-8	t(2;11)(p21;q23.3)	1
loss of Y*	5	inv(3)(q21.3;q26.2) /t(3;3)(q21.3;q26.2)	1
isochromosome 17q or t(17p)	3-5	t(6;9)(p23;q34.1)	1
del(11q)	3		
del(12p) or t(12p)	3		
loss of 13 or del(13q)	3		
del(9q)	1-2		
idic(X)(q13)	1-2		

Some abnormalities may be detected in individuals without evidence of hematologic disease & therefore are not MDS-defining; these are marked with an asterisk; note that a normal karyotype is found in 40%-50% of MDS cases
MDS, myelodysplastic syndrome

t8.3 Recurrent somatic gene mutations found in MDS, arranged by functional pathway & their clinical associations

Pathway	Gene	Frequency (%)	Clinical significance
Splicing	SF3B1*	20-30	Associated with ring sideroblasts; independently associated with favorable prognosis
	SRSF2*	15	Poorer prognosis
	U2AF1	5-10	Poorer prognosis
	ZRSR2	5-10	Prognostic impact uncertain
Epigenetics	TET2*	20-30	Prognostic impact uncertain; may predict increased response to hypomethylating agents
	ASXL1*	15-20	Independently associated with poor prognosis
	DNMT3A*	10	Prognostic impact uncertain; most common mutation found in individuals with CHIP
	IDH1/IDH2	5-10	Prognostic impact uncertain
	EZH2	5-10	Independently associated with poor prognosis
	BCOR	5	Poorer prognosis
Signaling	NRAS†	5-10	Poorer prognosis
	CBL*†	<5	Poorer prognosis
	JAK2*	3-4	Does not appear to affect prognosis
Transcription factor	RUNX1†	10	Independently associated with poor prognosis
	PPM1D	5-10	Associated with therapy-related MDS
	SETBP1	2-4	Poorer prognosis
	ETV6†	2-3	Independently associated with poor prognosis
	PHF6†	2-3	Poorer prognosis
Tumor suppressor	TP53*†	5-10	Independently associated with poor prognosis; associated with complex karyotype and therapy-related MDS, as well as resistance to lenalidomide in MDS with isolated del(5q); present in CHIP
Cohesin	STAG2	5-10	Poorer prognosis

These genes have been found in at least 1% of individuals with clonal hematopoiesis of indeterminate potential (CHIP) as discussed in Cases 7 & 17
†*Germline mutations in these genes may be associated with hematopoietic disease. In germline cases, detected mutations generally exhibit variant allele frequencies of 40%-50% & analysis of nonhematopoietic tissue is suggested to exclude a hereditary myeloid malignancy predisposition syndrome (see Case 11)*

The mutational landscape of MDS has been extensively studied and approximately 30-40 genes are mutated in 80%-90% of cases. These genes can be grouped by functional category **t8.3**. Mutations in genes associated with epigenetic regulation (*DNMT3A, TET2, ASXL1*) and the spliceosome complex (*SF3B1, SRSF2*) are commonly acquired during aging and are therefore frequently present in MDS patients, especially in early stages of disease. Late-occurring mutations include those involved in signaling, such as *RUNX1* or *NRAS*, and are postulated to contribute to disease progression. Although not necessarily required for diagnosis, the detection of somatic mutations in MDS patients provides evidence of clonal hematopoiesis and has prognostic and therapeutic implications. In particular, 5 genes (*ASXL1, EZH2, RUNX1, TP53, ETV6*) have been shown to be independently associated with inferior survival in multivariable models using IPSS-stratified groups. The presence of a mutation in 1 of these genes identifies patients whose survival is similar to that of patients in the next highest IPSS risk group. Many other genes are also associated with poorer prognosis in different studies **t8.3**, and a higher number of somatic mutations (>2) within the same patient also portends a worse prognosis. Of significance in relation to therapy, *TET2* mutations may predict increased response to therapy with hypomethylating agents (azacitidine and decitabine), while *TP53* mutations are associated with resistance to lenalidomide in MDS patients with isolated del(5q).

Given the prognostic and therapeutic implications of gene mutations in MDS, it is now standard in many academic centers to perform a targeted NGS panel analysis of ≥30 genes in all new cases. However, the presence of a mutation without appropriate morphologic criteria is not diagnostic of malignancy, because many of these mutations are found in clonal hematopoiesis associated with aging/CHIP. Therefore, cytogenetic and molecular results must always be interpreted in the context of clinical and morphologic findings.

Flow cytometry is useful in the diagnosis of MDS if abnormalities of granulocytes, monocytes, and/or blasts are found. These abnormalities include alterations in normal patterns of antigen expression or aberrant expression of antigens such as CD56 on granulocytes or monocytes, or expression of lymphoid antigens such as CD5 or CD7 on myeloid blasts. However, aberrant expression of antigens may also be seen in reactive or regenerative states. Therefore, caution should be exercised in the interpretation of flow cytometric abnormalities when evaluating a patient with cytopenias, and flow cytometry results should always be considered in context with other findings.

In this example case, the presence of trilineage dysplasia and 8% blasts in the bone marrow aspirate were morphologically diagnostic for MDS with excess blasts 1 (EB-1). The presence of iso(17q) by karyotype equated to a deletion of 17p, which was confirmed with FISH and indicated a poorer prognosis. Interestingly, isolated iso(17q) is a rare cytogenetic finding among myeloid neoplasms, and is more often found as a secondary event, especially in chronic myeloid leukemia (CML). The designation "myeloid neoplasms with isolated iso(17q)" has been used in the literature to describe these rare cases, which have a particularly aggressive clinical course and a median overall survival of 1-2 years. So far, these neoplasms have been described mainly as MDS/myeloproliferative neoplasm (MPN) or AML and only rarely as MDS or MPN. They frequently lack *TP53* mutations but demonstrate a high incidence of mutations in *SRSF2, SETBP1, ASXL1*, and *NRAS*, as seen in this case.

The patient declined therapy with hypomethylating agents and was initially treated supportively with regular blood transfusions and darbepoetin alfa for his anemia. He died 4 months after diagnosis as a result of cardiac complications aggravated by his cytopenias.

Diagnostic pearls/pitfalls

- Subclassification of MDS is based on the type of dysplasia, the presence of ring sideroblasts (with or without an *SF3B1* mutation), cytogenetic findings, and the blast percentage.
- A diagnosis of MDS generally requires morphologic dysplasia in at least 10% of cells within a single hematopoietic lineage; therefore, adequately prepared Wright-stained aspirate smears are essential. Knowledge of patient history is also critical because morphologic dysplasia may be seen in benign states such as nutritional deficiencies, reactive erythroid hyperplasia, toxin exposures, and with certain medications.
- Not all chromosomal abnormalities occurring in MDS patients are disease-defining. In particular, trisomy 8, del(20q), and loss of Y may be found in individuals without evidence of hematologic disease.

- Mutation analysis using targeted NGS panels plays an ever-increasing role in the evaluation of MDS cases because of potential prognostic and therapeutic implications.
- Somatic mutations in myeloid-associated genes are not disease-defining by themselves, as they are also found in age-related clonal hematopoiesis (also called *clonal hematopoiesis of indeterminate potential* or CHIP). The presence of somatic mutations must always be interpreted in the context of accompanying clinical and histologic findings.
- Flow cytometric detection of blasts, granulocytes, or monocytes with phenotypic atypia may aid in the diagnosis of MDS.

Readings

Bejar R. Clinical and genetic predictors of prognosis in myelodysplastic syndromes. Haematologica. 2014;99(6):956-64. **DOI: 10.3324/haematol.2013.085217**

Bejar R, Lord A, Stevenson K, Bar-Natan M, et al. TET2 mutations predict response to hypomethylating agents in myelodysplastic syndrome patients. Blood. 2014;124(17):2705-12. **DOI: 10.1182/blood-2014-06-582809**

Bejar R, Stevenson K, Abdel-Wahab O, et al. Clinical effect of point mutations in myelodysplastic syndromes. N Engl J Med. 2011;364(26):2496-506. **DOI: 10.1056/NEJMoa1013343**

Caponetti GC, Bagg A. Mutations in myelodysplastic syndromes: Core abnormalities and CHIPping away at the edges. Int J Lab Hematol. 2020 Dec;42(6):671-684. Epub 2020 Aug 5. **DOI: 10.1111/ijlh.13284**

Haferlach T, Nagata Y, Grossmann V, et al. Landscape of genetic lesions in 944 patients with myelodysplastic syndromes. Leukemia. 2014;28(2):241-7. **DOI: 10.1038/leu.2013.336**

Kanagal-Shamanna R, Luthra R, Yin CC, et al. Myeloid neoplasms with isolated isochromosome 17q demonstrate a high frequency of mutations in *SETBP1, SRSF2, ASXL1* and *NRAS*. Oncotarget. 2016;7(12):14251. **DOI: 10.18632/oncotarget.7350**

Kennedy JA, Ebert BL. Clinical implications of genetic mutations in myelodysplastic syndrome. J Clin Oncol. 2017;35(9):968-74. **DOI: 10.1200/JCO.2016.71.0806**

Malcovati L, Papaemmanuil E, Ambaglio I, et al. Driver somatic mutations identify distinct disease entities within myeloid neoplasms with myelodysplasia. Blood. 2014;124(9):1513-21. **DOI: 10.1182/blood-2014-03-560227**

McClure RF, Dewald GW, Hoyer JD, Hanson CA. Isolated isochromosome 17q: a distinct type of mixed myeloproliferative disorder/myelodysplastic syndrome with an aggressive clinical course. Br J Haematol. 1999;106(2):445-54. **DOI: 10.1016/j.jmoldx.2018.07.002**

McClure RF, Ewalt MD, Crow J, et al. Clinical significance of DNA variants in chronic myeloid neoplasms: a report of the Association for Molecular Pathology. J Mol Diagn JMD. 2018;20(6):717-37.

Mufti GJ, McLornan DP, van de Loosdrecht AA, Germing U, Hasserjian RP. Diagnostic algorithm for lower-risk myelodysplastic syndromes. Leukemia. 2018;32(8):1679-96. **DOI: 10.1038/s41375-018-0173-2**

Ogata K. Diagnostic flow cytometry for low-grade myelodysplastic syndromes. Hematol Oncol. 2008;26(4):193-8. **DOI: 10.1002/hon.857**

Papaemmanuil E, Gerstung M, Malcovati L, et al. Clinical and biological implications of driver mutations in myelodysplastic syndromes. Blood. 2013;122(22):3616-27; quiz 3699. **DOI: 10.1182/blood-2013-08-518886**

Stetler-Stevenson M, Arthur DC, Jabbour N, et al. Diagnostic utility of flow cytometric immunophenotyping in myelodysplastic syndrome. Blood. 2001;98(4):979-87. **DOI: 10.1182/blood.v98.4.979**

Swerdlow SH, Campo E, Harris NL, et al. World Health Organization Classification of Tumours of Haematopoietic and Lymphoid Tissues. 4th ed. Lyon, France: IARC Press; 2017. **ISBN: 9789283244943**

Valent P, Orazi A, Steensma DP, et al. Proposed minimal diagnostic criteria for myelodysplastic syndromes (MDS) and potential pre-MDS conditions. Oncotarget. 2017;8(43):73483-500. **DOI: 10.18632/oncotarget.19008**

Erika M Moore

9

Myelodysplastic syndrome with isolated del(5q)

History A 78-year-old woman presented for evaluation of prolonged macrocytic anemia. Serum vitamin B_{12} and folate levels were normal. CBC is shown at right.

A bone marrow biopsy with peripheral smear review was performed for further evaluation.

Morphology & flow cytometry The peripheral smear demonstrated macrocytic anemia and mild thrombocytosis **f9.1**. No overt dysplasia was noted. The bone marrow was mildly hypercellular for age with increased atypical megakaryocytes that were predominantly small and hypolobated, including many monolobated forms **f9.2a,b**. Blasts were not increased and there was no significant dyserythropoiesis or dysgranulopoiesis present in the aspirate smears, although a slightly increased myeloid:erythroid ratio was observed. Flow cytometric studies did not show any significant abnormalities.

Genetics/molecular results FISH studies were positive for del(5q) in 65% of nuclei examined and negative for abnormalities of 7/7q, 8, or 20q **f9.3a**. Karyotype also showed del(5q), without any other abnormalities **f9.3b**.

Based on the morphologic and cytogenetic findings, a diagnosis of **myelodysplastic syndrome with isolated deletion 5q** was rendered.

WBC	3.5×10^9/L
RBC	2.24×10^{12}/L
HGB	8.1 g/dL
HCT	26.7%
MCV	119 fL
RDW	17.1%
Platelets	488×10^9/L

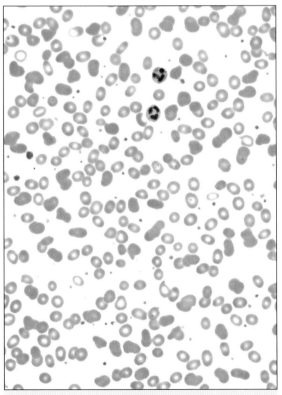

f9.1 Peripheral blood demonstrating macrocytic anemia & mild thrombocytosis

ISBN 978-089189-6814

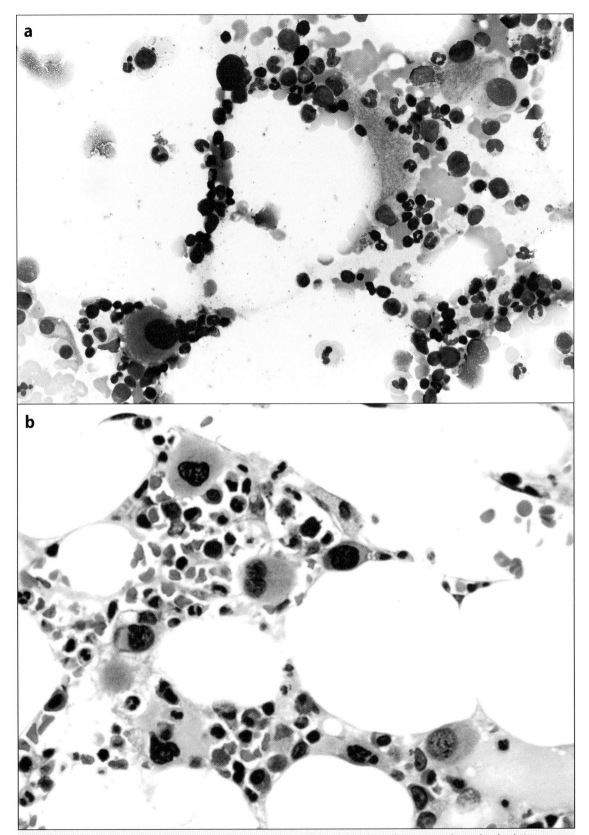

f9.2 Bone marrow aspirate **a** smear & **b** core biopsy demonstrating small, hypolobated megakaryocytes without other dysplasia

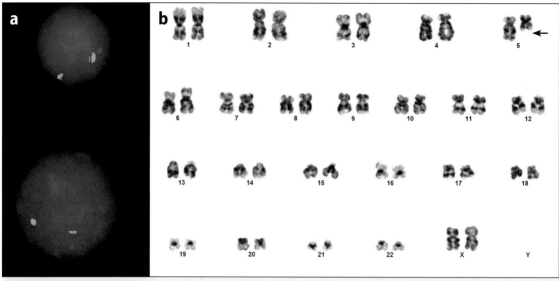

f9.3 **a** Single color FISH probes *D5S23* for 5p15.2 (green) & *EGR1* for 5q31 (orange) showing 2 green signals but only 1 orange signal, consistent with deletion 5q but not monosomy 5; **b** karyotype confirmed the presence of del(5q) (arrow) without any other chromosomal abnormalities

Discussion Myelodysplastic syndrome (MDS) with isolated del(5q) is a unique subcategory of MDS characterized by atypical, hypolobated megakaryocytes and the presence of a deletion in the long arm of chromosome 5 detected by FISH or karyotype. Historically, only cases with characteristic morphologic features and the presence of del(5q) as the only genetic abnormality fell into this category, but newer studies have shown that certain additional chromosomal abnormalities may be present and not affect overall prognosis or disease behavior. Thus, despite the name, a diagnosis of MDS with isolated del(5q) is still applicable in the presence of a second cytogenetic abnormality, as long as the abnormality is not monosomy 7 or del(7q). In addition, according to the World Health Organization criteria, blasts must comprise <5% of the cellularity in the bone marrow and <1% in the peripheral blood and no Auer rods can be present to make the diagnosis (**t8.1** of Case 8 outlines the subclassification of MDS).

Clinically, MDS with isolated del(5q) tends to affect older women, often presenting with macrocytic anemia but an intact white blood cell count. Thrombocytosis is common and occurs in up to half of cases. Pancytopenia is not typical of the disorder, and if present, should result in a diagnosis of MDS, unclassifiable, because the clinical behavior of such cases is unclear. The thalidomide analogue lenalidomide has been successfully used in affected patients to improve anemia and decrease transfusion dependence. Lenalidomide appears to directly suppress the abnormal stem cell clone, with reduction in the level of bone marrow cells having del(5q). Overall, MDS with del(5q) has a fairly good prognosis, with a median survival of ~5 years and <10% of cases will transform to acute myeloid leukemia (AML).

Histologically, the bone marrow of patients with MDS with isolated del(5q) generally demonstrates erythroid hypoplasia, whereas megakaryocytes are typically increased and small to normal in size, with characteristic hypolobated or monolobated nuclei. Mild dyserythropoiesis may be present but granulocytic dysplasia is unusual. Ring sideroblasts can be seen, and if identified, a diagnosis of MDS with isolated del(5q) should still be made if the appropriate morphologic and genetic criteria are present. FISH analysis will be positive for del(5q), with an intact 5 centromere, and karyotype analysis likewise demonstrates an interstitial deletion of chromosome 5, usually involving bands q31-q33. Mutation analysis may rarely show the presence of mutations in genes generally associated with other myeloid neoplasms, such as *JAK2*, *MPL*, or *SF3B1*; these mutations do not appear to affect prognosis. In contrast, the presence of a *TP53* mutation, identified in 15%-20% of cases, is associated with decreased response to lenalidomide, higher rate of transformation to AML, and decreased overall survival. Therefore, screening for *TP53* mutation using genetic analysis or immunohistochemistry has been suggested before treatment, because patients with a *TP53* mutation may require more careful monitoring or alternative therapies.

Diagnostic pearls/pitfalls

- Increased hypolobated megakaryocytes of decreased or near-normal size are the characteristic morphologic finding in MDS with isolated del(5q).

- A second cytogenetic abnormality may be present in MDS with isolated del(5q) and does not exclude the diagnosis unless the additional abnormality is monosomy 7 or del(7q).

- Ring sideroblasts and even *SF3B1* mutations may be present but a diagnosis of MDS with isolated del(5q), rather than MDS with ring sideroblasts, should still be made if genetic and morphologic criteria are met.

- Although this subtype of MDS has a fairly good prognosis, the presence of a coexisting *TP53* mutation may result in poor treatment response, inferior survival, and a higher likelihood of transformation to AML, and therefore, evaluating the *TP53* mutation status at diagnosis is recommended.

Readings

Geyer JT, Subramaniyam S, Jiang Y, et al. Bone marrow morphology predicts additional chromosomal abnormalities in patients with myelodysplastic syndrome with del(5q). Hum Pathol. 2015;44:346-56. **DOI: 10.1016/j.humpath.2012.05.022**

Gurney M, Patnaik MM, Hanson CA, et al. The 2016 revised World Health Organization definition of 'myelodysplastic syndrome with isolated del(5q)'; prognostic implications of single versus double cytogenetic abnormalities. Br J Haematol. 2017;178(1):57-60. **DOI: 10.1111/bjh.14636**

Ingram W, Lea NC, Cervera J, et al. The *JAK2* V617F mutation identifies a subgroup of MDS patients with isolated deletion 5q and a proliferative bone marrow. Leukemia. 2006;20:1319-21. **DOI: 10.1038/sj.leu.2404215**

Jädersten M, Saft L, Smith A, et al. *TP53* mutations in low-risk myelodysplastic syndromes with del(5q) predict disease progression. J Clin Oncol. 2011;29:1971-9. **DOI: 10.1200/JCO.2010.31.8576**

Malcovati L, Karimi M, Papaemmanuil E, et al. *SF3B1* mutation identifies a distinct subset of myelodysplastic syndrome with ring sideroblasts. Blood. 2015;126:233-41. **DOI: 10.1182/blood-2015-03-633537**

Saft L, Karimi M, Ghaderi M, et al. p53 protein expression independently predicts outcome in patients with lower-risk myelodysplastic syndromes with del(5q). Haematologica. 2014;99(6):1041-9. **DOI: 10.3324/haematol.2013.098103**

Swerdlow SH, Campo E, Harris NL, et al. World Health Organization Classification of Tumours of Haematopoietic and Lymphoid Tissues. 4th ed. Lyon, France: IARC Press; 2017. **ISBN: 9789283244943**

Rose C Beck

10

Myelodysplastic syndrome with ring sideroblasts & *SF3B1* mutation

History An 84-year-old male was referred by his primary care physician to an oncologist for evaluation of new onset anemia, low platelets, and unintentional weight loss over the past 6 months. CBC results are shown at right.

A bone marrow biopsy with peripheral smear review was performed for further evaluation.

Morphology & flow cytometry The peripheral smear showed mild poikilocytosis with few ovalocytes but otherwise no significant morphologic abnormalities. The bone marrow aspirate demonstrated left-shifted erythropoiesis with mild dysplasia consisting of megaloblastoid changes and rare nuclear irregularities **f10.1a**; no abnormalities in the granulocytes or megakaryocytes were seen. Blasts were counted in the aspirate smear at 2%, and iron staining showed many ring sideroblasts (>15%) **f10.1b**. The core biopsy demonstrated mild hypercellularity (40%) but otherwise normal marrow architecture; flow cytometric studies did not show any abnormalities. Based on the morphologic findings and clinical history, a tentative diagnosis of **myelodysplastic syndrome with ring sideroblasts** (MDS-RS) was rendered.

Genetics/molecular results Cytogenetics showed a normal 46,XY male karyotype. A targeted myeloid NGS panel revealed the presence of *SF3B1* p.R625C (c.1873C>T) at 37% variant allele frequency (VAF) **f10.2** and *DNMT3A* p.L905P (c.2714T>C) at 35% VAF. The molecular findings confirmed a diagnosis of MDS-RS.

WBC	4.2×10^9/L
RBC	3.11×10^{12}/L
HGB	10.7 g/dL
HCT	32.5%
MCV	105 fL
RDW	15.4%
Platelets	93×10^9/L

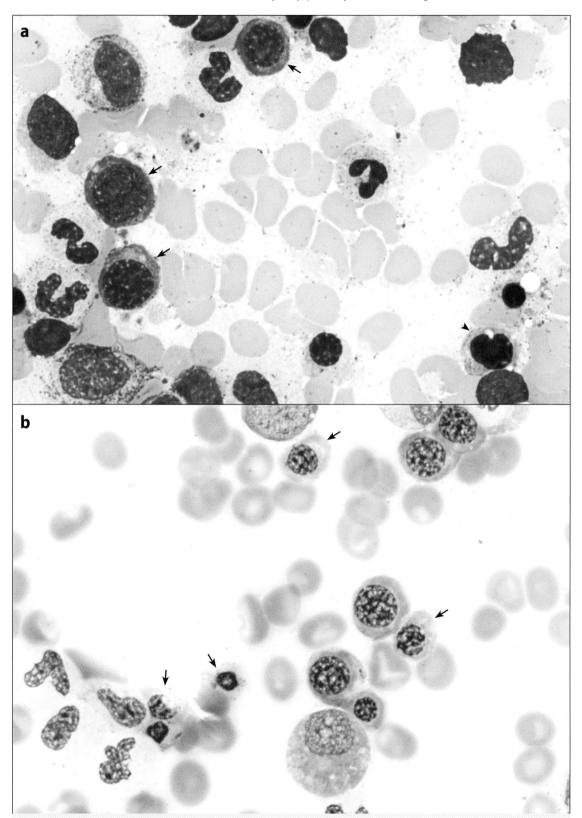

f10.1 a Erythroid precursors in the bone marrow aspirate with megaloblastoid changes (arrows) or nuclear irregularity (arrowhead); **b** iron staining of aspirate showing numerous ring sideroblasts (arrows)

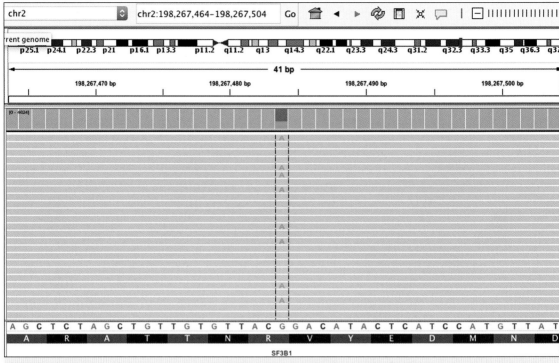

f10.2 Somatic variant analysis using a targeted myeloid NGS panel; annotated reads mapped to the *SF3B1* locus demonstrate p.R625C (c.1873C>T) at 37% variant allele frequency, highlighted in green (hg19, Integrative Genomics Viewer browser, showing the reverse strand) [see **fA.8**, p312]

t10.1 World Health Organization diagnostic criteria for myelodysplastic syndrome with ring sideroblasts (MDS-RS)

1. Cytopenia(s), with bone marrow showing at least erythroid dysplasia, with or without dysplasia in other lineages

2. Presence of at least 15% RS counted in erythroid precursors, or 5% RS if a pathogenic mutation in *SF3B1* is present; secondary causes of RS should be excluded

3. Blasts are <5% in marrow and <1% in peripheral blood; Auer rods are not present

4. Not meeting criteria for MDS with isolated del(5q)

Discussion Ring sideroblasts (RS) are red cell precursors having atypical iron deposits within mitochondria as a result of abnormal heme synthesis; mitochondria generally reside close to the nucleus, therefore, the iron deposits form a characteristic "strand of pearls" or ring pattern when visualized with Prussian blue (Perl) stain. RS have been defined as having at least 5 iron granules surrounding at least one-third or one-half of the cell nucleus. The presence of RS by itself is not diagnostic of malignancy but rather is an indicator of erythroid dysplasia; RS may be seen with lead poisoning, copper deficiency, ethanol toxicity, antibiotics (eg, isothiazide), hemoglobinopathies, congenital sideroblastic anemia, or myelodysplastic syndrome (MDS).

MDS-RS is a particular subtype of MDS typically presenting with isolated anemia and either single-lineage erythroid or multilineage dysplasia in the bone marrow. MDS-RS comprises ~20%-25% of all MDS cases and in the 2017 World Health Organization classification of hematopoietic neoplasms, encompasses the entities formerly known as refractory anemia with RS (RARS) and refractory cytopenia with multilineage dysplasia and RS (RCMD-RS; see **Case 8** for details on MDS subclassification). The presence of at least 15 RS out of 100 erythroid precursors is necessary for a diagnosis of MDS-RS unless a mutation in the spliceosome factor gene *SF3B1* is present, in which case only 5% RS are necessary for diagnosis **t10.1**. Even with these findings, a diagnosis of MDS-RS requires <5% blasts in bone marrow and <1% blasts in peripheral blood, as well as absence of criteria fitting MDS with isolated del(5q) (**t8.1** in **Case 8** outlines specific criteria used for subclassification of MDS). Patients with MDS-RS, especially those with single-lineage dysplasia, typically have a favorable prognosis with lower risk of progression to acute leukemia compared with other types of MDS. In particular, the presence of *SF3B1* mutation in MDS-RS is independently associated with significantly decreased rates of disease progression and increased overall survival.

ISBN 978-089189-6814   ©2021 ASCP

The protein SF3B1 is a component of the spliceosome complex responsible for processing of nascent mRNA transcripts. Mutations in *SF3B1* in hematopoietic disease are commonly seen in MDS, MDS/myeloproliferative (MPN) overlap neoplasms (Case 15), and chronic lymphocytic leukemia (Case 29); these mutations may also be present in clonal hematopoiesis associated with aging (Cases 7 & 17). In the context of a myeloid neoplasm, occurrence of an *SF3B1* mutation has a 97% positive predictive value for the presence of RS on histology. Specifically, mutations in exons 12-16, most commonly p.K700E (>50% of cases), occur in up to 90% of patients with MDS-RS exhibiting single-lineage dysplasia and up to 70% of those having multilineage dysplasia. These mutations appear directly involved in disease pathogenesis by causing abnormal splicing due to misrecognition of 3' splice sites, which results in increased mRNA decay. Although the exact relationship between mutated *SF3B1* and the formation of RS is unclear, studies indicate that the abnormal splicing machinery results in decreased heme synthesis, with subsequent abnormal iron accumulation.

Mutations in other spliceosome factor genes such as *SRFS2*, *U2AF1*, and *ZRSR2* are frequently found in MDS or other myeloid neoplasms and are usually mutually exclusive with *SF3B1* mutations. However, *SF3B1* mutations in MDS-RS may co-occur with mutations in other, non-spliceosome factor genes, as in this example case. In particular, the presence of co-occurring mutations in *TET2* or *DNMT3A* has been associated with multilineage dysplasia in MDS-RS, while concurrent *RUNX1* mutations are associated with significantly decreased overall survival. In cases of MDS-RS having wildtype *SF3B1*, usually a mutation in another spliceosome gene is present.

If an *SF3B1* mutation is present with a *JAK2* or *CALR* mutation, a diagnosis of MDS/MPN with RS and thrombocytosis (MDS/MPN-RS-T) should be suspected (see Case 15). In that disorder, the megakaryocytes are typically enlarged and hyperlobulated, as opposed to the small, hypolobate megakaryocytes that may be seen in MDS-RS. It is important to distinguish between these 2 entities, given the more favorable prognosis of MDS-RS.

Diagnostic pearls/pitfalls

- The presence of RS is indicative of erythroid dysplasia but is not specific to malignancy; RS may be caused by congenital syndromes, nutritional deficiencies, lead or ethanol toxicity, and antibiotic use. Among myeloid neoplasms, RS may be seen in MDS and MDS/MPN disorders.

- In the presence of an *SF3B1* mutation, only 5% RS (of erythroid precursors) is necessary to diagnose MDS-RS.

- If the iron stain is not adequate or the aspirate specimen is limited, the presence of RS may be missed when evaluating bone marrow morphology.

- The presence of RS with enlarged atypical megakaryocytes and peripheral thrombocytosis should raise suspicion for MDS/MPN-RS-T, especially if a *JAK2* or *CALR* mutation is present. MDS/MPN-RS-T has more aggressive clinical behavior than MDS-RS.

- *SF3B1* mutations are not specific to myeloid neoplasms with RS and occur in chronic lymphocytic leukemia as well as in older individuals without hematologic disease (clonal hematopoiesis of indeterminate potential). Therefore, the presence of an *SF3B1* mutation must always be interpreted together with the morphologic and clinical findings.

Readings

Haferlach T, Nagata Y, Grossmann V, et al. Landscape of genetic lesions in 944 patients with myelodysplastic syndromes. Leukemia. 2014;28(2):241-7. **DOI: 10.1038/leu.2013.336**

Malcovati L, Cazzola M. Recent advances in the understanding of myelodysplastic syndromes with ring sideroblasts. Br J Haematol. 2016;174(6):847-58. **DOI: 10.1111/bjh.14215**

Malcovati L, Della Porta MG, Pietra D, et al. Molecular and clinical features of refractory anemia with ringed sideroblasts associated with marked thrombocytosis. Blood. 2009;114(17):3538-45. **DOI: 10.1182/blood-2009-05-222331**

Malcovati L, Karimi M, Papaemmanuil E, et al. *SF3B1* mutation identifies a distinct subset of myelodysplastic syndrome with ring sideroblasts. Blood. 2015;126(2):233-41. **DOI: 10.1182/blood-2015-03-633537**

Malcovati L, Papaemmanuil E, Ambaglio I, et al. Driver somatic mutations identify distinct disease entities within myeloid neoplasms with myelodysplasia. Blood. 2014;124(9):1513-21. **DOI: 10.1182/blood-2014-03-560227**

Malcovati L, Papaemmanuil E, Bowen DT, et al. Clinical significance of SF3B1 mutations in myelodysplastic syndromes and myelodysplastic/myeloproliferative neoplasms. Blood. 2011;118(24):6239-46. **DOI: 10.1182/blood-2011-09-377275**

Papaemmanuil E, Cazzola M, Boultwood J, et al. Somatic *SF3B1* mutation in myelodysplasia with ring sideroblasts. N Engl J Med. 2011;365(15):1384-95. **DOI: 10.1056/NEJMoa1103283**

Papaemmanuil E, Gerstung M, Malcovati L, et al. Clinical and biological implications of driver mutations in myelodysplastic syndromes. Blood. 2013;122(22):3616-27; quiz 3699. **DOI: 10.1182/blood-2013-08-518886**

Yoshida K, Sanada M, Shiraishi Y, et al. Frequent pathway mutations of splicing machinery in myelodysplasia. Nature. 2011;478(7367):64-9. **DOI: 10.1038/nature10496**

John S Van Arnam & Olga K Weinberg

11

Myelodysplastic syndrome with germline *GATA2* mutation

History A 10-year-old girl with hemi-hypertrophy and progressive right lower extremity lymphedema was referred to hematology for incidental neutropenia noted on a routine CBC. The patient was lost to follow-up for 4 years and returned with a chief complaint of recurrent epistaxis. CBC results are shown at right.

A bone marrow biopsy was performed.

Morphology & flow cytometry The bone marrow aspirate **f11.1** demonstrated a marked increase in megakaryocytes with widely spaced nuclear lobes. The myeloid series demonstrated left-shifted maturation with aberrant nuclear lobation, while the erythroid series demonstrated forms with irregular nuclear contours. The core biopsy was hypercellular (95%), and immunohistochemistry for CD34 and CD117 showed myeloid blasts comprising 5% of the marrow cellularity **f11.2**. Flow cytometry demonstrated a population of myeloid blasts comprising 3.4% of viable events which coexpressed CD34, CD117, CD13, CD33 (dim), MPO, and HLA-DR. A myeloid neoplasm was strongly suspected based on the morphologic and immunophenotypic findings.

Genetics/molecular results The karyotype was 45,XX,-7[20], with loss of 1 copy of chromosome 7 in all 20 cells analyzed. FISH was positive for monosomy 7 in 95% of cells and negative for rearrangement or gain of 3q, monosomy 5, trisomy 8, partial deletions of chromosomes 5 and 7, and for *BCR-ABL1* rearrangement.

WBC	46×10^9/L
HGB	9.7 g/dL
Platelets	488×10^9/L

A targeted NGS panel demonstrated the following mutations:

GATA2 p.H51fs* (c.154_179delACGAGGTGGACGTCTTCTTCAATCAC) variant allele frequency (VAF) 32%
ASXL1 p.D879fs* (c.2636_2637insT) VAF 50%
SETBP1 p.G870S (c.2608G>A) VAF 50%
NRAS p.G13D (c.38G>A) VAF 23%
NRAS p.G12D (c.35G>A) VAF 9%
PTPN11 p.A72T (c.214G>A) VAF 11%

Based on the overall clinical, morphologic, and genetic findings, a diagnosis of **myeloid neoplasm with germline *GATA2* mutation** was rendered.

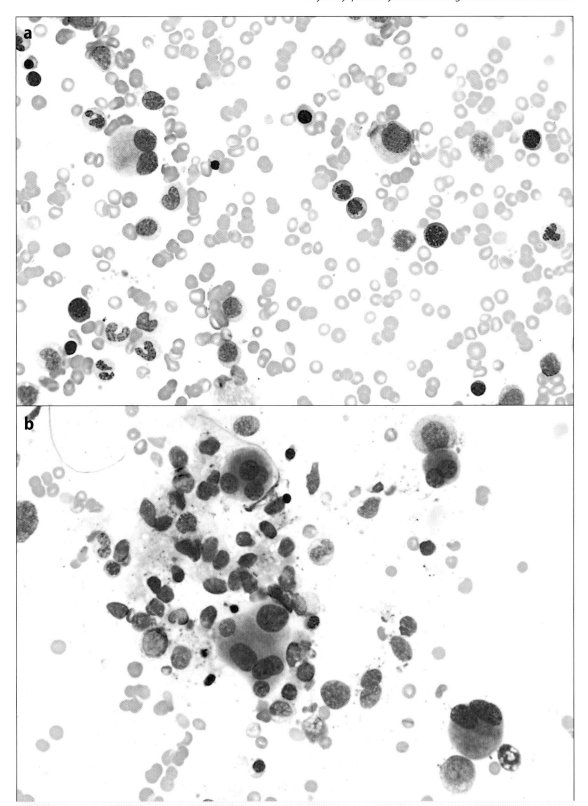

f11.1 **a** The bone marrow aspirate includes occasional erythroid dysplasia with nuclear contour irregularities, hypolobate neutrophils, and small megakaryocytic forms; **b** megakaryocytes are increased in number, with small & hypolobate forms, and others with widely separated nuclear lobes

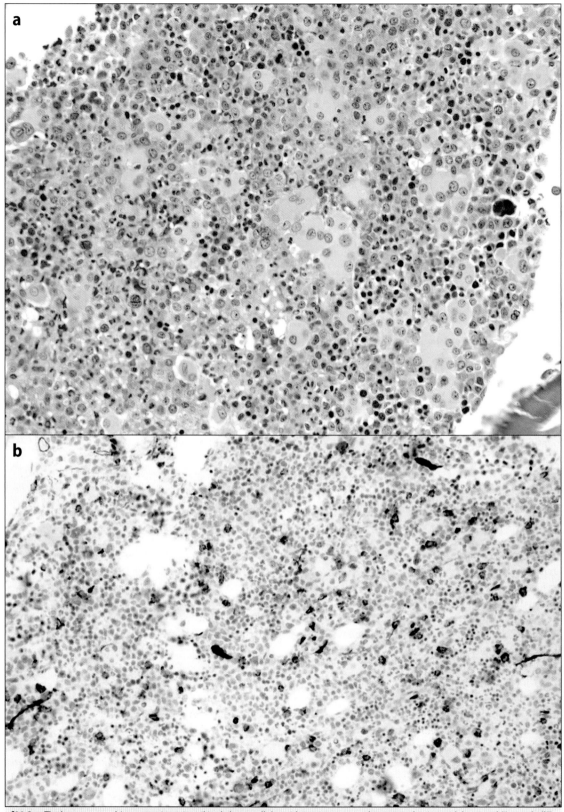

f11.2 **a** The bone marrow biopsy specimen is strikingly hypercellular with numerous megakaryocytes having widely spaced ("pawn ball") nuclear lobes; **b** CD34 staining highlights ~5% of the marrow cells, as well as increased megakaryocytes

ISBN 978-089189-6814   ©2021 ASCP

Discussion Extensive gene sequencing has demonstrated that the vast majority of myeloid neoplasms (>90%) have identifiable gene mutations that act as oncogenic drivers. The identification of these mutations is important for diagnosis, prognosis, and treatment, to the point that targeted gene sequencing is now standard of care in the evaluation of myeloid malignancies. Although most mutations found in myeloid neoplasms are somatically acquired, a small subset of cases contains inherited or germline mutations that confer predisposition to the development of hematologic malignancies and other diseases. Variable penetrance, lead time, and limited or protean manifestations prior to the development of malignancy may obscure the identification of syndromes caused by these mutations. In addition, some mutations associated with germline predisposition syndromes are also seen in sporadic malignancy, so their identification as germline is dependent on sequencing benign tissue such as fibroblasts. In the last decade, the expansion of knowledge surrounding these inherited or germline mutations, combined with the clinical importance of their identification, led to the creation of a separate category in the 2017 World Health Organization classification of hematologic neoplasms, namely "myeloid neoplasms with germline predisposition."

Identification of a hereditary mutation is critical for several reasons. It helps guide clinical management, both in terms of increased screening for hematopoietic malignancy but also for treatment of syndrome-related pathologies such as bleeding tendencies or elevated infection risk. In addition, the baseline blood count and bone marrow morphology in some patients with germline mutations may mimic a myeloid neoplasm such as myelodysplastic syndrome (MDS), but the presence of a germline disposition mutation does not change the diagnostic criteria for the myeloid neoplasm itself. Finally, identification of affected relatives is of obvious importance for their own treatment, but importantly, family members often represent potential allogeneic marrow donors for the proband, and engraftment failure and donor-derived malignancies have both been noted in the absence of appropriate screening. For patients with uncertain predisposition to malignancy, overall management is best accomplished by a synergy among the treating physicians, pathologists, and genetic counselors. The prognosis in many of these disorders is often poor, with allogeneic stem cell transplantation as the only potentially curative option.

Currently identified mutations found in myeloid neoplasms with germline predisposition are divided into three main categories based on other pre- or coexisting findings; these are summarized in **t11.1**. The presentation of MDS or chronic myeloid neoplasm in a child or young adult should prompt investigation for a germline predisposition syndrome. However, because some of these disorders can present later in life, any case of myeloid neoplasm having a germline-associated gene mutation with VAF closer to 50% should be further evaluated with molecular testing of nonaffected tissue, with cultured skin fibroblasts being recommended as having the least likelihood of blood contamination.

Myeloid neoplasms with germline *GATA2* mutation are often associated with other organ dysfunction. These mutations are monoallelic and variable in type, but all lead to loss of function of the affected allele with resultant haploinsufficiency. Clinical presentations are multifaceted, varying from mild cytopenias to syndromes having increased risk of infection, lymphedema, pulmonary dysfunction, autoimmunity, and both myeloid and nonhematopoietic malignancies. Flow cytometric analysis of otherwise healthy *GATA2*-mutant patients demonstrates progressive loss of monocytes, B cells, dendritic cells, and variable degrees of neutropenia. By late adulthood, MDS or acute myeloid leukemia develops in most cases.

In this patient, the initial presentation of leukocytosis, anemia, and thrombocytosis in the setting of dysplastic megakaryocytes and some dyspoiesis in the myeloid and erythroid lineages indicated both myelodysplastic and myeloproliferative features. Although germline testing was not available for this patient, her history of lymphedema, prior neutropenia, and dysplastic megakaryocytes with widely separated nuclear lobes, along with a predicted loss-of-function mutation in *GATA2*, are consistent with a germline *GATA2* mutation syndrome, specifically the variant formerly called Emberger syndrome **t11.1**, despite the presence of the mutation in only 30% of sequencing reads. Both *ASXL1* mutation and monosomy 7 are frequently identified in germline *GATA2*-mutated malignancies and are poor prognostic findings. The additional mutations in *NRAS* and *SETBP1* are often identified in MDS/ myeloproliferative neoplasm (MPN) overlap neoplasms and are consistent with the presentation of leukocytosis and thrombocytosis. Interestingly, a mutation in *PTPN11* was also identified; mutations in *PTPN11* are associated with Noonan syndrome and some cases

t11.1 Types of myeloid neoplasms with germline predispositions

Gene	Inheritance	Mutation type	Median age at diagnosis	CBC abnormality prior to neoplasm	Baseline marrow findings	Clinical association	Neoplasm predisposition	Additional mutations or genetic findings in neoplasms
Myeloid neoplasms with germline predisposition without a preexisting disorder or organ dysfunction								
CEBPA	AD	Germline mutations are FS	24.5 (2-46)	None	Uncertain	No pre-existing or organ dysfunction	AML	2nd hit (c-terminal), GATA1, WT1, EZH2
DDX41	AD	FS, MS, SS, Indel	69 (36-88)	Usually none; subset with variable cytopenias	Often hypocellular	Occasional autoimmune disease	MDS, AML (often erythroid), CML, CMML, MM	2nd hit, ASXL1, SRSF2, CUX1
Myeloid neoplasms with germline predisposition & preexisting platelet disorders								
RUNX1	AD	Del, SS, MS, FS	33 (6-76)	Plt↓	Hypo- or normocellular Megas small & hypolobate, disparate lobes; often eosinophilia	Subset with bleeding history, impaired plt aggregation, storage pool	MDS, AML, CMML, ALL, HCL	2nd hit, CDC25C, TET2, ASXL1,
ANKRD26	AD	MS	38 (1-84)	Plt↓	Hypercellular Increased megas, small & hypolobate	Mild or no bleeding	MDS, AML, CML, CMML	ASXL1
ETV6	AD	MS, SS, FS	Variable (ALL 2-37; myeloid neoplasm 8-82)	Plt↓	Megas small & hypolobate Some dysplasia in myeloid, erythroid lineages	Mild/moderate bleeding, impaired plt aggregation	MDS, AML, ALL, MPAL, MM, solid tumors	BCOR, RUNX1
Myeloid neoplasms with germline predisposition & other organ dysfunction								
GATA2	AD	MS, FS, Indel, SS	20 (<1-78)	Variable, often Plt↓, B cell↓, cytopenias	Hypocellular, variable dysplasia, megas small or with disparate lobes	Lymphedema, hearing loss (Emberger syndrome), infection risk, PAP	MDS, AML, CMML, aCML, ALL	ASXL1, STAG2, monosomy 7, trisomy 8
SAMD9/ SAMD9L	AD	MS, FS	Often in childhood (1-61)	Variable, often cytopenias	Variable, dyspoiesis in erythroid and mega lineages	MIRAGE syndrome	MDS, AML	Monosomy 7 (UPD), ETV6, SETBP1, RAS

Other myeloid disorders associated with congenital syndromes:

Myeloid neoplasms associated with bone marrow failure syndromes (eg, Fanconi anemia, severe congenital neutropenia, Schwachman-Diamond syndrome, Diamond-Blackfan anemia, telomere disorders such as dyskeratosis congenita)

Myeloid neoplasms associated with Down syndrome

Juvenile myelomonocytic leukemia associated with neurofibromatosis, Noonan(-like) syndrome

aCML, atypical chronic myeloid leukemia; AD, autosomal dominant transmission; ALL, acute lymphoblastic leukemia; AML, acute myeloid leukemia; CBC, complete blood cell count; CML, chronic myeloid leukemia; CMML, chronic myelomonocytic leukemia; Del, gene deletion; FS, frameshift mutation; HCL, hairy cell leukemia; Indel, insertion/deletion mutation; MDS, myelodysplastic syndrome; megas, megakaryocytes; MIRAGE syndrome, myelodysplasia, infection, restriction of growth, adrenal hypoplasia, genital abnormalities, enteropathy; MM, multiple myeloma; MPAL, mixed phenotype acute leukemia; MS, missense mutation; PAP, pulmonary alveolar proteinosis; Plt↓, thrombocytopenia; SS, splice site mutation; UPD, uniparental disomy

ISBN 978-089189-6814 ©2021 ASCP

of juvenile myelomonocytic leukemia with germline mutation (see **Case 13**).

Myeloid neoplasms with germline predisposition are rare, but more widespread recognition has resulted in increased diagnosis of these cases. Expanding efforts in gene sequencing in patients with idiopathic cytopenias/marrow failure and in those with early-onset or seemingly familial malignancy continue to identify candidate germline predisposition genes, including *ERCC6L2*, *XP-C*^{delTG}, and *MECOM*, though the molecular cause of some cases remains unknown even with whole genome sequencing.

Diagnostic pearls/pitfalls

– Although some mutations cause syndromes with prominent manifestations from birth or childhood, many mutations leading to myeloid neoplasms with germline predisposition have a very mild phenotype.

– The diagnostic criteria for the myeloid neoplasms with germline predisposition are the same as for sporadic cases of these neoplasms.

– Because many mutations in myeloid neoplasms with germline predisposition also occur somatically in sporadic neoplasms, verification of the germline mutation may require alternate samples for sequencing (eg, cultured skin fibroblasts, isolated T cells).

– Although disease in relatively young patients represents a significant proportion of myeloid neoplasms with germline predisposition, patients may present at nearly any age.

– The recognition of myeloid neoplasms with germline predisposition and their corresponding mutations is important for coordinated care of the proband, identification of affected relatives, and selection of potential marrow donors.

Readings

Collin M, Dickinson R, Bigley V. Haematopoietic and immune defects associated with *GATA2* mutation. Br J Haematol. 2015;169(2):173-87. **DOI: 10.1111/bjh.13317**

Dickinson RE, Milne P, Jardine L, et al. The evolution of cellular deficiency in *GATA2* mutation. Blood. 2014;123(6):863-74. **DOI: 10.1182/blood-2013-07-517151**

Ganapathi KA, Townsley DM, Hsu AP, et al. *GATA2* deficiency-associated bone marrow disorder differs from idiopathic aplastic anemia. Blood. 2015;125(1):56-70. **DOI: 10.1182/blood-2014-06-580340**

Ostergaard P, Simpson MA, Connell FC, et al. Mutations in *GATA2* cause primary lymphedema associated with a predisposition to acute myeloid leukemia (Emberger syndrome). Nat Genet. 2011;43(10):929-31. **DOI: 10.1038/ng.923**

Swerdlow SH, Campo E, Harris NL, et al. World Health Organization Classification of Tumours of Haematopoietic and Lymphoid Tissues. 4th ed. Lyon, France: IARC Press; 2017. **ISBN: 9789283244943**

University of Chicago Hematopoietic Malignancies Cancer Risk Team. How I diagnose and manage individuals at risk for inherited myeloid malignancies. Blood. 2016 Oct 6;128(14):1800-1813. Epub 2016 Jul 28. **DOI: 10.1182/blood-2016-05-670240**

West RR, Hsu AP, Holland SM, et al. Acquired *ASXL1* mutations are common in patients with inherited *GATA2* mutations and correlate with myeloid transformation. Haematologica. 2014 Feb;99(2):276-81. **DOI: 10.3324/haematol.2013.090217**

Wlodarski MW, Hirabayashi S, Pastor V, et al. Prevalence, clinical characteristics, and prognosis of *GATA2*-related myelodysplastic syndromes in children and adolescents. Blood. 2016;127(11):1387-97. **DOI: 10.1182/blood-2015-09-669937**

Herleen Rai & Rose C Beck

12

Chronic myelomonocytic leukemia with mutations in *TET2* & *SRSF2*

History A 73-year-old male with a past medical history of heart failure, end stage renal disease, and morbid obesity was seen by an oncologist for evaluation of severe anemia and persistent leukocytosis. CBC results are shown at right.

Review of the patient's prior blood counts showed a persistent absolute monocytosis for the last 2 years. A bone marrow biopsy with blood smear review was performed.

Morphology & flow cytometry The peripheral blood smear demonstrated monocytosis and neutrophilia with left shift and occasional morphologic atypia **f12.1**. The bone marrow aspirate smear showed granulocytic hyperplasia including rare hypogranular neutrophils, as well as an increased number of monocytes (10.5%) that morphologically appeared mature **f12.2**. The megakaryocytes and erythroid precursors were normal and blasts were not increased (1% in the aspirate differential). The core biopsy was markedly hypercellular for age (70%) and demonstrated similar findings as the aspirate **f12.3**. Overall, morphologic dysplasia was minimal.

Flow cytometry performed on the bone marrow identified immunophenotypic atypia in mature granulocytes (low CD177 expression) and aberrant CD56 expression on monocytes **f12.4**. Based on the clinical history of persistent monocytosis with anemia, together with the morphologic and flow cytometry findings, a diagnosis of "suspicious for myeloid neoplasm, such as chronic myelomonocytic leukemia (CMML-0)" was rendered and genetic and molecular studies were performed for further evaluation.

WBC	7.22×10^9/L
HGB	6.7 g/dL
HCT	23.8%
MCV	98 fL
Platelets	100×10^9/L
Absolute monocyte count	2.52×10^9/L
Differential: monocytes	34.9%

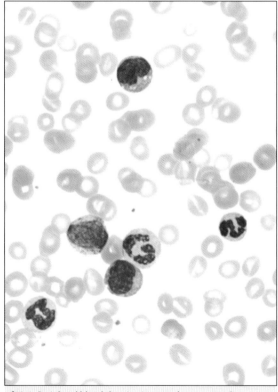

f12.1 Peripheral blood showing increased monocytes & granulocytic left shift

ISBN 978-089189-6814

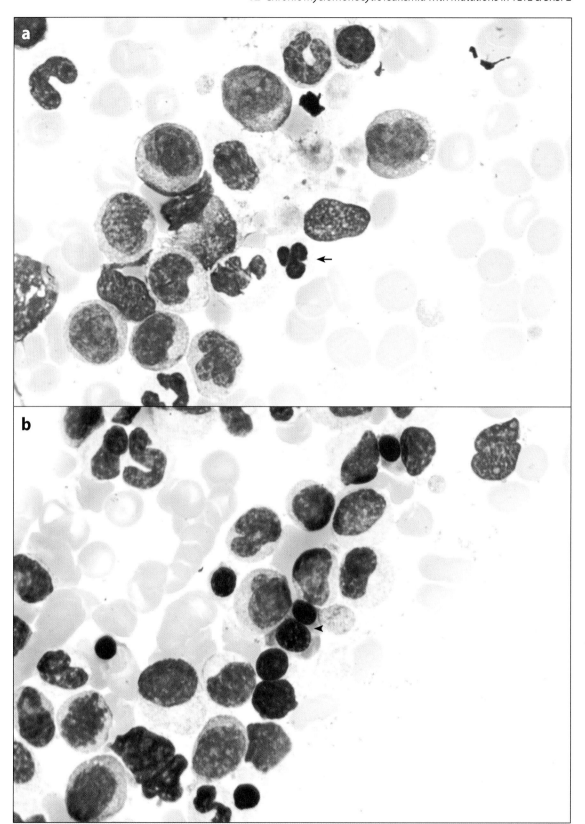

f12.2 a,b Monocytosis as well as granulocytic hyperplasia are also observed in the bone marrow aspirate, with few hypogranular neutrophils (arrow) & rare dysplastic erythroid cells (arrowhead), but otherwise minimal dysplasia

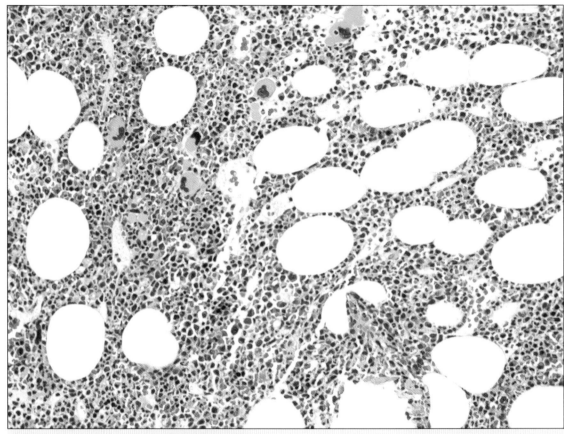

f12.3 The core biopsy specimen is significantly hypercellular for age

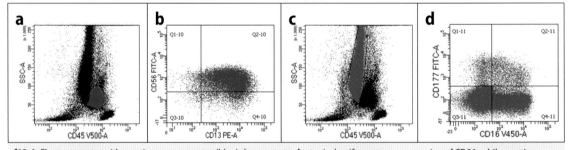

f12.4 Flow cytometry with **a** gating on monocytes (blue) demonstrates **b** atypical uniform strong expression of CD56, while **c** gating on granulocytes (purple) shows **d** decreased CD177 expression

Genetics/molecular results Quantitative polymerase chain reaction assay performed on blood for detection of *BCR-ABL1* fusion was negative. The bone marrow karyotype was normal and FISH was negative for *BCR-ABL1*. A targeted myeloid NGS panel was positive for the presence of 2 pathogenic variants: *TET2* p.Y1696* (c.5088T>G) at 50% variant allele frequency (VAF) and *SRSF2* p.P95R (c.284C>G) at 49% VAF **f12.5**. These findings along with the clinical history, morphology, and flow cytometry were consistent with a final diagnosis of **chronic myelomonocytic leukemia without increased blasts** (CMML-0).

Discussion Chronic myelomonocytic leukemia (CMML) is a rare hematopoietic neoplasm with features of dysplasia and myeloid proliferation; hence it is categorized in the myelodysplastic syndrome (MDS)/ myeloproliferative neoplasm "overlap" group of myeloid neoplasms in the 2017 World Health Organization (WHO) classification of hematopoietic neoplasms. CMML is characterized by persistent (at least 3 months' duration) absolute peripheral blood monocytosis of $\geq 1 \times 10^9$/L, in which monocytes constitute at least 10% of the total WBC count. CMML can be further divided into 3 categories based on the blast percentages

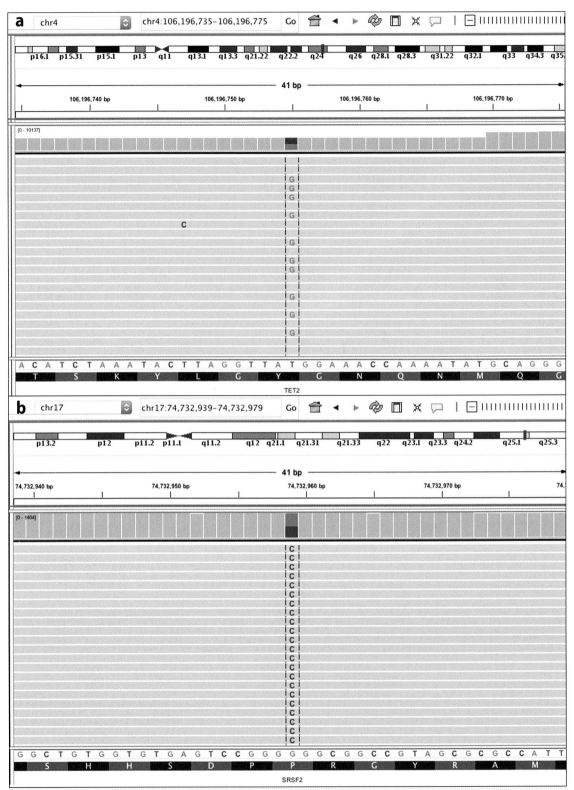

f12.5 Somatic variant analysis using a targeted myeloid NGS panel. Annotated reads demonstrate **a** *TET2* p.Y1696* (c.5088T>G, highlighted in orange) & **b** *SRSF2* p.P95R (c.284C>G), a common pathogenic variant of *SRSF2 (*highlighted in blue & showing the reverse strand). Among myeloid neoplasms, the combination of *TET2* & *SRSF2* mutations is highly suggestive of chronic myelomonocytic leukemia (hg19, IGV browser) [see **fA.8**, p312]

t12.1 World Health Organization (WHO) 2017 diagnostic criteria for chronic myelomonocytic leukemia

1. Persistent peripheral blood monocytosis (≥1 × 10⁹/L) with monocytes at least 10% of white blood cells

2. Not meeting WHO criteria for *BCR-ABL1*-positive chronic myeloid leukemia, primary myelofibrosis, polycythemia vera, or essential thrombocythemia

3. No rearrangement for *PDGFRA*, *PDGFRB* or *FGFR1* and no *PCM1-JAK2* fusion (these should be specifically excluded in cases with eosinophilia)

4. Blasts and blast equivalents (myeloblasts, monoblasts, and promoncytes) total <20% of the cells in the peripheral blood & bone marrow

5. Dysplasia involving ≥1 myeloid lineage or if myelodysplasia is absent or minimal, criteria 1-4 are met and:
   - An acquired, clonal cytogenetic or molecular genetic abnormality (eg, *TET2*, *SRSF2*, *ASXL*, *SETBP1*) is present in hematopoietic cells
   or
   - The monocytosis has lasted for ≥3 months and all other causes of monocytosis (eg, malignancy, infection & inflammation) have been excluded

in peripheral blood (PB) and bone marrow (BM): CMML-0 (<2% PB blasts, <5% BM blasts), CMML-1 (2%-4% PB blasts or 5%-9% BM blasts), and CMML-2 (5%-19% PB blasts or 10%-19% BM blasts). Blast equivalents in CMML include myeloblasts, monoblasts, and promonocytes (monocyte precursors), and increasing blast count portends transformation to acute myeloid leukemia.

Histologically, CMML is associated with granulocytic hyperplasia and monocyte proliferation which is especially prominent in blood. In the bone marrow, mature monocytes may be less conspicuous, and granulocytic dysplasia as well as atypical megakaryocytes with hypolobation are frequently seen. The absence of granulocytic dysplasia does not completely exclude CMML, and a diagnosis may still be made with minimal or lack of dysplasia in the presence of an acquired clonal cytogenetic or molecular genetic abnormality (most commonly *TET2*, *ASXL1*, *SRSF2*, and/or *SETBP1*, as discussed later). In this case, although dysplasia was minimally present, the presence of *TET2* and *SRSF2* mutations helped confirm the diagnosis. **t12.1** outlines the 2017 WHO diagnostic criteria for CMML.

Although at least half of all cases present with elevated WBC count, in the remaining cases the WBC count is normal or even decreased. Historically, a WBC count

of ≥13 × 10⁹/L has been used to distinguish the more myeloproliferative form (MP-CMML) from cases with more MDS-like features (MD-CMML); however, this distinction is controversial. MP-CMML is associated with increased incidence of splenomegaly and constitutional symptoms as compared to patients with MD-CMML, who tend to have more cytopenia-related symptoms.

Cytogenetic analysis demonstrates chromosomal abnormalities in about a third of CMML cases; these abnormalities are nonspecific and include trisomy 8, loss of Y, and monosomy 7 or del(7q). In contrast, the vast majority of cases (>90%) have detectable mutations in genes associated with myeloid neoplasms. These mutations can be divided into 5 major classes:

1. epigenetic control of transcription, including histone modification (*ASXL1*, *EZH2*) and DNA methylation genes (*TET2*, *DNMT3A*, *IDH1*, *IDH2*)
2. mutations in signaling genes (*JAK2*, *CBL*, *NRAS*, *KRAS*, *PTPN11*, *FLT3*)
3. mutations in mRNA splicing genes (*SRSF2*, *SF3B1*, *U2AF1*, *ZRSR2*)
4. mutations in transcription and nucleosome assembly genes (*RUNX1*, *SETBP1*)
5. DNA damage response gene mutations (*TP53*, *PHF6*).

Overall, the most commonly mutated genes identified in CMML are *TET2* (~60% of cases), *SRSF2* (~50%), *ASXL1* (~40%), and *NRAS* or *KRAS* (together, ~20%-30%).

CMML arises from the gain of multiple somatic genetic events in aging hematopoietic stem cells, which gives rise to malignant cell clones. In this context, *ASXL1* and *TET2* are considered early driver mutations that institute a preleukemic clonal hematopoietic phase and are able to give a selective advantage to a secondary clone that is needed for the development of overt disease. *TET2* mutations do not appear to influence prognosis in CMML, but *ASXL1* mutations, frame-shift and nonsense mutations specifically, have been shown to independently demonstrate a negative prognostic impact, being associated with decreased leukemia-free and overall survival. Other mutated genes that have been shown to have a negative impact on overall survival in CMML patients include *CBL*, *DNMT3A*, *EZH2*, *MPL*, *NPM1*, and *NRAS*.

Oncogenic RAS pathway mutations (*NRAS*, *KRAS*, *CBL*, *PTPN11*, and *NF1*) are secondary mutations that contribute to CMML progression. These mutations are more common in the myeloproliferative phenotype, MP-CMML, and patients tend to have a shorter life expectancy. *SRSF2* is the most commonly mutated spliceosome gene in CMML and has been associated with increasing age but is not an independent risk factor. Studies have shown that the co-occurrence of *SRSF2* and *TET2* mutations in a myeloid neoplasm is highly suggestive of CMML. In recent years, a pre-CMML condition has been recognized, termed "oligomonocytic CMML," with patients having characteristics of classic CMML but without an absolute monocyte count of 1×10^9/L. Cases of oligomonocytic CMML appear to have similar genomic findings as classic CMML, and most patients will progress to classic CMML or AML.

Flow cytometry can aid in the diagnosis of myeloid neoplasms by demonstrating aberrant expression of antigens such as CD56 by monocytes and granulocytes. Neoplastic monocytes express CD56 in most CMML cases, as exhibited by this example case. Other monocytic alterations observed in CMML include decreased CD14 and CD15 expression and increase in the proportion of CD14-positive, CD16-negative monocytes. Alterations in granulocyte antigens that have been associated with myelodysplasia include aberrations in the CD11b/CD16 maturation expression pattern, alterations in CD13 and CD33 expression, and decreased CD177 on mature granulocytes. However, aberrant expression of antigens may also be seen in reactive or regenerative states. Therefore, flow cytometry results should always be considered in context with other findings.

In this patient, the presence of both *TET2* and *SRSF2* mutations, in the context of persistent monocytosis with corroborating morphologic and flow cytometric findings, confirmed a diagnosis of CMML-0. Because of multiple health issues, the patient died several months after diagnosis.

Diagnostic pearls/pitfalls

- CMML is a clonal hematopoietic malignancy with overlapping myelodysplastic and myeloproliferative features that can be heterogeneous at initial presentation.
- A persistent (≥3 months) absolute peripheral blood monocytosis with a relative monocytosis (≥10% of total WBC count) must be present to diagnose CMML, and infectious as well as autoimmune causes of monocytosis must be ruled out.

- In suspect cases, *BCR-ABL1* fusion must be excluded, and if eosinophilia is present, fusions involving *PDGFRA*, *PDGFRB*, *FGFR1*, or *PCM1-JAK2* must also be ruled out with FISH testing.
- If there is minimal dysplasia, the presence of clonal genetic abnormalities can aid in a diagnosis of CMML, especially the presence of both *TET2* and *SRSF2* mutations.
- Flow cytometric detection of aberrant antigen expression by monocytes and granulocytes can be helpful in the evaluation of suspect CMML cases.

Readings

Coltro G, Patnaik MM. Chronic myelomonocytic leukemia: insights into biology, prognostic factors, and treatment. Curr Oncol Rep. 2019;21:101. **DOI: 10.1007/s11912-019-0855-6**

Geyer J, Tam W, Liu Y, et al, Oligomonocytic chronic myelomonocytic leukemia (chronic myelomonocytic leukemia without absolute monocytosis) displays a similar clinicopathologic and mutational profile to classical chronic myelomonocytic leukemia. Mod Pathol. 2017;30:1213-22. **DOI: 10.1038/modpathol.2017.45**

Harrington AM, Schelling LA, Ordobazari A, et al. Immunophenotypes of chronic myelomonocytic leukemia (CMML) subtypes by flow cytometry: a comparison of CMML-1 vs CMML-2, myeloproliferative vs dysplastic, de novo vs therapy-related, and CMML-specific cytogenetic risk subtypes. Am J Clin Pathol. 2016;146(2):170-81. **DOI: 10.1093/ajcp/aqw084**

Itzykson R, Duchmann M, Lucas N, et al. CMML: clinical and molecular aspects. Int J Hematol. 2017;105:711-9. **DOI: 10.1007/s12185-017-2243-z**

McCullough KB, Patnaik MM. Myelodysplastic syndrome/myeloproliferative neoplasm overlap syndromes: advances in treatment. Best Pract Res Clin Haematol. 2019;33(2):101130. **DOI: 10.1016/j.beha.2019.101130**

Patnaik MM, Lasho TL, Finke CM, et al. Spliceosome mutations involving SRSF2, SF3B1, and U2AF35 in chronic myelomonocytic leukemia: prevalence, clinical correlates, and prognostic relevance. Am J Hematol. 2013;88(3):201-6. **DOI: 10.1002/ajh.23373**

Patnaik MM, Tefferi A. Chronic myelomonocytic leukemia: 2020 update on diagnosis, risk stratification and management. Am J Hematol. 2020;95(1):97-115. **DOI: 95.10.1002/ajh.25684**

Ricci C, Fermo E, Corti S, et al. RAS mutations contribute to evolution of chronic myelomonocytic leukemia to the proliferative variant. Clin Cancer Res. 2010;16(8):2246-56. **DOI: 10.1158/1078-0432.CCR-09-2112**

Selimoglu-Buet D, Wagner-Ballon O, Saada V, et al. Characteristic repartition of monocyte subsets as a diagnostic signature of chronic myelomonocytic leukemia. Blood. 2015;125(23):3618-26. **DOI: 10.1182/blood-2015-01-620781**

Swerdlow SH, Campo E, Harris NL, et al. World Health Organization Classification of Tumours of Haematopoietic and Lymphoid Tissues. 4th ed. Lyon, France: IARC Press; 2017:82-86. **ISBN: 9789283244943**

Valent P, Orazi A, Savona MR, et al. Proposed diagnostic criteria for classical chronic myelomonocytic leukemia (CMML), CMML variants and pre-CMML conditions. Haematologica. 2019 Oct;104(10):1935-1949. Epub 2019 May 2. **DOI: 10.3324/haematol.2019.222059**

Sarah L Ondrejka & Erika M Moore

13

Juvenile myelomonocytic leukemia with *NRAS* mutation

History A 10-month-old female infant presented with leukocytosis and an enlarged spleen by abdominal ultrasound examination. CBC results are shown at right.

A peripheral blood smear was obtained and the manual differential count is shown at right.

Morphology & flow cytometry The peripheral blood smear demonstrated marked leukocytosis with occasional blasts and promonocytes, and a predominance of mature monocytes, some of which were atypical. Occasional hypogranular and/or hypolobated neutrophils were identified **f13.1**.

Flow cytometry of the peripheral blood confirmed absolute monocytosis and the presence of increased myeloblasts (7% of gated events) with phenotypic atypia including decreased expression of CD38 and HLA-DR **f13.2**.

A bone marrow biopsy was performed. The aspirate smears were hemodilute and similar to peripheral blood. The core biopsy showed hypercellular bone marrow (nearly 100%) with granulocytic hyperplasia and few abnormal-appearing megakaryocytes **f13.3**.

Genetics/molecular results Results of FISH were negative for t(9;22) *BCR-ABL1* and 11q23 *KMT2A* (*MLL*) rearrangements, and cytogenetic analysis showed a normal female karyotype. A myeloid NGS panel was performed and identified *NRAS* p.Q61R (c.182A>G), with 42% variant allele frequency **f13.4**.

WBC	131.3×10^9/L
Differential	
Neutrophils	4.5%
Lymphocytes	16%
Monocytes	70.5%
Eosinophils	3%
Basophils	0%
Blasts/promonocytes	6%
Nucleated RBCs	2/100 WBCs
RBC	2.81×10^{12}/L
HGB	5.2 g/dL
HCT	15.7%
MCV	84 fL
RDW	21.4%
Platelets	82×10^9/L

Based on the peripheral blood and bone marrow morphologic findings and molecular studies, a diagnosis of **juvenile myelomonocytic leukemia** (JMML) was rendered.

ISBN 978-089189-6814

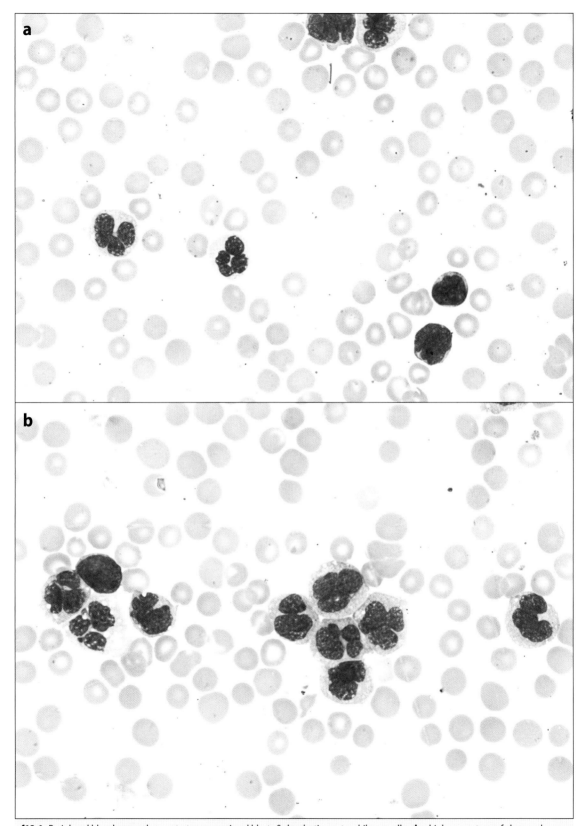

f13.1 Peripheral blood smear demonstrates **a** occasional blasts & dysplastic neutrophils, as well as **b** a high percentage of abnormal-appearing, mature monocytes

13 *Juvenile myelomonocytic leukemia with NRAS mutation*

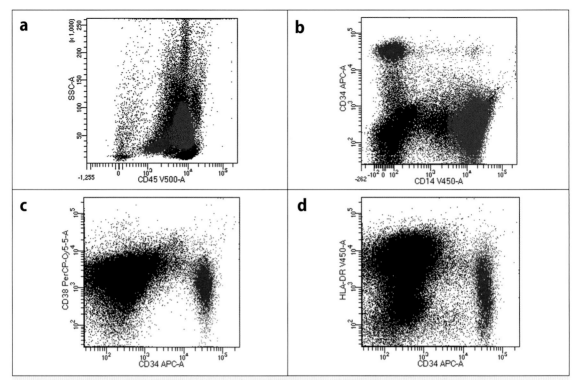

f13.2 Peripheral blood flow cytometry demonstrating **a** increased events in the blast & monocyte gates with **b** 7% CD34-positive myeloblasts in red & 60% CD14-positive monocytes in blue; the myeloblasts demonstrate phenotypic atypia with **c** decreased CD38 expression & **d** decreased HLA-DR expression

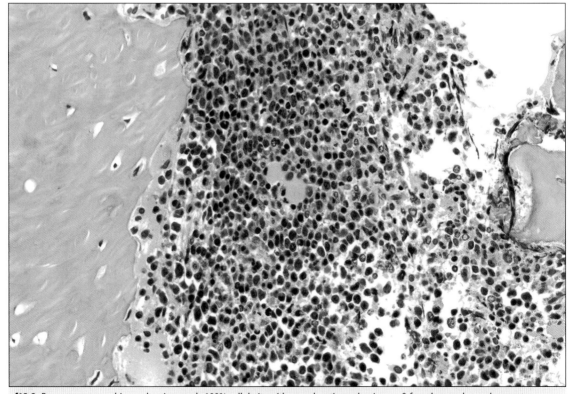

f13.3 Bone marrow core biopsy showing nearly 100% cellularity with granulocytic predominance & few abnormal megakaryocytes

ISBN 978-089189-6814   ©2021 ASCP

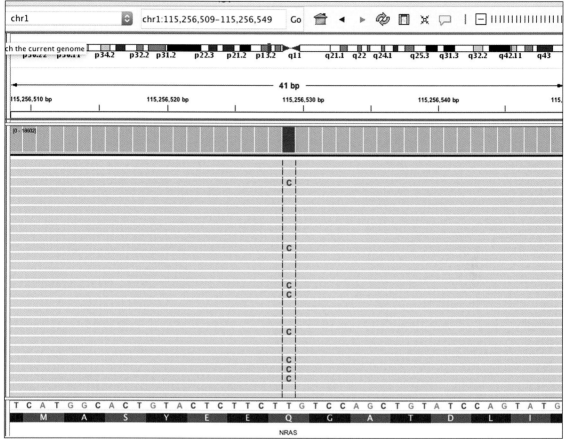

f13.4 Somatic variant analysis using a targeted myeloid NGS panel; annotated reads mapped to the *NRAS* locus demonstrate p.Q61R (c.182A>G) in 42% of reads, highlighted in blue (hg19, Integrative Genomics Viewer browser, showing the reverse strand) [see **fA.8**, p312]

Discussion JMML is a rare myeloid neoplasm occurring in childhood, usually presenting before 3 years of age, characterized by hyperproliferation of the granulocytic and monocytic lineages and <20% blasts in blood or bone marrow at the time of diagnosis. It is more common in males, and children with neurofibromatosis type 1 (NF1, with germline *NF1* mutation) have an increased risk of developing this disorder. Interestingly, patients with Noonan syndrome (germline mutations in *PTPN11* or other RAS pathway genes) can develop a JMML-like disorder with a highly variable disease severity. In addition, approximately 15% of JMML cases occur in infants with a Noonan syndrome-like disorder, caused by a germline *CBL* mutation.

Patients may present with constitutional symptoms such as fever and typically have marked hepatosplenomegaly, occasionally with lymphadenopathy. Laboratory features include increased synthesis of hemoglobin F, polyclonal hypergammaglobulinemia, and a positive result on direct Coombs test. Detection of a mutation in one of the 5 canonical RAS pathway genes (*PTPN11, NRAS, KRAS, NF1, CBL*) has largely supplanted other, more cumbersome diagnostic tools such as demonstration of in vitro hypersensitivity of the abnormal myeloid progenitors to granulocyte-macrophage colony-stimulating factor (GM-CSF). The most frequently detected driver mutations in JMML are somatic mutations in *PTPN11*, which occur in ~35% of patients.

RAS pathway hyperactivation is strongly implicated in the pathogenesis of JMML and evidence of a RAS pathway gene mutation along with the other characteristic features are now essential for making a diagnosis **t13.1**. Loss-of-function *NF1* mutations result in dysregulation of *RAS* activation, as do mutually exclusive gain-of-function mutations in *PTPN11, NRAS*, or *KRAS*. Other somatic mutations may be found in JMML patients, including *SETBP1* mutations, and the presence of at least 2 mutations has been associated with worse outcome.

t13.1 World Health Organization 2017 diagnostic criteria for juvenile myelomonocytic leukemia

Clinical & hematologic criteria (all 4 criteria must be met)

1. Peripheral blood monocyte count ≥1 × 10^9/L

2. Blast percentage in peripheral blood & bone marrow <20%

3. Splenomegaly

4. No Philadelphia chromosome or *BCR-ABL1* fusion

Genetic criteria (any 1 criterion is sufficient)

Somatic mutation in *PTPN11, KRAS*, or *NRAS*

Clinical diagnosis of neurofibromatosis type 1 or *NF1* mutation

Germline *CBL* mutation & loss of heterozygosity of *CBL*

Other criteria

Cases that do not meet any of the genetic criteria above must meet the following criteria in addition to the 4 clinical & hematologic criteria

Monosomy 7 or any other chromosomal abnormality

or

≥2 of the following:

   Increased hemoglobin F for age

   Myeloid or erythroid precursors on peripheral blood smear

   Granulocyte-macrophage colony-stimulating factor hypersensitivity in colony assay

   Hyperphosphorylation of STAT5

Cytogenetic studies show monosomy 7 as the most frequent recurrent chromosomal abnormality (25% of cases), although the majority of JMML patients (65%) have a normal karyotype. Monosomy 7 is not specific for JMML and can be seen in myelodysplastic syndromes of childhood as well as acute myeloid leukemia (AML).

The prognosis of JMML is variable. Some clinical and laboratory features including older age, increased fetal hemoglobin, and thrombocytopenia are associated with poorer outcomes. Currently, the only potentially curative therapy is hematopoietic stem cell transplantation. The patient in this case received an allogeneic stem cell transplant several months after diagnosis but unfortunately died of transplant-related complications shortly thereafter.

Diagnostic pearls/pitfalls

- The differential diagnosis for JMML includes benign leukemoid reaction as well as AML with monocytic differentiation. Children with viral or other infections can present with similar clinical and peripheral blood features, and benign causes for leukocytosis should be excluded. In AML with monocytic differentiation, distinguishing promonocytes (blast equivalents) from atypical mature monocytes may be difficult and requires quality smears with careful morphologic analysis.

- Cytogenetic and molecular analysis are pivotal to the evaluation of a child with suspected JMML. A RAS pathway gene mutation or clonal cytogenetic abnormality are useful in ruling out a reactive process. Because chronic myeloid leukemia can also occur in children, karyotype and/or FISH studies are required to exclude the presence of t(9;22) *BCR-ABL1* fusion.

– Identification of a mutation in *PTPN11*, *KRAS*, or *NRAS* in suspect JMML cases should prompt investigation for a germline syndrome such as Noonan syndrome. Occasionally, infants with Noonan syndrome develop a JMML-like, transient myeloproliferative disorder that may self-resolve. These cases should not be treated aggressively.

– Other syndromes can present with JMML-like clinical and pathologic features. These include Wiskott-Aldrich syndrome and infantile malignant osteopetrosis.

Readings

Baumann I, Bennett JM, Niemeyer CM, Thiele J. Juvenile myelomonocytic leukemia. In: World Health Organization Classification of Tumours of Hematopoietic and Lymphoid Tissues. 4th ed. Lyon, France: IARC Press; 2017. **ISBN: 978-9283224310**

Chan RJ, Cooper T, Kratz CP, et al. Juvenile myelomonocytic leukemia: a report from the 2nd International JMML Symposium. Leuk Res. 2009;33:355-62. **DOI: 10.1016/j.leukres.2008.08.022**

Locatelli F, Niemeyer CM. How I treat juvenile myelomonocytic leukemia. Blood 2015; 125:1083-90. **DOI: 10.1182/blood-2014-08-550483**

Niemeyer CM, Flotho C. Juvenile myelomonocytic leukemia: who's the driver at the wheel? Blood 2019;133(10):1060-1070. **DOI: 10.1182/blood-2018-11-844688**

Stieglitz E, Taylor-Weiner AN, Chang TY, et al. The genomic landscape of juvenile myelomonocytic leukemia. Nat Genet. 2015;47:1326-33. **DOI: 10.1038/ng.3400**

Rose C Beck

14

Atypical chronic myeloid leukemia with mutations in *SETBP1*, *SRSF2*, *ZRSR2* & *GATA2*

History A 70-year-old male with past medical history of coronary artery disease was referred to an oncologist for evaluation of increasing leukocytosis over the last year. He also complained of increasing fatigue for the past 3-6 months.

A peripheral blood smear was obtained and a bone marrow biopsy was performed for further evaluation.

Morphology & flow cytometry The peripheral smear demonstrated a granulocytic left shift and rare blasts, with a predominance of myelocytes, and occasional hypogranular or hypolobated neutrophils **f14.1**. The bone marrow aspirate showed a granulocytic predominance (myeloid:erythroid ratio 10:1), with 4% blasts as well as small, hypolobated megakaryocytes **f14.2a**. The core biopsy and clot section demonstrated similar findings as the aspirate, with 90% cellularity **f14.2b**.

Flow cytometry of the bone marrow aspirate identified 1.6% CD34-positive, CD117-positive myeloblasts which had atypical decreased CD45 expression and dim CD5 expression, consistent with a myeloid neoplasm **f14.3**. Based on the presence of peripheral leukocytosis with dysplasia and abnormal flow cytometry findings, a tentative diagnosis of myelodysplastic syndrome (MDS)/myeloproliferative neoplasm (MPN) was rendered, and results of genetic and molecular testing were reviewed before a final diagnosis was added to the surgical pathology report.

WBC	39.7×10^9/L
Differential	
Neutrophils	60%
Lymphocytes	4%
Myelocytes	16%
Metamyelocytes	19%
Blasts	1%
HGB	10.6 g/dL
HCT	35.6%
MCV	97.6 fL
Platelets	103×10^9/L

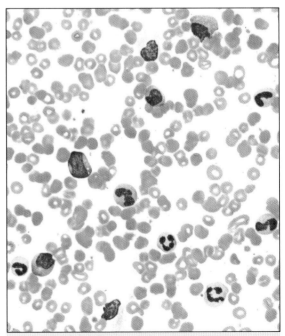

f14.1 Peripheral blood showing increased myelocytes & granulocytic left shift

ISBN 978-089189-6814 ©2021 ASCP

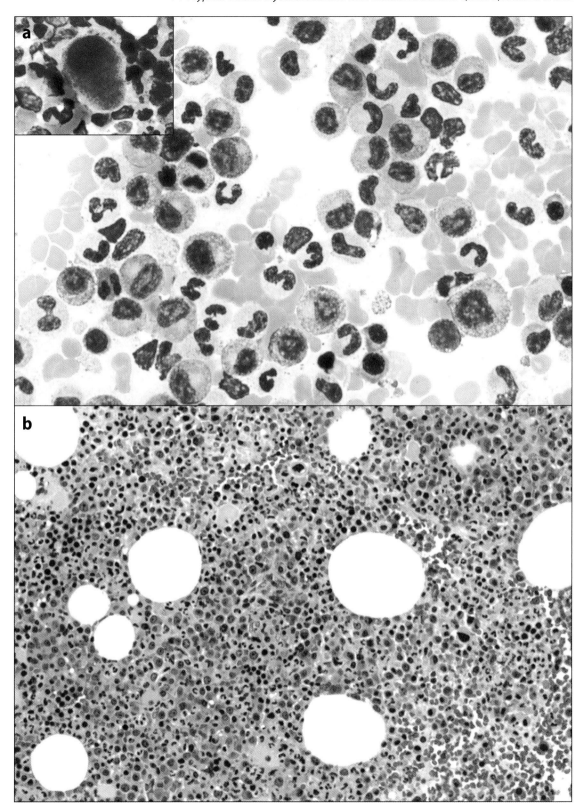

f14.2 **a** The bone marrow aspirate demonstrates granulocytic hyperplasia with hypogranular neutrophils & precursors, as well as hypolobated megakaryocytes (inset); **b** the clot section demonstrates hypercellularity, granulocyte predominance, and atypical, hypolobated megakaryocytes

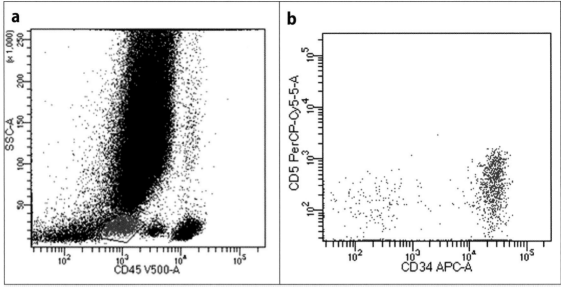

f14.3 Flow cytometry identified 1.6% CD34-positive, CD117-positive myeloblasts (highlighted in blue) having **a** decreased CD45 expression & **b** aberrant dim CD5

Genetics/molecular results The karyotype was normal and FISH was negative for *BCR-ABL1*, del(5q), monosomy 5, del(7q), monosomy 7, trisomy 8, del(17p), and del(20q). A myeloid NGS panel was positive for the presence of several pathogenic variants: *SETBP1* p.G870S (c.2608G>A) at 48% variant allele frequency (VAF) **f14.4**, *SRSF2* p.P95L (c.284C>T) at 49% VAF, *ZRSR2* p.Q273fs*13 (c.816_823del8) at 92% VAF, and *GATA2* p.L386fs*2 (c.1155_1156dupAC) at 41% VAF. Based on the absence of *BCR-ABL1* and presence of several myeloid-associated mutations including *SETBP1*, a final diagnosis of **atypical chronic myeloid leukemia** was rendered.

Discussion Atypical chronic myeloid leukemia (aCML), *BCR-ABL*-negative, is a rare myeloid disorder having both myelodysplastic and proliferative features, and hence is placed in the MDS/MPN category in the 2017 World Health Organization (WHO) classification of hematologic neoplasms. aCML is characterized by a high white blood cell (WBC) count (by definition at least 13×10^9/L) with granulocytic left shift, and blood morphology resembling that of *BCR-ABL*-positive CML, except for the presence of dysplasia and absence of basophilia in aCML. The neutrophils in aCML are often hypogranular, with dysplastic nuclear changes such as hypo- or hypersegmentation and/or abnormal chromatin clumping. The bone marrow often demonstrates megakaryocytic dysplasia and dyserythropoiesis may also be present.

The 2017 WHO criteria for diagnosing aCML are shown in **t14.1**. By definition, the t(9;22) *BCR-ABL1* translocation as well as any other disease-defining genetic lesions should be absent in aCML, with no recurring translocations being particular to this disorder. Cases of aCML may have cytogenetic abnormalities commonly associated with myeloid neoplasms, such as del(20q), trisomy 8, deletion 7/7q, or isochromosome 17q.

Clinically, patients diagnosed with aCML often have hepatosplenic involvement and a poor prognosis, with median survival of 1-2 years and a high risk of transformation to acute myeloid leukemia (AML). Adverse prognostic factors include higher WBC count, predominance of immature granulocytes in blood, female sex, and older age. At present there is no standard of treatment, and patients are often recommended for allogeneic stem cell transplantation. Hypomethylating agents and other therapies particular to MDS or MPN may be used on an individual basis.

Although the absence of a *BCR-ABL1* fusion excludes a diagnosis of CML, aCML may be difficult to distinguish from benign leukemoid reaction or other MDS/MPN or MPN with a prominent neutrophil component, such as chronic neutrophilic leukemia (CNL). **t14.2** compares features found in disorders presenting with granulocytic leukocytosis. The current availability of NGS testing for mutations associated with myeloid malignancy has enhanced the diagnosis

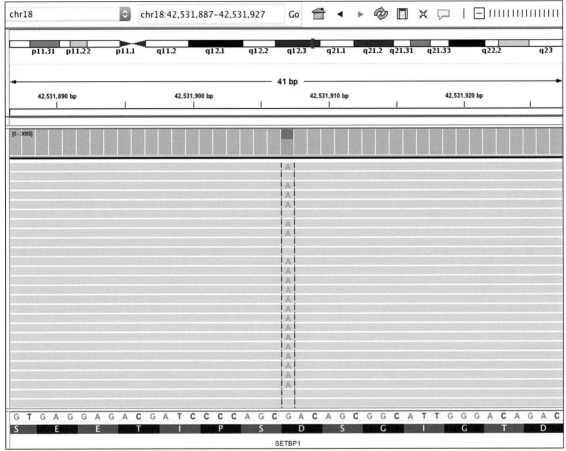

f14.4 Somatic variant analysis using a targeted myeloid NGS panel. Annotated reads mapped to the *SETBP1* locus demonstrate p.G870S (c.2608G>A), highlighted in green (hg19, Integrative Genomics Viewer browser) [see **fA.8**, p312]

t14.1 World Health Organization 2017 diagnostic criteria for atypical chronic myeloid leukemia

Blood leukocytosis ≥13 × 10⁹/L, with predominance of neutrophils and immature granulocytes (promyelocytes, myelocytes, and metamyelocytes); the immature forms comprise ≥10% of leukocytes
Dysgranulopoiesis
No or minimal absolute basophilia (basophils are usually <2% of leukocytes)
No or minimal absolute monocytosis (monocytes are <10% of leukocytes)
Hypercellular bone marrow with granulocytic hyperplasia and dysplasia, with or without erythroid and/or megakaryocytic dysplasia
<20% blasts in blood & bone marrow
No evidence of rearrangement of *PDGFRA*, *PDGFRB*, or *FGFR1*, or *PCM1-JAK2* fusion
Not meeting criteria for CML or other MPN; a prior history of MPN usually excludes a diagnosis of aCML
aCML, atypical chronic myeloid leukemia; MPN, myeloproliferative neoplasm

t14.2 Comparison between disorders presenting with granulocytic leukocytosis

	Reactive neutrophilia	Chronic myeloid leukemia	Chronic neutrophilic leukemia	Atypical chronic myeloid leukemia, BCR-ABL-negative
White blood cells	Usually <30 × 10⁹/L	Usually >50 × 10⁹/L	≥25 × 10⁹/L	≥13 × 10⁹/L
Toxic granulation	Often present	Usually absent	Often present	Usually absent
Granulocytic left shift	Few myelocytes, usually very rare promyelocytes, very rare blasts	Many myelocytes, frequent promyelocytes, variable blasts	Limited (<10% of granulocytic cells)	Present, at least 10% of granulocytic cells
Granulocytic dysplasia	Absent	Absent	Absent	Present
Basophilia	Absent	Present	Usually absent	Usually absent
Platelets	Variable	Often increased	Often normal	Normal or decreased
Nucleated red blood cells	Usually absent	Often present	Absent	May be present
Genetic findings	Normal	*BCR-ABL1* fusion in all cases	*CSF3R* mutation (>80% of cases)	Various mutation(s) in majority of cases (see text)

of aCML and can help distinguish aCML from other myeloid neoplasms. Although the presence of a myeloid-associated mutation by itself is not diagnostic of malignancy (see **Case 7 & 17**), the presence of particular gene mutations may corroborate or exclude a suspected diagnosis of aCML in the setting of appropriate morphologic findings. No single specific mutation is associated with aCML; however, a handful of genes are mutated in at least 10% of aCML cases: *ASXL1* (20%-66% of cases), *TET2* (30%-41%), *SRSF2* (40%), *SETBP1* (24%-32%), *NRAS* (27%-30%), *U2AF1* (13%), *EZH2* (13%-20%), and *KRAS* (10%). In particular, mutations in *SETBP1* and *ETNK1* appear enriched in aCML versus other chronic myeloid neoplasms and are associated with higher WBC counts and poorer prognosis among aCML patients. *SETBP1* mutations in aCML commonly occur in codons 858-871, corresponding to a 14-amino acid stretch of the protein usually targeted for ubiquitination, allowing for subsequent degradation of the SETBP1 protein. Mutations in this region result in decreased degradation and consequently increased binding to SET, a negative regulator of the tumor suppressor PP2A; thus, the overall consequence of pathogenic *SETBP1* mutations is enhanced cell proliferation. Although an early study reported that *CSF3R* T618I mutation occurs at a high frequency in aCML, larger studies have shown that this mutation occurs in <10% of cases, and its presence in patients with neutrophilic

leukocytosis should raise suspicion for CNL (**Case 4**). Similarly, the *JAK2* V617F mutation has been reported at low frequency in aCML (4%-8%), and its presence should prompt consideration of a *JAK2*-associated MPN such as primary myelofibrosis.

In this patient, the presence of *SETBP1* and other myeloid mutations, together with the morphologic findings and absence of *BCR-ABL1*, indicated a diagnosis of aCML. The presence of a *GATA2* mutation at a higher VAF (40%) also raised the possibility of myeloid neoplasm with germline *GATA2* (a germline predisposition syndrome; see **Case 11**); however, a germline mutation could not be verified in this patient without additional testing. The patient died of cardiac complications several months after diagnosis, and autopsy confirmed involvement by myeloid neoplasm in both the liver and spleen.

Diagnostic pearls/pitfalls

- Atypical CML is a rare chronic myeloid neoplasm with both myelodyspastic and myeloproliferative features and poorer prognosis vs other MDS/MPNs or MPNs.
- The diagnosis of aCML requires genetic testing to exclude *BCR-ABL*-positive CML and other myeloid neoplasms having specific chromosomal fusions.

– Mutations in *SETBP1* are particularly enriched in aCML vs other myeloid neoplasms and portend a poorer prognosis.

– *CSF3R* T618I and *JAK2* V617F mutations are only rarely found in aCML, and if identified in the presence of leukocytosis, should prompt consideration of a diagnosis of CNL or *JAK2*-associated MPN, respectively.

Readings

Gambacorti-Passerini CB, Donadoni C, Parmiani A, et al. Recurrent *ETNK1* mutations in atypical chronic myeloid leukemia. Blood. 2015 Jan 15;125(3):499-503. **DOI: 10.1182/blood-2014-06-579466**

Gotlib J. How I treat atypical chronic myeloid leukemia. Blood. 2017 16;129(7):838-45. **DOI: 10.1182/blood-2014-08-550483**

McClure RF, Ewalt MD, Crow J, et al. Clinical significance of DNA variants in chronic myeloid neoplasms: a report of the Association for Molecular Pathology. J Mol Diagn. 2018;20(6):717-37. **DOI: 10.1016/j.jmoldx.2018.07.002**

Meggendorfer M, Bacher U, Alpermann T, et al. *SETBP1* mutations occur in 9% of MDS/MPN and in 4% of MPN cases and are strongly associated with atypical CML, monosomy 7, isochromosome i(17)(q10), ASXL1 and CBL mutations. Leukemia. 2013;27(9):1852-60. **DOI: 10.1038/leu.2013.133**

Meggendorfer M, Haferlach T, Alpermann T, et al. Specific molecular mutation patterns delineate chronic neutrophilic leukemia, atypical chronic myeloid leukemia, and chronic myelomonocytic leukemia. Haematologica. 2014;99(12):e244-6. **DOI: 10.3324/haematol.2014.113159**

Piazza R, Valletta S, Winkelmann N, et al. Recurrent *SETBP1* mutations in atypical chronic myeloid leukemia. Nat Genet. 2013 Jan;45(1):18-24. **DOI: 10.1038/ng.2495**

Wang SA, Hasserjian RP, Fox PS, et al. Atypical chronic myeloid leukemia is clinically distinct from unclassifiable myelodysplastic/myeloproliferative neoplasms. Blood. 2014;123(17):2645-51. **DOI: 10.1182/blood-2014-02-553800**

Zoi K, Cross NCP. Molecular pathogenesis of atypical CML, CMML and MDS/MPN-unclassifiable. Int J Hematol. 2015;101(3):229-42. **DOI: 10.1007/s12185-014-1670-3**

Rose C Beck

15

Myelodysplastic/myeloproliferative neoplasm with ring sideroblasts & thrombocytosis, with mutations in *JAK2* & *SF3B1*

History A 69-year-old male presented to an oncologist for evaluation of prolonged thrombocytosis and anemia. CBC results are shown at right.

Morphology & flow cytometry A bone marrow biopsy specimen was obtained and the aspirate smear demonstrated erythroid predominance and dyserythropoiesis in the form of nuclear irregularities and megaloblastoid change **f15.1**, as well as enlarged atypical megakaryocytes that were clustered in the core biopsy **f15.2**. Iron staining showed many ring sideroblasts **f15.3**. Granulopoiesis was normal and myeloblasts were not increased. Mild to moderate reticulin fibrosis was also present in the core biopsy.

Flow cytometry was significant for 0.2% myeloblasts with slight phenotypic atypia including partial CD7 expression **f15.4**, concerning for myeloid neoplasm.

Based on the morphologic and flow cytometric findings, a diagnosis of **myelodysplastic/myeloproliferative neoplasm with ring sideroblasts and thrombocytosis** was rendered.

Genetics/molecular results Cytogenetics showed a normal male karyotype, and FISH studies were negative for deletion of 5/5q, 7/7q, 13q, and 20q and negative for trisomy 8. A myeloid NGS panel demonstrated the presence of *JAK2* p.V617F (c.1849G>T) with 43% VAF, *SF3B1* p.K700E (c.2098A>G) with 45% VAF, and *DNMT3A* p.R882H (c.2645G>A) with 28% VAF.

WBC	10.7×10^9/L
RBC	3.15×10^{12}/L
HGB	9.6 g/dL
HCT	30.4%
MCV	97 fL
RDW	26.2%
Platelets	637×10^9/L

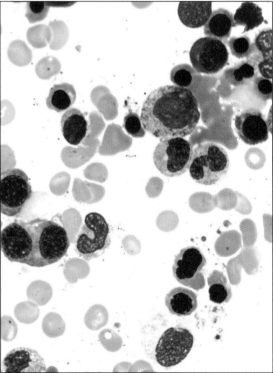

f15.1 Bone marrow aspirate showing erythroid predominance & dyserythropoiesis, including nuclear irregularities & megaloblastoid changes

ISBN 978-089189-6814

15 *Myelodysplastic/myeloproliferative neoplasm with ring sideroblasts & thrombocytosis, with mutations in JAK2 & SF3B1*

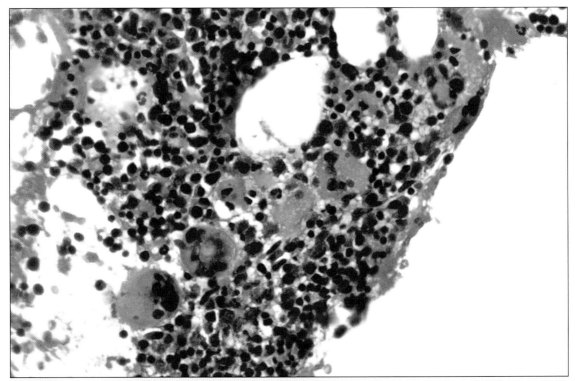

f15.2 Bone marrow core biopsy demonstrating hypercellularity with atypical, enlarged megakaryocytes with hyperlobation

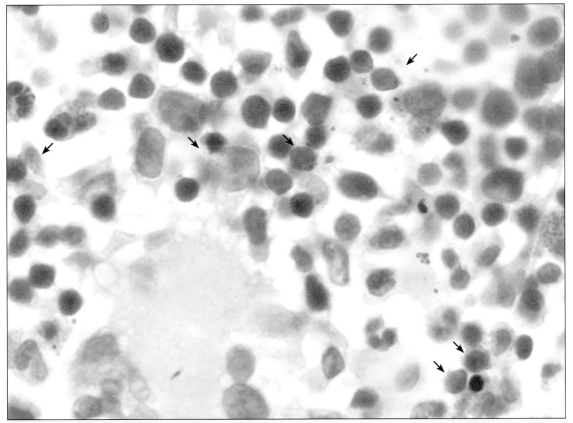

f15.3 Iron stain of the clot section showing numerous ring sideroblasts (arrows)

15 *Myelodysplastic/myeloproliferative neoplasm with ring sideroblasts & thrombocytosis, with mutations in JAK2 & SF3B1*

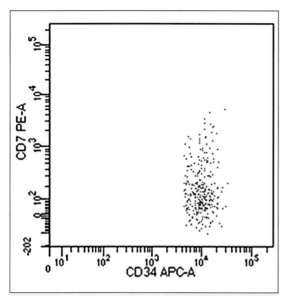

f15.4 Flow cytometry (gated on 0.2% CD34-positive CD117-positive myeloblasts) demonstrating partial CD7 expression by the blasts

t15.1 World Health Organization 2017 diagnostic criteria for MDS/MPN-RS-T
Anemia with erythroid dysplasia, with or without multilineage dysplasia, with ≥15% RS, as well as <1% blasts in peripheral blood & <5% blasts in bone marrow
Persistent thrombocytosis, with platelet count ≥450 ×10⁹/L
SF3B1 mutation, or in the absence of *SF3B1* mutation, no recent history of cytotoxic or growth factor therapy that would explain the morphologic findings
No genetic findings diagnostic for another myeloid neoplasm, including *BCR-ABL1*, *PCM1-JAK2*, inv(3), or rearrangement of *PDGRFA*, *PDGFRB*, or *FGFR1*
No history of other myeloid neoplasm, other than MDS-RS
MDS, myelodysplastic syndrome; MPN, myeloproliferative neoplasm; MDS/MPN-RS-T, MDS/MPN with ring sideroblasts & thrombocytosis; RS, ring sideroblasts

Discussion Myelodysplastic syndrome (MDS)/myeloproliferative neoplasm (MPN) with ring sideroblasts and thrombocytosis (MDS/MPN-RS-T) was formerly known as refractory anemia with ring sideroblasts and thrombocytosis (RARS-T), a provisional entity in the 2001 and 2008 versions of the World Health Organization (WHO) classification of hematologic neoplasms. More recent studies have shown MDS/MPN-RS-T to be a distinct neoplasm with characteristic morphologic and genetic findings and clinical behavior, and it is now formally included in the 2017 WHO classification as a distinct entity. MDS/MPN-RS-T is characterized clinically by thrombocytosis with anemia in older patients, with occasional splenomegaly; WHO 2017 diagnostic criteria for MDS/MPN-RS-T are listed in **t15.1**. In the bone marrow, cases of MDS/MPN-RS-T demonstrate dyserythropoiesis, including ring sideroblasts, as well as atypical megakaryocytes that are morphologically similar to those seen in non-*BCR-ABL1* MPNs, ie, enlarged and clustered megakaryocytes with hyperlobated, bulbous ("cloudlike"), or hyperchromatic nuclei.

Over 80% of MDS/MPN-RS-T patients have similar *SF3B1* mutations as seen in MDS with ring sideroblasts (**Case 10**), with *SF3B1* K700E being the most common. The SF3B1 protein is part of the mRNA spliceosome complex, and pathogenic mutations in *SF3B1* cause abnormal mRNA splicing due to misrecognition of 3' splice sites, resulting in increased mRNA decay. The role of mutated SF3B1 in the pathogenesis of ring sideroblasts is not completely understood. Interestingly, approximately 50%-60% of MDS/MPN-RS-T cases also harbor concurrent *JAK2* V617F mutations, while rare cases have concurrent mutations in *CALR* or *MPL*. Thus, this disorder represents a true hybrid myelodysplastic/myeloproliferative neoplasm in pathophysiology. In fact, rare cases of *SF3B1*-mutated MDS-RS have been shown to evolve to MDS/MPN-RS-T with the acquisition of *JAK2* V617F mutation. About 90% of MDS/MPN-RS-T cases have a normal karyotype, and the majority of cases will also have other myeloid-associated gene mutations, such as the *DNMT3A* mutation in this case.

MDS/MPN-RS-T is a low-grade myeloid neoplasm, with patients having a median overall survival of 6-10 years; factors that have a negative impact on survival include the absence of either *JAK2* or *SF3B1* mutation, advanced age, and an abnormal karyotype. Patients with MDS/MPN-RS-T have a prognosis that is more favorable than patients with MDS-RS but less favorable than patients with essential thrombocytosis (ET). Therefore, accurate diagnosis of this rarer entity is necessary for correct prognostication. There is no specific treatment for this disorder and therapies used in either MDS or MPN may be beneficial.

ISBN 978-089189-6814   ©2021 ASCP

Diagnostic pearls/pitfalls

– If the iron stain is not adequate or ring sideroblasts are not readily identified, a misdiagnosis of ET or primary myelofibrosis (PMF) may be made, especially because fibrosis occasionally occurs in MDS/MPN-RS-T, as seen in this case. The presence of dyserythropoiesis would not be typical for ET or PMF at presentation, although dysplastic changes may be seen in late-stage PMF. The distinction from ET or PMF is necessary because overall survival is shorter for patients with MRD/MPN-RS-T vs those with ET, but longer than those with PMF.

– MDS/MPN-RS-T may be misdiagnosed as myelodysplastic syndrome with ring sideroblasts (MDS-RS; see **Case 10**), given the presence of ring sideroblasts and *SF3B1* mutation. However, the megakaryocyte morphology in MDS/MPN-RS-T resembles that seen in non-chronic myeloid leukemia MPNs and does not resemble the small, hypolobated forms typically present in pure MDS. The *JAK2* V617F mutation may occur very rarely in MDS but the presence of both *SF3B1* mutation and mutation in *JAK2*, *CALR*, or *MPL* would not be consistent with a diagnosis of MDS-RS. In addition, patients with MDS/MPN-RS-T generally have higher white blood cell counts than patients with MDS-RS.

– *SF3B1* mutations are not specific to myeloid neoplasms with RS and occur in other hematopoietic neoplasms, such as chronic lymphocytic leukemia, and can be found in older individuals without hematologic disease as part of age-related clonal hematopoiesis of indeterminate potential (see **Case 17**). The presence of an *SF3B1* mutation must always be interpreted together with the morphologic and clinical findings.

Readings

Broséus J, Alpermann T, Wulfert M, et al. Age, *JAK2*(V617F) and *SF3B1* mutations are the main predicting factors for survival in refractory anaemia with ring sideroblasts and marked thrombocytosis. Leukemia. 2013;27(9):1826-31. **DOI: 10.1038/leu.2013.120**

Broséus J, Florensa L, Zipperer E, et al. Clinical features and course of refractory anemia with ring sideroblasts associated with marked thrombocytosis. Haematologica. 2012;97(7):1036-41. **DOI: 10.3324/haematol.2011.053918**

Malcovati L, Della Porta MG, Pietra D, et al. Molecular and clinical features of refractory anemia with ringed sideroblasts associated with marked thrombocytosis. Blood. 2009;114(17):3538-45. **DOI: 10.1182/blood-2009-05-222331**

Malcovati L, Papaemmanuil E, Bowen DT, et al. Clinical significance of *SF3B1* mutations in myelodysplastic syndromes and myelodysplastic/myeloproliferative neoplasms. Blood. 2011;118(24):6239-46. **DOI: 10.1182/blood-2011-09-377275**

Patnaik MM, Lasho TL, Finke CM, et al. Predictors of survival in refractory anemia with ring sideroblasts and thrombocytosis (RARS-T) and the role of next-generation sequencing. Am J Hematol. 2016;91(5):492-98. **DOI: 10.1002/ajh.24332**

Swerdlow SH, Campo E, Harris NL, et al. World Health Organization Classification of Tumours of Haematopoietic and Lymphoid Tissues. 4th ed. Lyon, France: IARC Press; 2017. **ISBN: 978-9283224310**

Sarah L Ondrejka & Erika M Moore

16 Myeloid neoplasm with eosinophilia & *FIP1L1-PDGFRA*

History A 47-year-old male presented to an oncologist for evaluation of persistent leukocytosis. He was noted to also have both elevated erythrocyte sedimentation rate and C-reactive protein. CBC results are shown at right.

A bone marrow biopsy was performed with peripheral blood smear review.

Morphology & flow cytometry There were 4% eosinophils, resulting in a slight absolute eosinophilia (1.44×10^9/L), and some of the eosinophils showed atypical features **f16.1**.

The bone marrow aspirate smears and core biopsy were hypercellular (90%-100%) with slight granulocytic hyperplasia (myeloid:erythroid ratio 4:1) and relative eosinophilia (12% eosinophils in the aspirate differential) **f16.2**. Dysplasia was not evident.

WBC	10.7×10^9/L
Differential	
Neutrophils	41%
Metamyelocytes	22%
Myelocytes	20%
Blasts	1%
Eosinophils	4%
HGB	11.0 g/dL
HCT	33.2%
MCV	101 fL
RDW	26.2%
Platelets	171×10^9/L

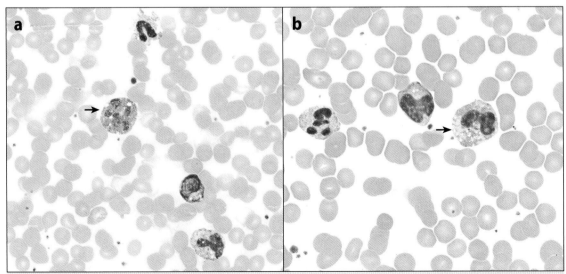

f16.1 Eosinophils in the peripheral blood smear are occasionally abnormal, with **a** nuclear hypersegmentation (arrow) or **b** sparse granulation with clear areas of cytoplasm (arrow)

  ISBN 978-089189-6814 ©2021 ASCP

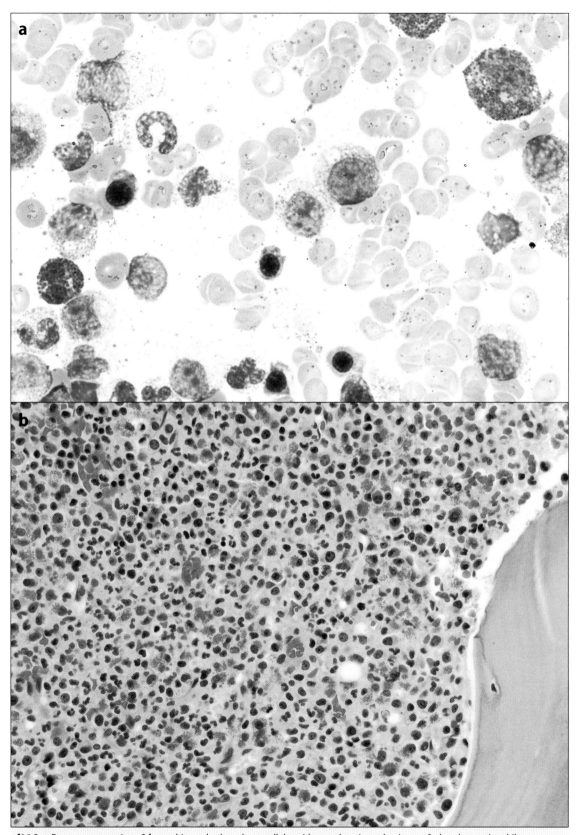

f16.2 a Bone marrow aspirate & **b** core biopsy; both are hypercellular with granulocytic predominance & abundant eosinophils

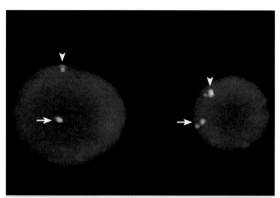

f16.3 Three-color FISH for detection of *FIP1L1-PDGFRA* (4q12) fusion. An intact, normal pattern is indicated by a green probe for *FIP1L1* fused to an orange probe for *CHIC2* and fused to an aqua probe for *PDGFRA* (denoted by the white arrows); deletion of the orange probe with resultant fusion of green & aqua indicates *CHIC2* deletion (denoted by the white arrowheads), which occurs in the presence of *FIP1L1-PDGFRA*

Flow cytometry did not reveal a specific phenotypic abnormality.

Based on the peripheral blood and bone marrow morphologic findings, a myeloid stem cell disorder was favored over a reactive condition. The process was somewhat difficult to classify, and atypical chronic myeloid leukemia was noted to be in the differential diagnosis. Additional cytogenetic and molecular genetic testing was recommended.

Genetics/molecular results The karyotype was normal. A FISH panel for hypereosinophilia workup was negative for *PDGFRB* or *FGFR1* rearrangement. However, FISH analysis was positive for *CHIC2* deletion consistent with *PDGFRA-FIP1L1* rearrangement **f16.3**. Based on the supplemental genetic information, the diagnosis was revised to **myeloid neoplasm with *PDGFRA* rearrangement**.

Discussion Myeloid/lymphoid neoplasms with *PDGFRA* rearrangement arise from a pluripotent stem cell capable of differentiating to lymphoblastic neoplasms, myeloid neoplasms, and clonal eosinophilias. Rearranged *PDGFRA* produces a constitutively active tyrosine kinase receptor, platelet-derived growth factor receptor α (PDFGRA), as a result of disruption to its autoinhibitory domain. The most common rearrangement is the *FIP1L1-PDGFRA* gene fusion, occurring as a result of a cytogenetically cryptic interstitial deletion of chromosome 4q12. This fusion gene was initially identified in patients with idiopathic hypereosinophilic syndrome by Cools and colleagues, who demonstrated sensitivity to imatinib in patients having this fusion. Other genetic variants have been described including

several cases with *BCR-PDGFRA*, which may have disease characteristics overlapping chronic eosinophilic leukemia (CEL) and chronic myeloid leukemia with or without eosinophilia. Other rare fusion partners include *ETV6*, *KIF5B*, *STRN*, *TNKS2*, and *CDK5RAP2*. Very rarely, the disease can also result from an activating point mutation in *PDGFRA*.

Hematologic neoplasms with *FIP1L1-PDGFRA* occur more commonly in men, with a peak incidence during the fourth decade. Patients may present with nonspecific symptoms including fatigue and pruritis. Splenomegaly is common. The peripheral blood typically shows cytopenias (anemia, thrombocytopenia) and neutrophilia with coexisting eosinophilia (eosinophil count generally $1.4\text{-}17.2 \times 10^9/\text{L}$). Characteristic elevations in vitamin B_{12} and serum tryptase are frequent. The bone marrow is usually hypercellular and often mast cell proliferation is observed in cases presenting as CEL. In addition to CEL, which is the most common disease presentation, other phenotypes include T-lymphoblastic leukemia/lymphoma and acute myeloid leukemia. Damage to any number of organs from cytokine release and the release of eosinophil granules may occur, with cardiac tissue damage being a particularly ominous feature.

The 800-kb interstitial deletion that leads to *FIP1L1-PDGFRA* is typically not seen on standard karyotyping (ie, it is "cryptic"), but is detectable with FISH analysis for deletion of *CHIC2*, which lies in between *FIPIL1* and *PDGFRA* at 4q12 **f16.3**. This genetic aberration can also be detected with comparative genomic hybridization or single-nucleotide polymorphism arrays (**Appendix A**), or nested reverse transcriptase polymerase chain reaction.

It is important to identify these cases because patients often respond very well to imatinib therapy, with only rare instances of resistance mutations, as opposed to the generally poor prognosis of most myelodysplastic/myeloproliferative overlap neoplasms or myeloproliferative neoplasm, not otherwise specified. Notably in this case, the eosinophilia was not a particularly prominent feature in the peripheral blood and yet was critical in leading to the diagnosis with appropriate FISH testing.

Myeloid/lymphoid neoplasms with *PDGFRA* rearrangement belong to a group of rare hematologic neoplasms generally presenting with eosinophilia, in which a specific cytogenetic abnormality results

t16.1 World Health Organization 2017 diagnostic criteria for myeloid/lymphoid neoplasms with eosinophilia associated with *FIP1L1-PDGFRA* or a variant fusion gene

A myeloid or lymphoid neoplasm, usually with prominent eosinophilia

and

The presence of *FIP1L1-PDGFRA* fusion gene or a variant fusion gene with rearrangement of *PDGFRA* or an activating mutation of *PDGFRA*

t16.2 Comparison of myeloid/lymphoid neoplasms with eosinophilia & specific gene rearrangements*

Genetic abnormality	Common fusion(s)	Method of detection	Typical disease presentation	Response to kinase inhibitor
PDGFRA rearrangement[†]	*FIP1L1-PDGFRA* from cryptic del(4q12)	FISH (typically probe for *CHIC2* deletion)	CEL (often with proliferation of mast cells); rarely AML, T-ALL	imatinib
PDGFRB	*ETV6-PDGFRB* t(5;12)(q32;p13.2)	FISH (*PDGFRB* breakapart) and/or karyotype	CMML; rarely aCML, CEL	imatinib or similar
FGFR1	Various involving *FGFR1* at 8p11	FISH (*FGFR1* breakapart) and/or karyotype	MPN, MDS/MPN, AML, T- or B-ALL	none consistent
PCM1-JAK2[‡]	*PCM1-JAK2* t(8;9) (p22;p24.1)	FISH (*JAK2* breakapart, not specific to this disorder) and/or karyotype	MPN, MDS/MPN, rarely AML, T- or B-ALL	ruxolitinib

aCML, atypical chronic myeloid leukemia; AML, acute myeloid leukemia; B-ALL, B-lymphoblastic leukemia/lymphoma; CEL, chronic eosinophilic leukemia; CMML, chronic myelomonocytic leukemia; MDS, myelodysplastic syndrome; MPN, myeloproliferative neoplasm; T-ALL, T-lymphoblastic leukemia/lymphoma
*Each entity in this group is characterized by a specific cytogenetic abnormality resulting in expression of an abnormal tyrosine kinase
[†]Rare cases result from an activating mutation of PDGFRA
[‡]Provisional entity in the 2017 WHO classification of hematopoietic neoplasms

in expression of an abnormal tyrosine kinase. **t16.1** lists 2017 World Health Organization criteria for the myeloid/lymphoid neoplasms associated with eosinophilia and specific gene fusions. **t16.2** shows a comparison of these rare disorders.

Diagnostic pearls/pitfalls

- Cytogenetic analysis alone is insufficient for the evaluation of eosinophilia with suspected *FIP1L1-PDGFRA* rearrangement, which is not seen on standard karyotyping but is detectable with FISH. A typical FISH test uses a 3-color approach to demonstrate deletion of the *CHIC2* region at 4q12.
- Mast cell proliferation is a feature of *FIP1L1-PDGFRA*-associated MPN and can lead to an erroneous diagnosis of systemic mastocytosis. Mast cells in the bone marrow may be in loose, noncohesive clusters and may be atypical and spindled. The absence of a *KIT* mutation and appropriate FISH testing can resolve the diagnosis.
- Some cases with *FIP1L1-PDGFRA* may show elevated eosinophil counts above the reference range but below the defined threshold for idiopathic hypereosinophilic syndrome ($>1.5 \times 10^9$/L)
- The clinical presentation of myeloid/lymphoid neoplasm with *FIP1L1-PDGFRA* is varied and

may include a myeloproliferative neoplasm, acute myeloid leukemia, or lymphoblastic leukemia/ lymphoma, so a high degree of suspicion is necessary to diagnose these cases.

Readings

Cools J, DeAngelo DJ, Gotlib J, et al. A tyrosine kinase created by fusion of the *PDGFRA* and *FIP1L1* genes as a therapeutic target of imatinib in idiopathic hypereosinophilic syndrome. N Engl J Med 2003;348(13):1201-14. **DOI: 10.1056/NEJMoa025217**

Gotlib J. World Health Organization-defined eosinophilic disorders: 2017 update on diagnosis, risk stratification, and management. Am J Hematol. 2017;92:1243-59. **DOI: 10.1002/ajh.24196**

Pardanani A, Brockman SR, Paternoster SF, et al. *FIP1L1-PDGFRA* fusion: prevalence and clinicopathologic correlates in 89 consecutive patients with moderate to severe eosinophilia. Blood 2004;104:3038-45. **DOI: 10.1182/blood-2004-03-0787**

Reiter A, Gotlib J. Myeloid neoplasms with eosinophilia. Blood. 2017;129:704-14. **DOI: 10.1182/blood-2016-10-695973**

Swerdlow SH, Campo E, Harris NL, et al. World Health Organization Classification of Tumours of Haematopoietic and Lymphoid Tissues. 4th ed. Lyon, France: IARC Press; 2017. **ISBN: 978-9283224310**

Vandenberghe P, Wlodarska I, Michaux L, et al. Clinical and molecular features of *FIP1L1-PDFGRA* (+) chronic eosinophilic leukemias. Leukemia. 2004;18(4):734-42. **DOI: 10.1038/sj.leu.2403313**

Vega F, Medeiros LJ, Bueso-Ramos CE, Arboleda P, Miranda RN. Hematolymphoid neoplasms associated with rearrangements of *PDGFRA, PDGFRB*, and *FGFR1*. Am J Clin Pathol. 2015;144:377-92. **DOI: 10.1309/AJCPMORR5Z2IKCEM**

Rose C Beck

17

Secondary polycythemia with *JAK2* V617F clonal hematopoiesis of indeterminate potential

History A 64-year-old male with a past medical history of obesity, hypertension, diabetes mellitus, and hyperlipidemia was referred to an oncologist for evaluation of polycythemia, with hemoglobin concentrations ranging from 15-17 g/dL over the last 2 years. A new CBC was obtained and results are shown at right.

WBC	8.2×10^9/L
RBC	5.86×10^{12}/L
HGB	17.9 g/dL
HCT	54.0%
MCV	92 fL
RDW	14.1%
Platelets	255×10^9/L

The patient admitted to having mild fatigue, although physically he felt well overall; the oncologist also noted a prior diagnosis of obstructive sleep apnea found on sleep study. A serum erythropoietin (EPO) level was 13.0 mIU/mL (normal 2.6-18.5 mIU/mL). Result of a qualitative PCR assay for *JAK2* V617F performed on the blood was positive. A bone marrow biopsy with genetic studies was then ordered for a suspected myeloproliferative neoplasm, presumed polycythemia vera, and the patient was given a prescription for hydroxyurea therapy.

Morphology & flow cytometry The peripheral blood smear showed no morphologic abnormalities. The bone marrow aspirate smears were aspicular and hemodilute, but the touch prep showed normal erythropoiesis and granulopoiesis **f17.1**, with a slightly decreased myeloid:erythroid ratio of 1:1; megakaryocytes were not seen on the touch prep. The bone marrow core biopsy was normocellular for age (30%-40%) with adequate megakaryocytes that lacked atypia **f17.2**. Flow cytometry revealed no definite abnormalities.

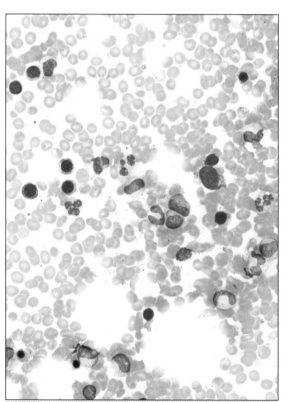

f17.1 Bone marrow touch prep showing normal erythropoiesis & granulopoiesis

17 *Secondary polycythemia with JAK2 V617F clonal hematopoiesis of indeterminate potential*

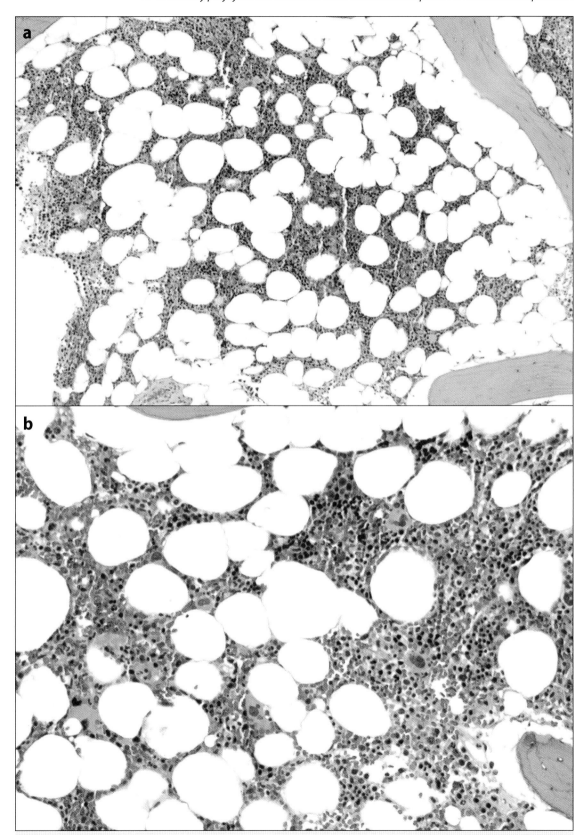

f17.2 a, b Sections of the core biopsy show normocellular bone marrow with scattered normal-appearing megakaryocytes

Genetics/molecular results Chromosome analysis showed a normal male karyotype; FISH was not performed. A targeted myeloid NGS panel was positive for a *JAK2* p.V617F (c.1849G>T) mutation with 3% variant allele frequency (VAF) (see **Case 2** for an illustration of this mutation).

Because no significant morphologic or chromosomal abnormalities were found, a diagnosis of myeloproliferative neoplasm was not rendered, and the low-level *JAK2* V617F mutation was considered to be consistent with **clonal hematopoiesis of indeterminate potential**.

Discussion Throughout life, humans continually acquire somatic mutations and/or clonal chromosomal abnormalities, including specific genetic abnormalities associated with neoplastic disorders. When these aberrations occur in the hematopoietic compartment in individuals without evidence of hematologic disease, this process is termed age-related clonal hematopoiesis or clonal hematopoiesis of indeterminate potential (CHIP). The prevalence of CHIP increases to ~10% of individuals by age 70, and the presence of CHIP carries increased risk for the development of a hematologic neoplasm as well as cardiovascular disease.

Although chromosomal abnormalities such as trisomy 8 and del(20q) may be evidence of CHIP, somatic mutations are more commonly identified, with the most frequent mutations occurring in 3 genes related to epigenetic regulation: *DNMT3A*, *TET2*, and *ASXL1*. Mutations in any of these three genes are found in approximately 60%-70% of individuals with CHIP. It is important to note, however, that mutations usually associated with overt neoplasia also occur in CHIP, including mutations in *JAK2*, *SF3B1*, *SRSF2*, and *TP53*, among other cancer-associated genes. The types of mutations in these genes occurring in CHIP are the same as those found in hematologic neoplasms, such as the *JAK2* V617F observed in this case, leading to the hypothesis that CHIP mutations represent precursor lesions to hematologic malignancy (see **Case 7** for further discussion of CHIP and clonal hematopoiesis found in the setting of cytopenias). The overall rate of conversion to overt hematologic neoplasia in individuals with CHIP is approximately 1% per year. Several studies indicate individuals with CHIP having *JAK2* V617F are predisposed to developing myeloproliferative neoplasms.

The *JAK2* V617F mutation is present in >95% of polycythemia vera (PV) cases as well as ~50%-60% of cases of essential thrombocytosis and primary myelofibrosis. The presence of this mutation by itself is not sufficient to diagnose one of these neoplasms, each of which is defined by specific World Health Organization (WHO) criteria. Although this patient had elevated hemoglobin and hematocrit values, the serum EPO level, which should be low in PV, was normal, and the bone marrow did not demonstrate hypercellularity or atypical, clustered megakaryocytes. Therefore, the patient did not meet WHO diagnostic criteria for PV (see **Case 2**). In addition, the low VAF of 3% was not highly suggestive of overt neoplasia, although it should be noted that WHO criteria do not specify a cut-off for allelic burden and histologically-evident PV has been found in some patients with very low levels of *JAK2* V617F (2% or less). While most single-gene *JAK2* assays are qualitative and only indicate the presence of mutation, not its frequency, NGS methods are able to quantitate the relative level of the mutation using the VAF, which is the percentage of variant sequences (or "reads") out of the total read number. VAF is an approximation, not a direct measurement, of the level of mutation in a given sample and is impacted not only by the starting number of mutated copies but also by variances in primer binding and other assay characteristics unique to any given targeted region. In the setting of overt neoplasia, the VAF of *JA2K* V617F varies considerably and may reach 100% in cases with loss of heterozygosity.

Due to the lack of histologic evidence for PV, the plan for hydroxyurea for this patient was discontinued and it was felt that sleep apnea likely contributed to his erythrocytosis. One year after the marrow biopsy, a new CBC showed a hemoglobin level of 17.6 g/dL and a hematocrit of 52.7%, with the *JAK2* V617 mutation present in blood at 4% VAF, as measured by an NGS assay. He continues to be closely followed by his oncologist.

Diagnostic pearls/pitfalls
– The presence of pathologic mutations in blood or bone marrow, even with abnormalities found on CBC, is not enough to diagnose a hematologic malignancy in many cases. The finding of a mutation must be considered in context with all clinical and pathologic studies.

ISBN 978-089189-6814 ©2021 ASCP

– The mutations found in individuals with CHIP are the same as those detected in hematologic malignancy but are generally of lower VAF (eg, ≤10%), whereas mutations found in the context of overt malignancy are typically higher.

– VAF is reported with NGS methods, but not qualitative PCR assays, which only indicate presence or absence of a mutation and may have a lower or higher sensitivity than NGS depending on the primers used.

Readings

Alvarez-Larrán A, Angona A, Ancochea A, et al. Masked polycythaemia vera: presenting features, response to treatment and clinical outcomes. Eur J Haematol. 2016 Jan;96(1):83-9. Epub 2015 Apr 17. **DOI: 10.1111/ejh.12552**

Genovese G, Kähler AK, Handsaker RE, et al. Clonal hematopoiesis and blood-cancer risk inferred from blood DNA sequence. N Engl J Med. 2014;371(26):2477-87. **DOI: 10.1056/NEJMoa1409405**

Jaiswal S, Fontanillas P, Flannick J, et al. Age-related clonal hematopoiesis associated with adverse outcomes. N Engl J Med. 2014;371(26):2488-98. **DOI: 10.1056/NEJMoa1408617**

Jaiswal S, Natarajan P, Silver AJ, et al. Clonal hematopoiesis and risk of atherosclerotic cardiovascular disease. N Engl J Med. 2017;377(2):111-21. **DOI: 10.1056/NEJMoa1701719**

McKerrell T, Park N, Chi J, et al. *JAK2* V617F hematopoietic clones are present several years prior to MPN diagnosis and follow different expansion kinetics. Blood Adv 2017;1(14): 968-971. **DOI: 10.1182/bloodadvances.2017007047**

McKerrell T, Park N, Moreno T, et al. Leukemia-associated somatic mutations drive distinct patterns of age-related clonal hemopoiesis. Cell Rep. 2015 Mar 3;10(8):1239-45. Epub 2015 Feb 26. **DOI: 10.1016/j.celrep.2015.02.005**

Nielsen C, Bojesen SE, Nordestgaard BG, et al. *JAK2* V617F somatic mutation in the general population: myeloproliferative neoplasm development and progression rate. Haematologica. 2014 Sep;99(9):1448-55. Epub 2014 Jun 6. **DOI: 10.3324/haematol.2014.107631**

Perricone M, Polverelli N, Martinelli G, et al. The relevance of a low *JAK2* V617F allele burden in clinical practice: a monocentric study. Oncotarget. 2017 Jun 6;8(23):37239-37249. **DOI: 10.18632/oncotarget.16744**

Shlush LI. Age-related clonal hematopoiesis. Blood. 2018;131(5):496-504. **DOI: 10.1182/blood-2017-07-746453**

Swerdlow SH, Campo E, Harris NL, et al. World Health Organization Classification of Tumours of Haematopoietic and Lymphoid Tissues. 4th ed. Lyon, France: IARC Press; 2017. **ISBN: 9789283244943**

Szybinski J, Meyer SC. Genetics of Myeloproliferative Neoplasms. Hematol Oncol Clin North Am. 2021 Apr;35(2):217-236. Epub 2021 Jan 29. **DOI: 10.1016/j.hoc.2020.12.002**

Vainchenker W, Kralovics R. Genetic basis and molecular pathophysiology of classical myeloproliferative neoplasms. Blood. 2017;129(6):667-79. **DOI: 10.1182/blood-2016-10-695940**

Howard Meyerson

18

Aplastic anemia with clonal hematopoiesis

History A 52-year-old man with a 20-year history of nonsevere aplastic anemia (AA) presented with progressive cytopenia of 6 months' duration. No constitutional cause for the aplasia was previously identified. CBC results are shown at right.

A bone marrow biopsy with genetic studies was performed.

Morphology & flow cytometry The bone marrow aspirate was markedly hypocellular, consisting predominantly of mature lymphocytes with few hematopoietic precursors. There was mild dyserythropoiesis, with occasional nucleated red cells (<10%) demonstrating nuclear irregularities **f18.1a**. Granulocytic maturation was normal and megakaryocytes were not observed on the aspirate. The trephine core biopsy was markedly hypocellular (5% cellularity) **f18.1b**. Bone marrow flow cytometry demonstrated no specific abnormality and no increase in myeloblasts. Peripheral blood flow cytometry for paroxysmal nocturnal hemoglobinuria (PNH) revealed a small PNH clone at 1% **f18.2**.

Genetics/molecular results Cytogenetics showed a normal 46,XY karyotype in 10/10 metaphases (low cell yield), and FISH studies were negative for deletion of 5/5q, 7/7q, 17p, and 20q and negative for trisomy 8. A myeloid NGS panel demonstrated an *ASXL1* p.D616Efs*17 (c.1848_1852delCATTA) mutation with variant allele frequency (VAF) of 19% and a *RUNX1* p.R174Q (c.521G>A) mutation with VAF of 11%. Based on the history, morphology, flow cytometry, and genetic/molecular findings, a diagnosis of **aplastic anemia with clonal hematopoiesis** was rendered.

WBC	2.2×10^9/L
RBC	3.06×10^{12}/L
HGB	10.9 g/dL
HCT	31.4%
MCV	103 fL
RDW	14.7%
Platelets	40×10^9/L
Absolute reticulocyte count	0.073×10^{12}/L

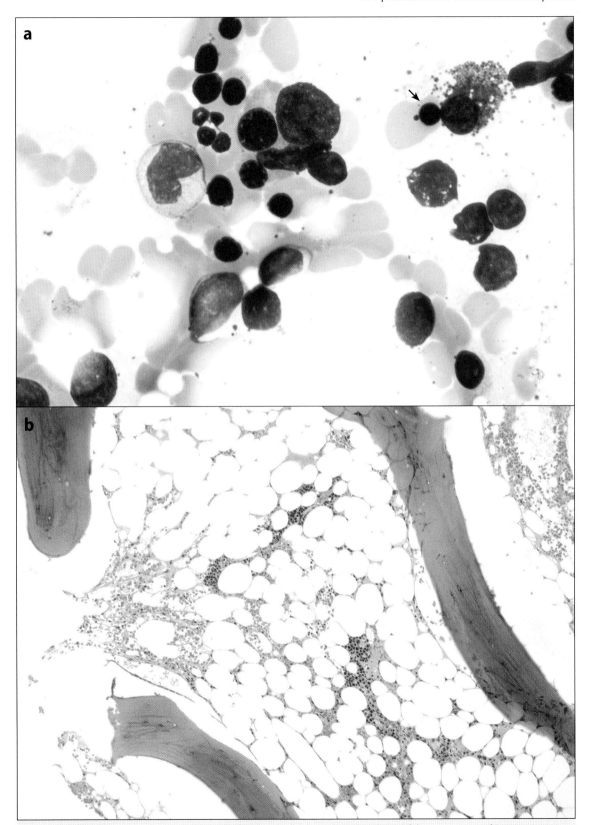

f18.1 a Bone marrow aspirate showing mild (<10% of erythroid cells) dyserythropoiesis (arrow); **b** bone marrow core biopsy demonstrating marked hypocellularity (~5% cellular)

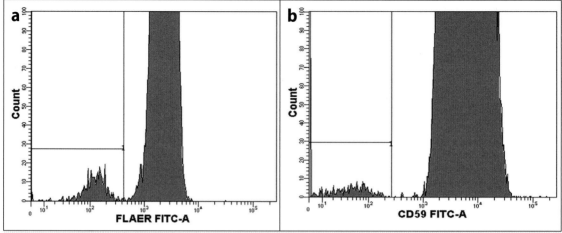

f18.1 **a** Flow cytometric analysis performed on blood demonstrates a small (1%) paroxysmal nocturnal hemoglobinuria clone detected by the absence of staining with **a** fluorescein-labeled aerolysin (FLAER) on granulocytes & **b** CD59 on red cells (denoted by events in the boxed region on the left for each plot). FLAER binds to glycosylphosphatidylinositol (GPI) residues and CD59 is a GPI-linked protein. The finding indicates the presence of a small GPI-deficient hematopoietic cell population because of a mutation in the *PIG-A* gene, a common clonal abnormality in acquired, immune-mediated aplastic anemia

Discussion The main differential diagnosis in this case is between aplastic anemia (AA) and hypoplastic myelodysplastic syndrome (MDS). Distinguishing between the two can be difficult, especially because AA can evolve into AML/MDS. Cytogenetic and molecular studies can be helpful but must be evaluated in the context of the clinical and morphologic findings. Although mutations were detected, the morphologic criteria for MDS were not present, with only mild dyserythropoiesis in <10% of erythroid cells. In addition, an MDS-defining karyotypic or FISH abnormality was not seen. Therefore, a diagnosis of hypoplastic MDS could not be rendered. It is not uncommon for mild dyserythropoiesis to be present in AA, manifesting primarily as nuclear irregularities. However, the number of dysplastic erythroid cells does not meet the 10% threshold required for diagnosing MDS. This case could also be considered a clonal cytopenia of uncertain significance (CCUS; see **Case 7**); however, the patient had a 20-year, well-documented history of AA. The overall findings therefore fit best with a diagnosis of AA with clonal hematopoiesis.

AA may be the result of inherited bone marrow failure (IBMF) syndrome or secondary to drug or toxin exposure or an idiopathic, immune-mediated process. IBMF syndromes have multiple underlying genetic causes and are summarized in **t18.1**. Most of these disorders are associated with increased risk for MDS/AML, frequently associated with monosomy 7. Screening NGS panels for most or all of the known mutations associated with IBMF are available at reference laboratories and should be considered in a young patient presenting with bone marrow aplasia.

Genetic alterations occur in ~50% of patients with acquired, immune-mediated AA, with structural cytogenetic abnormalities occurring in approximately 10%-25%. The most common cytogenetic findings include −7/del(7q) and trisomy 8, with less common alterations being del(13q), trisomy 6, trisomy 15, and trisomy 21. Monosomy 7/del(7q) is deleterious, exhibiting a low response rate to immunosuppression and greater risk for progression to MDS. Trisomy 8 and deletion 13q are associated with more favorable prognosis. In rare cases, cytogenetic abnormalities may be lost with marrow response to immunotherapy.

The selective pressure of the immune attack on marrow stem cells leads to mechanisms of molecular escape in acquired AA. In particular, loss of HLA class I alleles via uniparental disomy of 6p (6pUPD) occurs in ~10% of cases (note that the 6pUPD assay is generally not performed by clinical laboratories), and loss of glycosylphosphatidylinositol (GPI)-anchored proteins, resulting from somatic mutations in the *PIG-A* gene, are seen in ~12%-40% of cases. The latter results in

t18.1 Inherited bone marrow failure syndromes

Disorder	Mutated gene(s)	Inheritance	Frequency	Mechanism	Clinical features	AML/MDS
Congenital amegakaryocytic thrombocytopenia	*MPL*	AR	>95%	growth factor receptor	thrombocytopenia with decreased or absent megakaryocytes	rare
Diamond-Blackfan anemia	*RPL5,11, 15, 23, 26, 27, 31, 35a, 36*	AD	10%	ribosome assembly & function	macrocytic anemia, marrow red cell aplasia; increased RBC adenosine deaminase; short stature, webbed neck, thumb abnormalities; Klippel-Feil anomaly; heart & genitourinary defects; cleft lip	<2%
	RPS7, 10, 15, 17, 19, 24, 26, 27, 27A, 28, 29	AD	40% (25% RPS19)			
	GATA1	X-linked	rare			
Dyskeratosis congenita	*CTC1, NHP2, NOP10, WRAP53*	AR	<1%	telomere maintenance	short telomeres, reticular skin pigmentation, nail abnormalities, oral leukoplakia; pulmonary fibrosis; stenosis of esophagus, urethra, lacrimal ducts; liver disease, premature gray hair, avascular necrosis	200-2,000 fold risk
	TERC,TINF2	AD	15-25%			
	ACD, PARN, RTEL1, TERT	AR,AD	10-15%			
	DKC	X-linked	~30%			
Fanconi anemia	*FANCA,C,D1/ BRAC2, D2, E, F, G, I, J, L, N, O, P, Q, S, T, U, V*	AR	98% (60% *FANCA*)	DNA repair	radius, thumb abnormalities, short stature, microcephaly, café au lait spots, renal, cardiac anomalies; increased chromosome breaks with clastogenic agents	>500 fold risk
	FANCR/RAD51	AD	<1%			
	FANCB	X-linked	2%			
GATA2 deficiency	*GATA2*	AD	>95%	transcription factor necessary for hematopoeitic cell survival	monocytopenia & mycobacterial infection (MonoMAC); warts; dendritic, monocyte, B & NK lymphoid deficiency; lymphedema, deafness, pulmonary alveolar proteinosis	~9% childhood MDS, ~40% with monosomy 7
Schwachman-Diamond syndrome	*SBDS*	AR	95%	ribosome assembly & function	neutropenia, exocrine pancreatic insufficiency, failure to thrive, short stature, developmental delay; low serum trypsinogen, isoamylase	~10% at 20 years
Thrombocytopenia absent radii	1q21 deletion with *RMB8A* deletion	AR	>90%	mRNA maturation	thrombocytopenia, bilateral radial hypoplasia, preservation of thumbs, skeletal abnormalities, congenital heart disease	rare
Severe congenital neutropenia	*ELANE, TCIRG1*	AD	30-60% (ELANE)	multiple mechanisms affecting granulocyte maturation	severe neutropenia early in life, granulocyte maturation arrest in bone marrow	~20% at 10 years
	HAX1, G6PC3, GFI1, JAGN1, CSF3R	AR	2-35% (G6PC3)			
	WAS	X-linked	<1%			

AD, autosomal dominant; AML, acute myeloid leukemia; AR, autosomal recessive; MDS, myelodysplastic syndrome
Adapted from [Wegman-Ostrosky 2017]

t18.2 Clonal hematopoiesis in hematopoietic stem cell disorders

	Aplastic anemia	MDS	Age-related CHIP
mutation frequency	~50%	~90%	increases with age (~10% by age 70 years)
mutations, age <40 y	20-40%	~90%	<1%
mutations, age >70 y	~50%	~90%	>10%
commonly mutated genes	*BCOR/BCORL1, PIGA, DNMT3A, ASXL1*	*TET2, SF3B1, ASXL1, SRSF2, DNMT3A, RUNX1, TP53*	*DNMT3A, TET2, ASXL1, JAK2, TP53, SF3B1*
typical VAF of mutated genes	<10%	20%-50%	<10%
cytogenetics	−7/del(7q), +8, +6, +15, del(13q)	−5/del(5q), −7/del(7q), +8, del(20q), del(17p)	del(20q), del(13q), del(11q), del(17p), +8, +12

CHIP, clonal hematopoiesis of indeterminate potential; MDS, myelodysplastic syndrome; VAF, variant allele frequency
Adapted in part from [Ogawa 2016]

the frequent occurrence of low-level PNH clones in acquired AA **f18.2**. The detection of a PNH clone in AA, as seen in this case, is indirect evidence of an immune-mediated process affecting the marrow stem cell. Therefore, PNH testing is useful in the evaluation of a patient suspected of having marrow aplasia.

Myeloid-associated somatic mutations occur in ~20% of individuals with AA. These mutations are most frequently seen in *BCOR/BCORL1*, *DNMT3A*, and *ASXL1*, while other AML/MDS-associated mutations such as *RUNX1* mutation, occur at lower frequency. In fact, compared to mutation patterns in AML/MDS, *BCOR/BCORL1* mutations are overrepresented and mutations in *TET2*, *TP53*, *RUNX1*, and splicing factors are underrepresented **t18.2**. Myeloid-associated mutations are more common in older AA patients and in those having long-standing disease, both features in this case. In contrast to AML/MDS, the VAFs of mutated genes in AA are generally low. Mutations in *DNMT3A*, *ASXL1*, *TP53*, and *RUNX1* are unfavorable and associated with faster progression to MDS/AML, shorter overall survival, and poor response to immune suppressive therapy, as compared to the favorable *PIG-A* and *BCOR/BCORL1* mutations in AA patients.

The patient in this case was given a trial of immunosuppressive therapy without improvement. Due to the presence of high-risk mutations and lack of response to therapy, he underwent allogeneic stem cell transplantation.

Diagnostic pearls/pitfalls
– IBMF syndromes have a high propensity to evolve into AML/MDS. Genetic/molecular evaluation should be performed for any younger patient with marrow aplasia to exclude an IBMF syndrome.
– Distinguishing hypoplastic both MDS from AA is difficult and requires integrating clinical, morphologic, and genetic data. A diagnosis of MDS requires morphologic dysplasia in at least 10% of cells of a hematopoietic lineage.
– Similar cytogenetic abnormalities and somatic mutations can occur in both MDS and in idiopathic (immune-mediated) AA.
– The presence of −7/del(7q) is highly suggestive of either MDS or AA evolving into MDS.
– In the setting of bone marrow failure (BMF), the presence of a small PNH clone is evidence of immune-mediated AA rather than other causes of BMF, although small PNH clones can also occur in MDS.

– In a patient with AA, mutations in *BCOR/BCORL1* or a PNH clone portend a favorable course whereas mutations in *ASXL1*, *DMT3A*, *TP53*, and *RUNX1* are unfavorable.

Readings

Babushok DV. A brief, but comprehensive, guide to clonal evolution in aplastic anemia. Hematology Am Soc Hematol Educ Program. 2018 Nov 30;2018(1):457-466. **DOI: 10.1182/asheducation-2018.1.457**

Boddu PC, Kadia TM. Molecular pathogenesis of acquired aplastic anemia. Eur J Haematol. 2019 Feb;102(2):103-110. **DOI: 10.1111/ejh.13182.**

Foglesong JS, Bannon SA, DiNardo CD. Inherited bone marrow failure syndromes, focus on the hematological manifestations: a review. Eur Med J. 2017;2(3):105-12. **https://www.emjreviews.com/hematology/article/inherited-bone-failure-syndromes-focus-on-the-haematological-manifestations-a-review/**

Gálvez E, Vallespín E, Arias-Salgado EG, et al. Next-generation sequencing in bone marrow failure syndromes and isolated cytopenias: experience of the spanish network on bone marrow failure syndromes. Hemasphere. 2021 Mar 9;5(4):e539. **DOI: 10.1097/HS9.0000000000000539**

Imi T, Katagiri T, Hosomichi K, et al. Sustained clonal hematopoiesis by HLA-lacking hematopoietic stem cells without driver mutations in aplastic anemia. Blood Adv. 2018 May 8;2(9):1000-1012. **DOI: 10.1182/bloodadvances.2017013953**

Maciejewski JP, Risitano A, Sloand EM, et al. Distinct clinical outcomes for cytogenetic abnormalities evolving from aplastic anemia. Blood. 2002;99(9):3129-35. **DOI: 10.1182/blood.v99.9.3129**

Mufti GJ, Marsh JCW. Somatic Mutations in Aplastic Anemia. Hematol Oncol Clin North Am. 2018 Aug;32(4):595-607. **DOI: 10.1016/j.hoc.2018.03.002**

Ogawa S. Clonal hematopoiesis in acquired aplastic anemia. Blood. 2016;128(3):337-47. **DOI: 10.1182/blood-2016-01-636381**

Shallis RM, Ahmad R, Zeidan AM. Aplastic anemia: Etiology, molecular pathogenesis, and emerging concepts. Eur J Haematol. 2018 Dec;101(6):711-720. **DOI: 10.1111/ejh.13153**

Skibenes ST, Clausen I, Raaschou-Jensen K. Next-generation sequencing in hypoplastic bone marrow failure: What difference does it make? Eur J Haematol. 2021 Jan;106(1):3-13. **DOI: 10.1111/ejh.13513**

Skokowa J, Dale DC, Touw IP, et al. Severe congenital neutropenias. Nat Rev Dis Primers. 2017;3:17032. **DOI: 10.1038/nrdp.2017.32**

Stanley N, Olson TS, Babushok DV. Recent advances in understanding clonal haematopoiesis in aplastic anaemia. Br J Haematol. 2017;177:509-25. **DOI: 10.1111/bjh.14510**

Sun L, Babushok DV. Secondary myelodysplastic syndrome and leukemia in acquired aplastic anemia and paroxysmal nocturnal hemoglobinuria. Blood. 2020 Jul 2;136(1):36-49. **DOI: 10.1182/blood.2019000940**

Yoshizato T, Dumitriu B, Hosokawa K, et al. Somatic mutations and clonal hematopoiesis in aplastic anemia. N Engl J Med. 2015;373(1):35-47. **DOI: 10.1056/NEJMoa1414799**

Wegman-Ostrosky T, Savage S. The genomics of inherited bone marrow failure: from mechanism to the clinic. Br J Haematol. 2017;177:526-42. **DOI: 10.1111/bjh.14535**

Priyatharsini Nirmalanantham, Rose C Beck & Kwadwo A Oduro

19

Acute myeloid leukemia with t(8;21)(q22;q22) *RUNX1-RUNX1T1* & *KIT* mutation

History A 56-year-old female with a past medical history of hypertension presented with oral pain after dental extraction, palpitations, and increased bruising in her legs. Selected CBC results are shown at right. A peripheral blood smear review with subsequent bone marrow biopsy was performed.

Morphology & flow cytometry The blood smear showed marked leukocytosis with granulocytic left shift and 59% blasts, which appeared variable in size and had occasional granulation including Auer rods **f19.1a**; some of the blasts as well as neutrophilic precursors displayed an atypical "hazy" pink cytoplasm **f19.1b**. The bone marrow aspirate smear and core biopsy showed many blasts with occasional coarse granules and rare Auer rods as well as occasional myelocytes with similar salmon-colored, "hazy" cytoplasm as seen in the blood **f19.2a, b**. Flow cytometry demonstrated 31% myeloblasts, which were positive for CD34, CD117, CD13, and HLA-DR, CD33 dim to negative, and partially positive for CD19 **f19.3**. Based on the morphologic and flow cytometry findings, a diagnosis of acute myeloid leukemia (AML) was rendered, with morphology consistent with AML with maturation (FAB M2) and suspicion for t(8;21) *RUNX1-RUN1T1* based on morphology.

Genetics/molecular results An AML FISH panel was positive for t(8;21) *RUNX1-RUNX1T1* **f19.4** and negative for inv(3), t(3;3), t(6;9), t(9;22), *KMT2A* (*MLL*) rearrangement, inv(16), and del(17p). Chromosome analysis revealed 46,XX,t(8;21) (q22;q22)[20]. Molecular analysis was negative for *FLT3-ITD* and *NPM1* mutations but was positive for a *KIT* p.N822Y (c.2464A>T) mutation, predicted to be gain of function **f19.5**. The genetic findings were consistent with a final diagnosis of **AML with t(8;21) (q22;q22.1)** *RUNX1-RUNX1T1*, **with** *KIT* **mutation**.

WBC	105.4×10^9/L
HGB	6.9 g/dL
Platelets	9×10^9/L

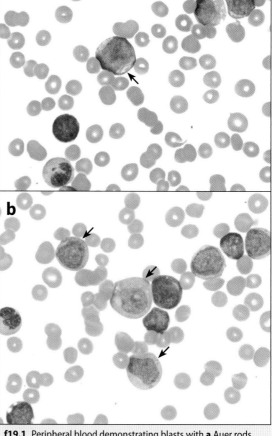

f19.1 Peripheral blood demonstrating blasts with **a** Auer rods (arrow) as well as blasts & **b** neutrophil precursors with hazy pink cytoplasm (arrows)

ISBN 978-089189-6814

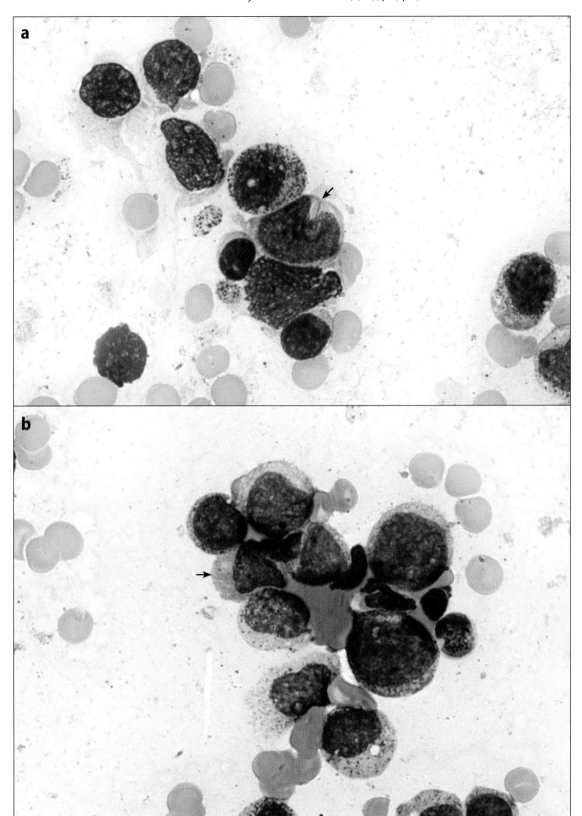

f19.2 The bone marrow aspirate also showed **a** rare blasts with Auer rods (arrow) & **b** myelocytes with hazy pink cytoplasm (arrow)

19 *Acute myeloid leukemia with t(8;21)(q22;q22) RUNX1-RUNX1T1 & KIT mutation*

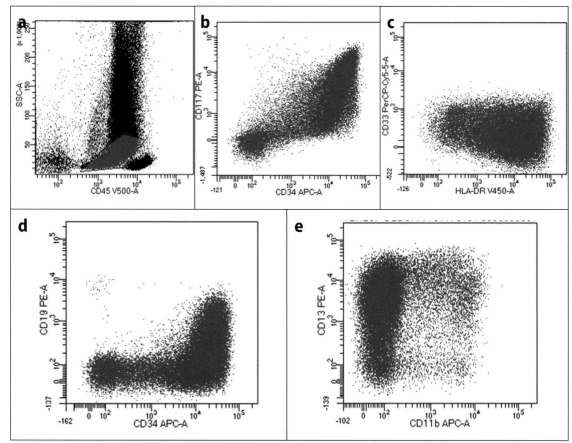

f19.3 Flow cytometry performed on the bone marrow demonstrates **a** CD45-dim blast population with slightly increased side scatter (highlighted in blue); the blasts are **b** positive for CD34 & CD117, **c** HLA-DR & CD33 (dim to negative), **d** CD19 (partial), & **e** CD13

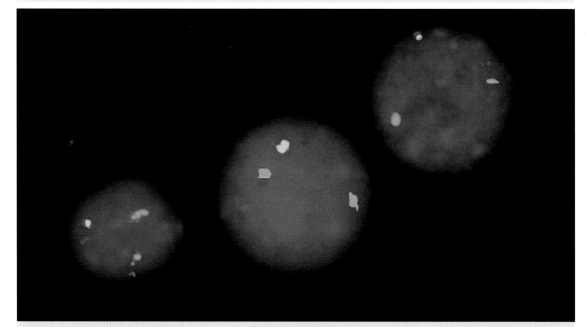

f19.4 Dual fusion FISH probes for *RUNX1* (21q22, green) & *RUNX1T1* (8q22, orange) showing 1 green, 1 orange, & 2 juxtaposing (sometimes yellow) signals, consistent with the presence of *RUNX1-RUNX1T1* translocation (note that in some cells, 1 of the reciprocal fusion events appears as slightly separated, smaller red & green signals)

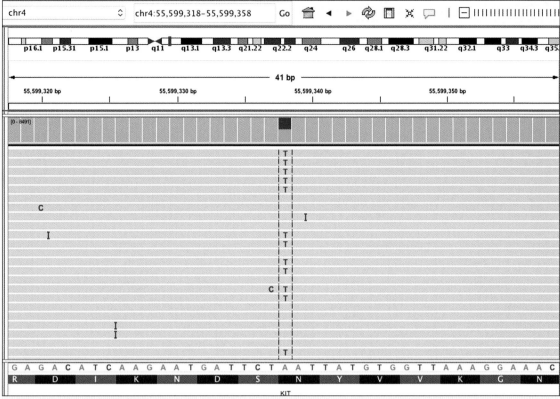

f19.5 Somatic variant analysis using a targeted myeloid NGS panel. Annotated reads mapped to the *KIT* locus demonstrate p.N822Y (c.2464A>T), highlighted in red (hg19, IGV browser) [see **fA.8**, p312]

Discussion AML with t(8;21) *RUNX1-RUNX1T1* accounts for 8% of adult AML and 12% of childhood AML cases and is classified within AML with recurrent genetic abnormalities by the World Health Organization. AML with t(8;21) is morphologically associated with the French-American-British (FAB) M2 ("with maturation") subtype, with maturation specifically along the neutrophil pathway and manifested by at least 10% of bone marrow cells composed of granulocytic precursors and mature neutrophils. The maturing granulocytic cells often show atypia with abnormal nuclear segmentation in neutrophils and a characteristically hazy, salmon-pink cytoplasm, especially prominent in myelocytes. The blasts in AML with t(8;21) are typically medium to large in size and may contain numerous azurophilic granules, and Auer rods are often present. Few blasts may show larger granules (pseudo-Chédiak-Higashi granules) indicative of abnormal granule fusion.

The blasts in AML with t(8;21) typically express CD34, CD117, HLA-DR, MPO, and CD13, with relatively dim expression of CD33. Aberrant expression of lymphocyte antigens by the blasts is often present. In particular,

the B-cell markers CD19 and/or PAX5 are frequently expressed, and some cases may express cytoplasmic CD79a. CD56 expression may also be seen and has been reported especially in cases of AML t(8;21) with mutated *KIT*.

AML with t(8;21), together with AML with inv(16)/t(16;16) *CFBB-MYH*, comprise the core binding factor (CBF) AML, so called because both have fusions involving the genes encoding subunits of CBF, a transcription factor having a critical role in granulocyte differentiation. The *CBF* gene fusions cause a block in transcription of genes related to stem cell differentiation, resulting in an excess of immature blasts. *RUNX1* encodes an α-CBF subunit (CBFA 2), and the translocation fuses *RUNX1* (formerly called *AML1*) on chromosome 21 with *RUNX1T1* (formerly *ETO*) on chromosome 8. The presence of either t(8;21) *RUNX1-RUNX1T1* or inv(16)/t(16;16) in a myeloid neoplasm is diagnostic of AML, regardless of the blast count in bone marrow or blood.

Overall, patients with t(8;21) AML have a favorable prognosis, with a high rate of complete remission and prolonged duration of complete remission, especially after consolidation chemotherapy with high-dose cytarabine. However, 30%-50% of patients with CBF AML experience relapse, with 5-year survival of ~50%. This discrepancy in prognosis is caused by additional chromosomal or molecular aberrations, such as *KIT* mutations. Adults with AML with t(8;21) who also have mutation of *KIT* in exon 17 have higher relapse rates, with shorter overall survival and event-free survival, than those without a mutation. The *KIT* proto-oncogene encodes for a class III transmembrane receptor tyrosine kinase (KIT receptor or CD117) which binds to stem cell factor, a cytokine essential for the development of bone marrow stem cells. Mutations in *KIT* occur with relatively high incidence in adult (12.8%-46.1%) and pediatric (19.0%-37.0%) patients having either of the 2 types of CBF AML. These mutations occur most frequently at D816 within exon 17, which encodes the activation loop in the kinase domain, and in exon 8, which encodes the extracellular portion of the receptor. The current recommendation is that all adult AML patients with t(8;21) or inv(16) be analyzed for *KIT* mutations in exon 17 for prognostication purposes, although more recent studies have demonstrated that the adverse prognostic impact of *KIT* mutation is more pronounced in AML with t(8;21).

KIT is mutated in various neoplasms, including systemic mastocytosis (see **Case 6**). A few studies have reported an association of AML t(8;21) in particular with concurrent systemic mastocytosis; the neoplastic mast cells become especially prominent after induction chemotherapy clears the AML blast population. These studies recommend assessing for neoplastic mast cell populations in all cases of t(8;21) AML with *KIT* mutation, because of poor outcomes observed in patients having both disorders. If atypical mast cells are detected in association with AML t(8;21), allogeneic hematopoietic stem cell transplantation should be considered early in treatment planning.

Myeloid sarcoma, an extramedullary tumor composed of leukemic blasts, has been reported in up to 15% of patients with t(8;21) AML and can involve almost any site, including the head and neck soft and subcutaneous tissue, orbits, lymph nodes, and skin. Myeloid sarcoma may be the first presentation of disease and precede bone marrow involvement by several months, or it can represent the first manifestation of a relapse.

In CBF AML, newer guidelines recommend monitoring of minimal residual disease (MRD) using quantitative

reverse transcriptase polymerase chain reaction (RT-PCR) for fusion genes, to allow for risk stratification based on treatment responses after chemotherapy, because sequential monitoring during follow-up can accurately predict relapse. A consensus document from the European LeukemiaNet MRD Working Party recommends that patients with CBF AML have an initial assessment of MRD after 2 cycles of chemotherapy, followed by serial measurement every 3 months for at least the first 2 years after the end of treatment, in bone marrow and peripheral blood.

Quantitative RT-PCR was performed on the bone marrow of this patient approximately 1 month after diagnosis and showed persistent *RUNX1-RUNX1T1* fusion transcript, with ratio of fusion transcript to internal control transcript (*ABL1*) of 0.013. However, peripheral blood tested approximately 3 months at the end of treatment was negative, as was bone marrow biopsy performed 6 months after diagnosis.

Diagnostic pearls/pitfalls

– Myeloid neoplasms with t(8;21)(q22;22.1) or inv(16)(p13.1q22)/t(16;16)(p13.1;q22) (ie, CBF translocations) are considered to be AML regardless of blast cell count.

– CBF AML typically have favorable prognosis. However, the presence of a *KIT* mutation (particularly in exon 17) confers higher relapse risk and adversely affects overall survival. Testing for a *KIT* mutation is recommended for all new cases of CBF AML.

– Unique features often found in t(8;21) AML include blasts with large fused granules (pseudo–Chediak-Higashi granules), thin elongated Auer rods, homogeneous salmon-pink cytoplasm in neutrophils and their precursors, and CD19 and/or CD56 expression by leukemic blasts.

– Evaluation for a neoplastic mast cell population has been recommended at diagnosis and subsequent follow-up of patients with t(8;21) AML with *KIT* mutation, because of the poor outcomes among these patients.

– MRD testing for *RUNX1-RUNX1T1* transcript by quantitative RT-PCR at the end of treatment and during follow-up can be used to help predict relapse and overall survival.

Readings

Cairoli R, Beghini A, Grillo G, et al. Prognostic impact of c-KIT mutations in core binding factor leukemias: an Italian retrospective study. Blood. 2006;107(9):3463-8. **DOI: 10.1182/blood-2005-09-3640**

De J, Zanjani R, Hibbard M, Davis BH. Immunophenotypic profile predictive of KIT activating mutations in AML1-ETO leukemia. Am J Clin Pathol. 2007;128(4):550-7. **DOI: 10.1309/JVALJNL4ELQMD536**

Ishikawa Y, Kawashima N, Atsuta Y, et al. Prospective evaluation of prognostic impact of *KIT* mutations on acute myeloid leukemia with *RUNX1-RUNX1T1* and *CBFB-MYH11*. Blood Adv. 2020;4(1):66-75. **DOI:10.1182/bloodadvances.2019000709**

Intzes S, Wiersma S, Meyerson HJ. Myelomastocytic leukemia with t(8;21) in a 3-year-old child. J Pediatr Hematol Oncol. 2011;33(8):e372-5. **DOI: 10.1097/MPH.0b013e3182329b80**

Johnson RC, Savage NM, Chiang T. Hidden mastocytosis in acute myeloid leukemia with t(8;21)(q22;q22). Am J Clin Pathol. 2013;140(4):525-35. **DOI: 10.1309/AJCP1Q0YSXEAHNKK**

Park SH, Chi HS, Min SK, Park BG, Jang S, Park CJ. Prognostic impact of c-KIT mutations in core binding factor acute myeloid leukemia. Leuk Res. 2011;35(10):1376-83. **DOI: 10.1016/j.leukres.2011.06.003**

Paschka P, Marcucci G, Ruppert AS, et al; Cancer and Leukemia Group B. Adverse prognostic significance of KIT mutations in adult acute myeloid leukemia with inv(16) and t(8;21): a Cancer and Leukemia Group B Study. J Clin Oncol. 2006;24(24):3904-11. **DOI: 10.1200/JCO.2006.06.9500**

Schnittger S, Kohl TM, Haferlach T, et al. KIT-D816 mutations in AML1-ETO-positive AML are associated with impaired event-free and overall survival. Blood. 2006;107(5):1791-9. **DOI: 10.1182/blood-2005-04-1466**

Schuurhuis GJ, Heuser M, Freeman S, et al. Minimal/measurable residual disease in AML: a consensus document from the European LeukemiaNet MRD Working Party. Blood. 2018;131(12):1275-91. **DOI: 10.1182/blood-2017-09-801498**

Swerdlow SH, Campo E, Harris NL, et al. World Health Organization Classification of Tumours of Haematopoietic and Lymphoid Tissues. 4th ed. Lyon, France: IARC Press; 2017:130-3. **ISBN: 9789283244943**

Yin JA, O'Brien MA, Hills RK, Daly SB, Wheatley K, Burnett AK. Minimal residual disease monitoring by quantitative RT-PCR in core binding factor AML allows risk stratification and predicts relapse: results of the United Kingdom MRC AML-15 trial. Blood. 2012;120(14):2826-35. **DOI: 10.1182/blood-2012-06-435669**

Kwadwo Oduro

20

Acute promyelocytic leukemia with subsequent therapy-related myeloid neoplasm (myelodysplastic syndrome)

History (part 1) A 29-year-old female with no significant past medical history presented to an urgent care facility for sore throat and a petechial rash. Pertinent CBC results are shown at right and were notable for leukocytosis and thrombocytopenia. The patient was admitted and further workup revealed: prothrombin time 16 sec (elevated), international normalized ratio 1.56 (elevated), partial thromboplastin time 23 sec (normal), and fibrinogen <50 mg/dL (<1.47 g/L; low).

Morphology & flow cytometry (part 1) Peripheral blood smear review revealed a predominance of immature, medium-sized atypical cells with scant to moderately abundant cytoplasm and bi-lobed or butterfly shaped nuclei, comprising about 80% of total leukocytes **f20.1**. Most of these atypical cells appeared agranular or hypogranular. Overall the morphology was compatible with hypogranular atypical promyelocytes, characteristic of the microgranular variant of **acute promyelocytic leukemia** (APL). Bone marrow biopsy showed complete replacement of the marrow by these cells **f20.2**. Flow cytometry performed on the peripheral blood revealed a large atypical population that was CD34 partial positive, CD117 dim, CD33 positive, HLA-DR heterogeneous, CD2 partial positive, CD56 negative, CD11b negative, and myeloperoxidase (MPO) positive, comprising 76% of total events **f20.3**.

Genetics/molecular results (part 1) FISH for *PML-RARA* fusion was performed emergently on the peripheral blood, based on the high morphologic and clinical suspicion for APL, and was positive **f20.4**, confirming the diagnosis. AML molecular testing was positive for *FLT3-ITD* mutations (48bp and 60bp ITDs identified).

WBC	49.1 × 10⁹/L
Platelets	18 × 10⁹/L

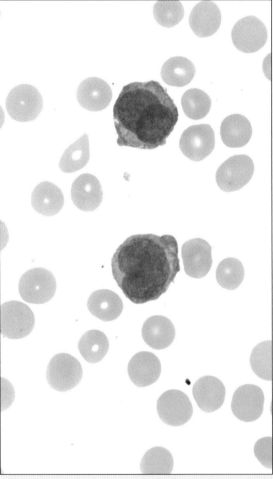

f20.1 Circulating atypical promyelocytes having bilobed nuclei without obvious granulation

ISBN 978-089189-6814 ©2021 ASCP

20 *Acute promyelocytic leukemia with subsequent therapy-related myeloid neoplasm (myelodysplastic syndrome)*

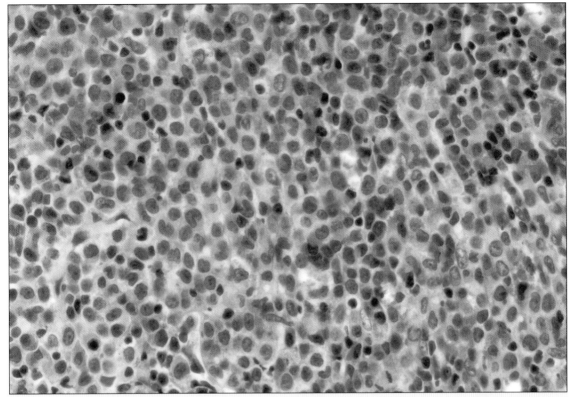

f20.2 Sheets of atypical promyelocytes in the bone marrow core biopsy

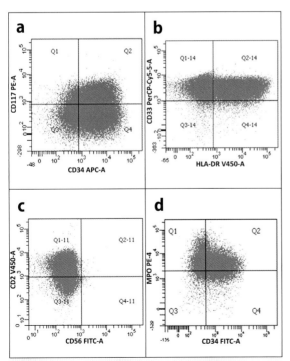

f20.3 Flow cytometry performed on peripheral blood demonstrates an atypical blast population with high side scatter & partial expression of **a** CD34, CD117, **b** HLA-DR & **c** CD2, but **d** fairly uniform expression of MPO

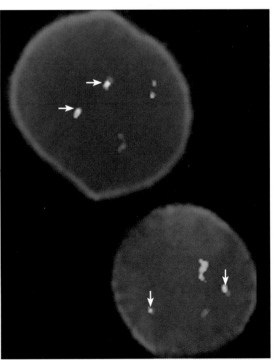

f20.4 Dual fusion FISH probes for *PML* (15q24, orange) & *RARA* (17q21, green) demonstrate the presence of *PML-RARA* fusion; the presence of 2 yellow signals (arrows) is consistent with reciprocal translocation

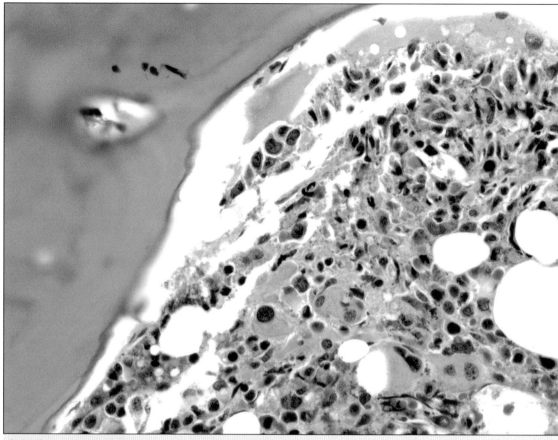

f20.5 The core biopsy contains clusters of dysplastic, hypolobated megakaryocytes

History (part 2) The patient was treated with induction chemotherapy plus all-trans retinoic acid (ATRA), followed by consolidation chemotherapy and then maintenance therapy. She successfully achieved morphologic and sustained molecular remission based on multiple peripheral blood quantitative PCR assays for *PML-RARA*. However, approximately 2 years after completion of consolidation chemotherapy, during routine follow-up, the patient was noted to have decreasing platelet counts over a 2-month period, with platelets at 120×10^9/L, then 71×10^9/L, without clinical explanation. The peripheral blood was then reviewed and a new bone marrow biopsy specimen was obtained.

Morphology & flow cytometry (part 2) The peripheral blood smear was unremarkable except for thrombocytopenia. The bone marrow core biopsy showed normocellularity with increased megakaryocytes, many of which were small with nuclear hypolobation, as well as occasional forms with separated nuclear lobes, indicative of dysplasia **f20.5**. Blasts were increased in the bone marrow (~3%-5% based on touch prep evaluation and CD34 staining on the core biopsy). The blasts showed round nuclei with scant cytoplasm, and were morphologically distinct from the patient's APL blasts **f20.6**. Flow cytometry identified 3% blasts that were CD34 bright, CD117 positive, HLA-DR positive, and CD2 negative, with aberrant partial CD56 expression **f20.7**. These findings were indicative of development of therapy-related myelodysplastic syndrome (MDS).

ISBN 978-089189-6814 ©2021 ASCP

20 *Acute promyelocytic leukemia with subsequent therapy-related myeloid neoplasm (myelodysplastic syndrome)*

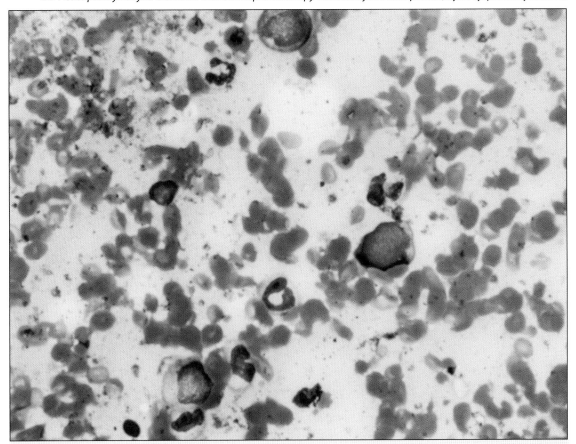

f20.6 Touch prep demonstrating hypogranular neutrophils as well as occasional blasts with oval nuclei & high nuclear:cytoplasmic ratios

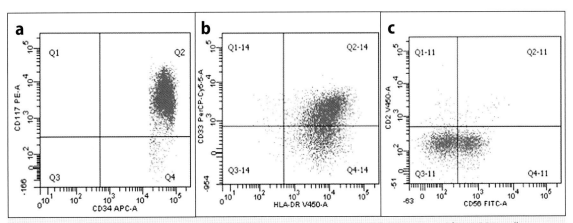

f20.7 Flow cytometry demonstrates an atypical blast population with uniform expression of **a** CD34, CD117 & **b** HLA-DR as well as **c** aberrant expression of CD56 & lack of CD2, distinct from the patient's original acute promyelocytic leukemia blasts

Genetics/molecular results (part 2) Quantitative reverse-transcriptase PCR for *PML-RARA* was negative, confirming the absence of residual/recurrent APL. However, chromosome analysis revealed a 45,XX,–7[5]/46,XX[2] karyotype **f20.8**. A myeloid NGS panel was positive for a *CBL* p.R420Q (c.1259G>A) variant in 25% of reads and no *FLT3-ITD* mutation was detected. These genetic/molecular findings, in particular the presence of monosomy 7, confirmed a new diagnosis of **MDS**, ie, **therapy-related myeloid neoplasm** (TRMN) based on the 2017 World Health Organization (WHO) criteria.

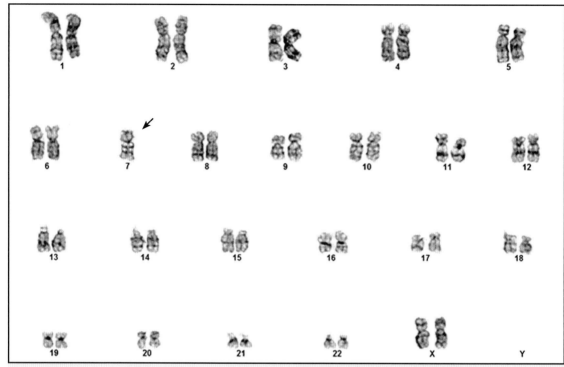

f20.5 Karyotype demonstrating monosomy 7 (arrow); the formerly present t(15;17) *PML-RARA* was not identified

Discussion APL is a unique type of AML characterized by proliferation of atypical promyelocytes that are considered to be blast equivalents. APL was designated as AML M3 in the French-American-British (FAB) AML classification, and as acute promyelocytic leukemia with *PML-RARA* in the 2017 WHO classification of hematologic neoplasms. Rapid diagnosis is crucial because patients are at high risk of developing and dying of disseminated intravascular coagulation (DIC). This unique subtype of AML is highly responsive to differentiation therapy with ATRA, and in low-risk cases (those with a WBC count $\leq 10 \times 10^9$/L), chemotherapy can be avoided altogether by combined usage of ATRA and arsenic trioxide.

Morphologically, 2 main variants are recognized. In the classic variant, leukemic cells show cytoplasmic hypergranulation and Auer rods, with high side scatter detected by flow cytometry. In contrast, the microgranular variant demonstrates bilobed or butterfly-shaped nuclei similar to the classic variant, but lacks morphologically evident cytoplasmic granules and Auer rods. However, flow cytometry or cytochemical stains demonstrate strong MPO positivity in the microgranular variant, hence its name. On flow cytometry, the leukemic cells in either variant show a characteristic immunophenotype that is CD117 positive, CD34 negative, HLA-DR negative, with variable positivity for other myeloid markers such as CD33 and CD13. The microgranular variant in particular

may be confused morphologically with AML having monocytic differentiation, and flow cytometry can be helpful in challenging cases. It is worth noting that the microgranular variant, as in the current case, is more likely to demonstrate a nonclassic APL immunophenotype, such as expression of CD34 or CD2 and thus may be more difficult to recognize by flow cytometry. Interestingly, CD2 expression in APL has been associated with the presence of *FLT3-ITD* mutations.

The characteristic translocation in either APL variant is t(15;17)(q22;q11-12) *PML-RARA*, a fusion between the promyelocytic leukemia gene (*PML*, a tumor suppressor) and the retinoic acid receptor α gene (*RARA*, a modulator of cell differentiation); the resulting fusion product causes a myeloid differentiation block at the promyelocyte stage. Several variant translocations with *RARA* are recognized, some of which are associated with resistance to ATRA, namely translocations involving *ZBTB16* at 11q23.2 or *STAT5B* at 17q21.2. Genetic or molecular confirmation of a *RARA* translocation is crucial to establish a diagnosis of APL and should be ordered whenever there is clinical, morphologic, or immunophenotypic suspicion. Testing for specific gene mutations, typically recommended for other AML cases, currently has limited use in the management of APL cases. Although *FLT3* mutations (both internal tandem duplication [ITD] and tyrosine kinase domain [TKD] types) are common

ISBN 978-089189-6814

in APL, occurring in 30%-40% of cases, the prognostic significance of these mutations in APL is controversial, with some studies suggesting an increased relapse rate in patients having these mutations. The presence of *FLT3-ITD* or *FLT3-TKD* mutations may be helpful for clinicopathologic correlation, however, because they tend to associate with the microgranular morphologic variant, high WBC count, bcr3 breakpoint of PML, and CD2 expression.

A new cytopenia in a patient with a history of hematologic neoplasm raises concern for disease relapse or progression. However, if the patient was previously treated with chemotherapy, then a therapy-related myeloid neoplasm is also in the differential diagnosis. In this case with a non-APL blast population detected several years after treatment, a therapy-related MDS was confirmed with molecular and genetic results showing a distinct mutational and chromosomal profile. In particular, the absence of *PML-RARA* and newly identified monosomy 7 indicated TRMN characteristic of alkylating agent therapy (for further discussion on genetic findings in TRMN, see **Cases 25 & 26**). After the diagnosis of TRMN, this young patient underwent stem cell transplantation rather than APL-related therapy, underscoring the importance of confirming the diagnosis with ancillary studies in this setting.

Diagnostic pearls/pitfalls

- The classic blasts of APL have a distinctive immunophenotype that is typically positive for CD117 and negative for CD34 and HLA-DR, with strong expression of MPO.
- The microgranular variant of APL has morphologic and/or immunophenotypic features that are distinct from classic APL and may be confused with AML with monocytic differentiation.
- Pathologists should have a low threshold for ordering *PML-RARA* FISH testing, if there is any suspicion for APL based on clinical, morphologic, or flow cytometric findings.
- qRT-PCR for *PML-RARA* is commonly used for monitoring of minimal residual disease in APL patients.
- *FLT3* mutations (ITD or TKD) occur in about one third of APL cases but the prognostic impact of these mutations is unclear.
- TRMN can occur secondary to treatment for any hematologic disease, and genetic/molecular studies can confirm the presence of a clonal myeloid process distinct from the original neoplasm.

Readings

Breccia M, Loglisci G, Loglisci MG, et al. *FLT3-ITD* confers poor prognosis in patients with acute promyelocytic leukemia treated with AIDA protocols: long-term follow-up analysis. Haematologica. 2013;98(12):e161-3. **DOI: 10.3324/haematol.2013.095380**

De Rossi G, Avvisati G, Coluzzi S, et al. Immunological definition of acute promyelocytic leukemia (FAB M3): a study of 39 cases. Eur J Haematol. 1990;45(3):168-71. **DOI: 10.1111/j.1600-0609.1990.tb00446.x**

Fan Y, Cao Y, Bai X, Zhuang W. The clinical significance of *FLT3-ITD* mutation on the prognosis of adult acute promyelocytic leukemia. Hematology. 2018;23(7):379-84. **DOI: 10.1080/10245332.2017.1415717**

Lehmann-Che J, Bally C, Letouzé E, et al. Dual origin of relapses in retinoic-acid resistant acute promyelocytic leukemia. Nat Commun. 2018;9(1):2047. **DOI: 10.1038/s41467-018-04384-5**

Lo-Coco F, Avvisati G, Vignetti M, et al. Retinoic acid and arsenic trioxide for acute promyelocytic leukemia. N Engl J Med. 2013;369(2):111-21. **DOI: 10.1056/NEJMoa1300874**

National Comprehensive Cancer Network. Acute myeloid leukemia (version 3.2020). **https://www.nccn.org/professionals/physician_gls/pdf/aml.pdf**

Paietta E, Andersen J, Gallagher R, et al. The immunophenotype of acute promyelocytic leukemia (APL): an ECOG study. Leukemia. 1994;8(7):1108-12. **PMID: 8035602**

Piedras J, López-Karpovitch X, Cárdenas R. Light scatter and immunophenotypic characteristics of blast cells in typical acute promyelocytic leukemia and its variant. Cytometry. 1998;32(4):286-90. **PMID: 9701397**

Renneville A, Attias P, Thomas X, et al. Genetic analysis of therapy-related myeloid neoplasms occurring after intensive treatment for acute promyelocytic leukemia. Leukemia. 2018;32(9):2066-9. **DOI: 10.1038/s41375-018-0137-6**

Swerdlow SH, Campo E, Harris NL, et al. World Health Organization Classification of Tumours of Haematopoietic and Lymphoid Tissues. 4th ed. Lyon, France: IARC Press; 2017. **ISBN: 9789283244943**

Zompi S, Viguié F. Therapy-related acute myeloid leukemia and myelodysplasia after successful treatment of acute promyelocytic leukemia. Leuk Lymphoma. 2002;43(2):275-80. **DOI: 10.1080/10428190290006044**

Theresa Spivey & Kwadwo Oduro

21

Acute myeloid leukemia with mutated *NPM1* & *FLT3-ITD*

History A 68-year-old female with a long history of smoking and chronic obstructive pulmonary disease presented with decreased appetite, fatigue, and gradual weight loss over several months. CBC results are shown at right. A peripheral blood smear was reviewed and a subsequent bone marrow biopsy was performed.

Morphology & flow cytometry The peripheral blood demonstrated frequent blasts, some with Auer rods, and promonocytes (blast equivalents), together comprising >80% of the white cell differential. Some of the blasts had a cup-shaped indentation of the nucleus **f21.1**. Also, an abnormal monocytosis was noted. The bone marrow aspirate smear differential revealed 71% blasts and promonocytes **f21.2**. Occasional erythroid forms with nuclear budding and atypical megakaryocytic forms with discrete, separate nuclear lobes were also seen. The bone marrow core biopsy was 90% cellular and was composed predominantly of sheets of immature monocytic cells and blasts.

Bone marrow flow cytometry showed 8% myeloblasts in the CD45dim region; the blasts had moderate expression of CD13, CD33, HLA-DR, and CD163, with heterogenous expression of CD117 and partial myeloperoxidase (MPO) positivity (in 6% of these cells), and were negative for CD34, CD14, and CD56. In addition, there were 71% cells in the monocyte-gated region, with brighter CD45 expression and higher side scatter. These cells showed partial aberrant CD117 and CD56 expression and aberrant partial loss of CD14. They were also negative for CD34 **f21.3**.

Based on the morphologic and flow cytometry findings, a diagnosis of **acute myeloid leukemia** (AML) **with evidence of myelomonocytic differentiation**, pending genetic/molecular studies for World Health Organization (WHO) classification, was rendered.

WBC	76.1 × 10⁹/L
RBC	3.14 × 10¹²/L
HGB	8.6 g/dL
HCT	27.8%
MCV	89 fL
RDW	17.8%
Platelets	73 × 10⁹/L

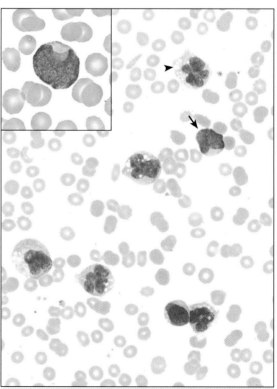

f21.1 Peripheral blood demonstrating increased & abnormal monocytes (arrowhead), promonocytes, and blasts (arrow); the inset shows a blast with a nuclear invagination resembling a cup

ISBN 978-089189-6814 ©2021 ASCP

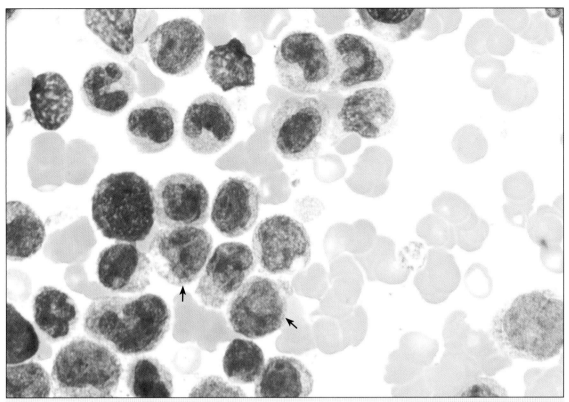

f21.2 Bone marrow aspirate demonstrating blasts & promonocytes (blast equivalents). The promonocytes (some highlighted by arrows) have irregular nuclei with open chromatin & delicate folds

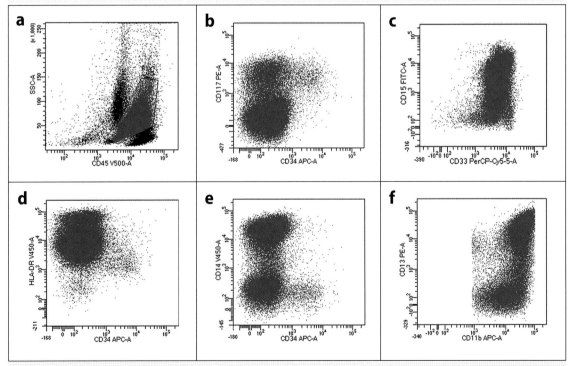

f21.3 **a** Flow cytometry performed on the bone marrow demonstrates an atypical combined blast/monocytic population (highlighted in blue); **b** the atypical population has partial expression of CD117 but not CD34; **c-f** the expression of CD15 (partial), CD33, HLA-DR, CD14 (partial), CD11b, and CD13 (partial) are all consistent with monocytic differentiation

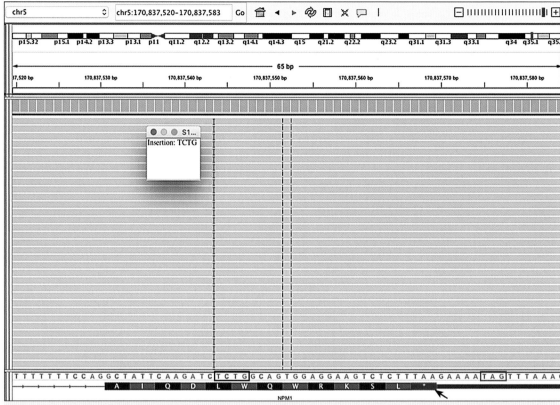

f21.4 Somatic variant analysis using a targeted myeloid NGS panel demonstrates type "A" mutation of *NPM1* (hg19, Integrative Genomics Viewer browser). Annotated reads mapped to *NPM1* exon 12 demonstrate a 4-bp insertion, a duplicate TCTG (noted in small white box) which starts at the purple "I." The original TCTG in the germline sequence is boxed in black. The duplication/insertion causes a frameshift that disrupts the normal TAA stop codon (red box, arrow) & generates a new stop codon (TAG, outlined in red) just downstream. This mutation results in an elongated nucleophosmin protein with abnormal cellular localization [see **fA.8**, p312]

Genetics/molecular results The karyotype was normal and an AML FISH panel was negative for inv(3), t(3;3), t(8;21), del(5q), monosomy 7, del(7q), trisomy 8, inv(16), *KMT2A* (*MLL*) rearrangement, del(17q), and del(20q). A targeted myeloid NGS panel was positive for the following pathogenic variants:

NPM1 p.W288CFS*12 (c.860_863dupTCTG) at 45% variant allele frequency (VAF) **f21.4**
DNMT3A p.R882C (c.2644C>T) at 47% VAF
IDH2 p.R140Q (c.419G>A) at 45% VAF
U2AF p.Q157R (c. 470A>G) at 46% VAF
PTPN11 p.A72V (c.215C>T) at 38% VAF
FLT3-ITD (p.Y597_E598insDYVDFREY) at 0.03 variant allelic ratio (VAR)

Based on the molecular findings of mutated *NPM1*, a final WHO diagnosis of **AML with mutated *NPM1*** was rendered.

The patient was treated with standard induction chemotherapy. The day 31 count recovery bone marrow biopsy showed no morphologic or flow cytometric evidence of disease. However, NGS-based minimal residual disease (MRD) assays for both *NPM1* and *FLT3-ITD* were both positive at a VAR of 1.93×10^{-4} and 1.2×10^{-5}, respectively. Bone marrow biopsy after 2 cycles of consolidation showed persistent molecular residual disease (mutated *NPM1* at 1.08×10^{-3} VAR and *FLT3-ITD* at 1.36×10^{-4} VAR), despite normal morphology and flow cytometry findings

Discussion AML with mutated *NPM1* is now recognized as a distinct entity in the 2017 WHO classification of hematopoietic neoplasms. As the name suggests, it is defined by the presence of a mutation in the *NPM1* gene, which encodes for nucleophosmin, a nuclear protein that functions to shuttle proteins from the nucleus to the cytoplasm. Typically, the mutation is a 4-bp insertion (rarely a deletion) occurring in the terminal exon 12,

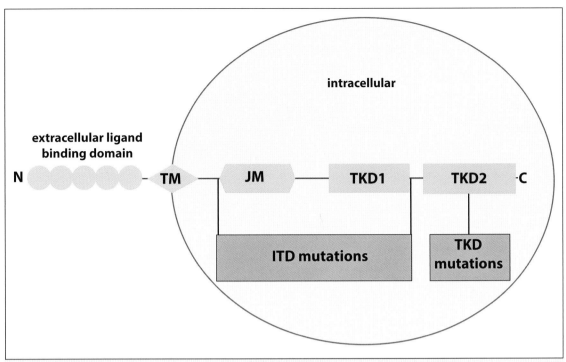

f21.5 Schematic demonstration of the location of mutations in the *FLT3* gene. Internal tandem duplications (ITD) occur either in the juxtamembrane domain (JM) or in the first tyrosine kinase domain (TKD) & are highly variable in length, ranging in size from a few to hundreds of base pairs. By contrast, "TKD" mutations are gain-of-function mutations that occur in the second tyrosine kinase domain & consist of either single nucleotide point mutations or small deletions. JM, juxtamembrane domain; TM, transmembrane domain

causing a frameshift and resulting in a dysfunctional, abnormally localized and elongated protein **f21.4**. The aberrant cytoplasmic localization of mutated NPM1 protein is postulated to disrupt normal tumor suppressor activity, among other functions, and can be detected with immunohistochemistry (although this is not routinely performed). At least 10 different types of pathogenic *NPM1* mutations have been described in AML and the c.860_863dupTCTG ("type A") seen in this patient is the most frequent, occurring in >75% of cases.

NPM1 is one of the most commonly mutated genes found in AML, occurring in 28%-35% of all AML cases. *NPM1* mutation is most frequently associated with monocytic (or myelomonocytic) differentiation of blasts, which sometimes demonstrate distinctive "cuplike" or "fish mouth" invagination of the nucleus (**f21.1**, inset). The blasts are frequently negative for CD34 and may also be negative for CD117, features common in AML with monocytic differentiation. Some cases without overt monocytic differentiation can show an immunophenotype that is negative for CD34 and HLA-DR and strongly positive for MPO, which can raise suspicion for acute promyelocytic leukemia, but testing for t(15;17) *PML-RARA* will exclude this diagnosis.

In general, *NPM1* mutation in AML with normal karyotype confers a favorable prognosis. This appears to be true even in the setting of significant background dysplasia, such that these cases are classified as AML with mutated *NPM1* rather than AML with myelodysplasia-related changes. However, in many patients, including this example case, mutation in *NPM1* co-occurs with other mutations that may affect prognosis, in particular internal tandem duplication (ITD) of *FLT3*, the gene encoding fms-like tyrosine kinase 3. *FLT3-ITD* is the most common abnormality of *FLT3* found in AML and results from an in-frame head-to-tail duplication, with a length of 3 to several hundred base pairs, leading to constitutive activation of this tyrosine kinase receptor. Other mutations in *FLT3* occur mostly in the second tyrosine kinase domain, so called *FLT3-TKD* mutations **f21.5**, and have not been shown to have the same impact on prognosis as *FLT3-ITD*. The co-occurrence of *FLT3-ITD* present at high VAR (defined as ratio of *FLT3-ITD* to normal *FLT3* >0.5) elevates prognostic risk from favorable to intermediate. Therefore, based on current National Comprehensive Cancer Network (NCCN) risk stratification, this patient's disease was favorable because of the *FLT3-ITD* VAR being <0.5. Undoubtedly, there are other less well-characterized molecular risk modifiers in *NPM1* mutant AML, with some recent studies suggesting, for instance, adverse outcomes with co-occurring *DNMT3A* and *IDH* mutations, as seen in this patient. Based on clonal studies, *NPM1* is a secondary mutation to *DNMT3A*, *IDH1*, *IDH2*, and *TET2*, but in contrast precedes *FLT3* mutations.

In addition to potentially altering the risk stratification of *NPM1* mutant AML, the presence of *FLT3-ITD* has therapeutic significance. AML with *FLT3-ITD* responds to the kinase inhibitor midostaurin. Addition of this drug to standard induction chemotherapy is now recommended for *FLT3-ITD* mutant AML, specifically in cases having VAR of at least 0.05. This patient received standard chemotherapy without midostaurin specifically because of the low FLT3-ITD VAR (0.03). Based on her follow-up samples, the *FLT3-ITD* clone persisted, concerning for increased risk of relapse.

The frequent absence of CD34 and CD117 on blasts in *NPM1*-mutant AML may cause difficulty in identifying residual leukemic blasts using flow cytometry during follow-up, independent of the inherent sensitivity of the flow cytometry method. Fortunately, a quantitative reverse transcriptase PCR assay able to detect low levels of mutant *NPM1* (sensitivity of 10^{-4} allelic ratio) has been developed and shown to be effective not only in detecting residual disease but also in predicting future relapse. This initial assay is RNA-based and detects only type A *NPM1* mutation. The advent of DNA-based NGS platforms allows detection of MRD independent of *NPM1* mutation type, using direct sequencing methods. Future studies will determine which molecular MRD assays are most robust in AML patients with multiple mutations, and at what specific time points these assays should be used.

This patient had a relapse with leukemia cutis 6 months after initial diagnosis, 1 month after completing 4 cycles of high-dose ara-C (HIDAC) consolidation. Frank marrow relapse was demonstrated 2 weeks later, with relapsed disease being positive for both *FLT3-ITD* (VAR of 0.08) and mutated *NPM1* (VAF of 6%). She was treated with gilteritinib, a FLT3 inhibitor recently approved by the Food and Drug Administration, which has proven to be effective in relapsed or refractory AML with *FLT3* mutation. If she continues to be refractory, the patient may be treated with IDH2-targeted therapy (enasidenib), given the presence of *IDH2* mutation at diagnosis and relapse.

Diagnostic pearls/pitfalls

- AML with mutated *NPM1* is a distinct entity in the 2017 WHO classification of hematopoietic tumors. *NPM1* is one of the most frequently mutated genes in AML, and such cases typically have a normal karyotype and monocytic differentiation, with *NPM1* mutation being found in >80% of acute monocytic leukemias.
- Multilineage dysplasia may be seen in up to 25% of AML cases with mutated *NPM1*, and these cases should not be diagnosed as AML with myelodysplasia-related changes unless an MDS-associated karyotypic abnormality is detected.
- *NPM1* mutation in AML is associated with cup-shaped nuclei of blasts and loss of CD34 expression. The mutant NPM1 protein can be detected with immunohistochemistry using an anti-NPM1 antibody based on aberrant cytoplasmic localization.
- *FLT3-ITD* mutations are the most common *FLT3* mutations found in AML and are important for prognostication and use of targeted therapy.
- In the presence of a normal karyotype, *NPM1* mutation in AML is associated with a favorable prognosis compared to AML with normal karyotype and wildtype *NPM1*. However, co-occurrence of *FLT3-ITD* at VAR >0.5 adversely affects prognosis.
- With current molecular assays, both mutated *NPM1* and *FLT3-ITD* can be used as biomarkers for MRD and prediction of relapse.

ISBN 978-089189-6814

Readings

Chen W, Konoplev S, Medeiros L, et al. Cuplike nuclei (prominent nuclear invaginations) in acute myeloid leukemia are highly associated with *FLT3* internal tandem duplication and *NPM1* mutation. Cancer. 2009;115(23):5481-9. **DOI: 10.1002/cncr.24610**

Dunlap JB, Leonard J, Rosenberg M, et al. The combination of *NPM1*, *DNMT3A*, and *IDH1/2* mutations leads to inferior overall survival in AML. Am J Hematol. 2019;94(8):913-20. **DOI: 10.1002/ajh.25517**

Falini B, Macijewski K, Weiss T, et al. Multilineage dysplasia has no impact on biologic, clinicopathologic, and prognostic features of AML with mutated nucleophosmin (*NPM1*). Blood. 2010;115(18):3776-86. **DOI:10.1182/blood-2009-08-240457**

Falini B, Mecucci C, Tiacci E, et al. Cytoplasmic nucleophosmin in acute myelogenous leukemia with a normal karyotype. N Engl J Med. 2005;352(3):254-66. **DOI: 10.1056/NEJMoa041974**

Freeman SD, Hourigan CS. MRD evaluation of AML in clinical practice: are we there yet? Hematology Am Soc Hematol Educ Program. 2019 Dec 6;2019(1):557-569. **DOI: 10.1182/hematology.2019000060**

Ivey A, Hills R, Simpson A, et al. Assessment of minimal residual disease in standard-risk AML. N Engl J Med. 2016;374(5):422-33. **DOI:10.1056/NEJMoa1507471**

Schnittger S1, Bacher U, Kern W. Prognostic impact of *FLT3-ITD* load in *NPM1* mutated acute myeloid leukemia. Leukemia. 2011;25(8):1297-304. **DOI:10.1038/leu.2011.97**

Stone R, Mandrekar S, Sanford B, et al. Midostaurin plus chemotherapy for acute myeloid leukemia with a *FLT3* mutation. N Engl J Med. 2017;377(5):454-64. **DOI: 10.1056/NEJMoa1614359**

Thiede C, Koch S, Creutzig E, et al. Prevalence and prognostic impact of *NPM1* mutations in 1485 adult patients with acute myeloid leukemia (AML). Blood. 2006;107(10):4011-20. **DOI: 10.1182/blood-2005-08-3167**

Mason EF, Kuo FC, Hasserjian RP, et al. A distinct immunophenotype identifies a subset of *NPM1*-mutated AML with *TET2* or *IDH1/2* mutations and improved outcome. Am J Hematol. 2018;93(4):504-10. **DOI: 10.1002/ajh.25018**

Perl AE, Altman JK, Cortes J, et al. Selective inhibition of *FLT3* by gilteritinib in relapsed or refractory acute myeloid leukaemia: a multicentre, first-in-human, open-label, phase 1-2 study. Lancet Oncol. 2017;18(8):1061-1075. **DOI:10.1016/S1470-2045(17)30416-3**

Megan O Nakashima & Rose C Beck

22

Acute myeloid leukemia with biallelic mutation of *CEBPA*

History A 66-year-old male was found to have pancytopenia with circulating blasts on a CBC performed for routine follow-up for prostate cancer. Results of CBC are shown at right. A peripheral smear was reviewed and a bone marrow biopsy obtained.

WBC	1.45×10^9/L
HGB	11.2 g/dL
HCT	34%
MCV	86.1 fL
Platelets	77×10^9/L

Morphology & flow cytometry The peripheral blood smear demonstrated 12% circulating blasts, which were intermediate in size and had scant to moderate cytoplasm and fine chromatin, often with one prominent nucleolus **f22.1**. The aspirate smears showed 25% blasts morphologically similar to these seen in peripheral blood. There was also dyserythropoiesis in the form of nuclear budding, binucleation, and megaloblastoid change **f22.2**. The trephine core and clot sections showed a mildly hypercellular marrow for age (50%). Trilineage hematopoiesis was present with a decreased myeloid:erythroid ratio. Mononuclear cells were variably increased, consistent with blasts, sometimes forming large interstitial clusters **f22.3**.

Flow cytometric analysis performed on peripheral blood before the biopsy specimen was obtained showed increased myeloid blasts positive for CD7, CD13, CD33, CD34, CD38, CD45, CD64 (subset), CD65, CD117, and HLA-DR **f22.4**.

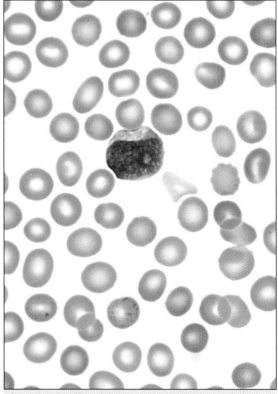

f22.1 Peripheral blood showing a blast in a background of pancytopenia

   ISBN 978-089189-6814

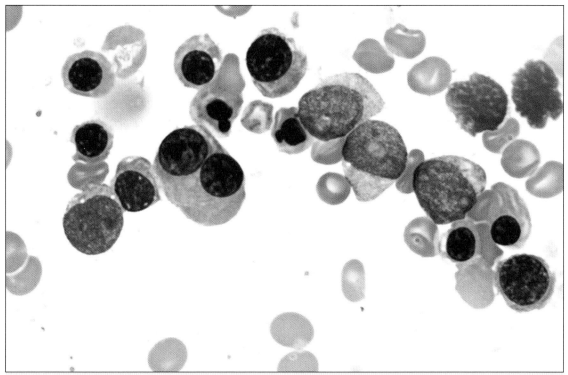

f22.2 Blasts increased in the aspirate smear (25%); there is also erythroid dysplasia in the form of budding & binucleation with relatively decreased maturing granulopoiesis

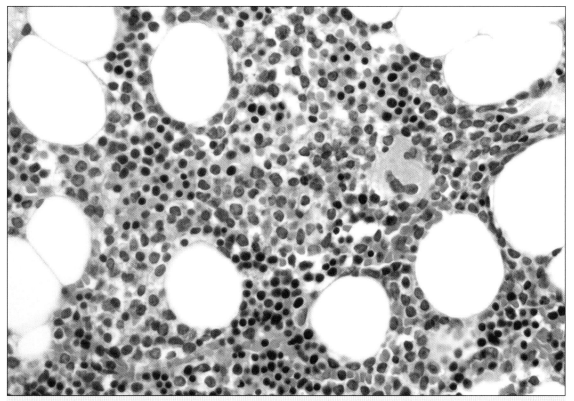

f22.3 Increased cellularity in the core biopsy due to increased mononuclear cells having fine chromatin & visible nucleoli, consistent with blasts; erythroid maturation is prominent; maturing granulopoiesis is reduced, but megakaryocytes are present

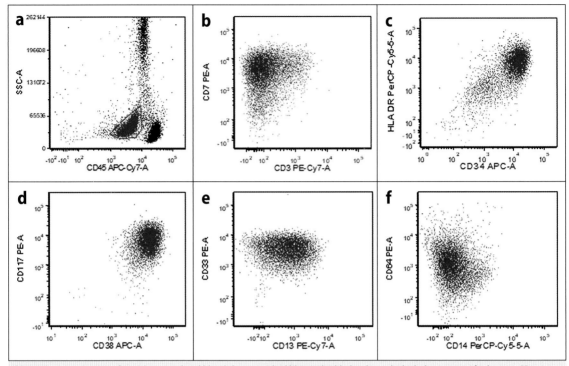

f22.4 Flow cytometry performed on peripheral blood shows myeloid blasts **a** highlighted in red which demonstrate **b** aberrant CD7 expression & are positive for **c** CD34, HLA-DR, **d** CD117, **e** CD33, CD13 & **f** CD64 (subset)

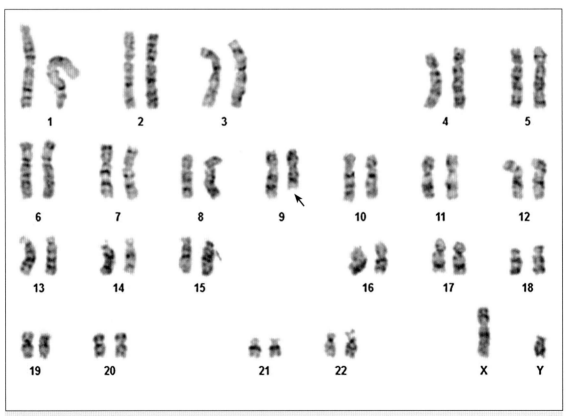

f22.5 Karyotype showing del(9)(q13q22) as the only chromosomal abnormality (arrow)

f22.6 Diagrammatic representation of *CEBPA* with its 2 normal protein isoforms (p42 and p30); location of N-terminal (red arrows) & C-terminal (black arrows) mutations are shown: N-terminal mutations result in a truncated p42 isoform, whereas C-terminal mutations interfere with normal DNA binding; bZIP, basic leucine zipper; TAD, transactivation domain

Genetics/molecular results FISH studies for recurrent abnormalities found in acute myeloid leukemia (AML) were negative. Karyotype showed: 46,XY,del(9) (q13q22)[8]/46,XY[12] **f22.5**.

An NGS panel showed the following variants:

CEBPA p.K313_L317dup c.938_952dup15 at 31.2% variant allele frequency (VAF)
CEBPA p.Q83Pfs*25 c.247dupC at 38.6% VAF
GATA2 p.L321F c.961C>T at 40.9% VAF

Based on the morphologic, flow cytometric, and molecular genetic findings, a final diagnosis of **AML with biallelic mutations in *CEBPA*** was rendered.

Discussion The 2008 World Health Organization (WHO) classification of hematopoietic neoplasms included the provisional entity, AML with mutations in the CCAAT enhancer binding protein α gene (*CEBPA*), based on data showing that AML patients with this abnormality typically had a more favorable prognosis. Additional studies showed that cases specifically harboring biallelic, double *CEBPA* mutations have the more favorable prognosis. Biallelic *CEBPA* mutations have a characteristic

pattern: frameshift mutations in the N-terminal region and in-frame mutations in the C-terminal region of the opposite allele. AML cases with this pattern of mutations have a distinct gene expression profile and better prognosis than either cases with wild-type *CEBPA* or singly-mutated cases. Thus, AML with biallelic mutations in *CEBPA* is a confirmed diagnostic category in the 2017 WHO classification, with a prognosis similar to that of AML with inv(16)(p13.1q22) or t(8;21)(q22;q22.1).

AML with biallelic mutations in *CEBPA* typically occurs in children and young adults, among whom it represents 4%-9% of AML cases. Patients typically present with higher hemoglobin, lower platelet count, and lower lactate dehydrogenase than patients with other subtypes of AML. Extramedullary disease is uncommon. There is no distinctive morphology and these cases usually present as AML with or without maturation, as seen in this case; rare cases may have monocytic differentiation. Multilineage dysplasia is found in a quarter of cases but does not itself confer a worse prognosis, and therefore cases with dysplasia should not be classified as AML with myelodysplasia-related changes (AML-MRC) based on morphology alone. The blasts express typical myeloid antigens, and there is often aberrant expression of CD7

(~75% of cases), as seen in this case. HLA-DR is usually positive. CD15 is also commonly expressed while CD56 is infrequent (10%).

CEBPA encodes a transcription factor necessary for myeloid differentiation and growth arrest; the gene transcript is translated into 2 isoforms, p42 and p30. *CEBPA* mutations occurring in AML are clustered in the N-terminal region and in the C-terminal basic leucine zipper region (part of the DNA-binding domain; **f22.6**. The N-terminal mutations are generally out of frame and lead to a truncated form of p42, whereas the C-terminal mutations are in-frame and interfere with homo- and heterodimerization required for binding to DNA by either isoform. These mutations can be quite variable, and detection requires sequencing all relevant portions of the gene. Although initial studies confirmed the biallelic nature of these mutations by sub-cloning and sequencing, in clinical practice, cases with this pattern of N-terminal and C-terminal mutations are generally assumed to be biallelic. Evaluation of *CEBPA* mutations using NGS methods may be challenging because of the high GC content of the gene, and other assays may use Sanger sequencing with or without fragment length analysis.

Additional genetic abnormalities that can be seen include *GATA2* zinc finger mutations in up to 40% of cases, similar to this case. *FLT3-ITD* is relatively uncommon, present in 5%-9% of patients, and its presence has a negative impact on survival, while co-occurring *NPM1* mutations are very rare. Most cases of AML with biallelic mutation of *CEBPA* (70%) have normal karyotype. In the cases that do have abnormal karyotype, del(9q) is one of the more common abnormalities, again as seen in this case. In this context, presence of del(9q) does not appear to be associated with a worse prognosis, and so these cases are considered AML with biallelic *CEBPA* mutations and not classified as AML-MRC. However, less is known about the behavior of cases with other karyotypic abnormalities, so cases with other myelodysplasia-defining lesions should be considered AML-MRC, at least until more data are compiled.

The diagnosis of AML with biallelic mutations in *CEBPA* is reserved for cases with purely somatic mutations.

AML with germline *CEBPA* mutation is a separate entity in the 2017 WHO classification. These patients inherit an N-terminal mutation and develop AML after acquiring a C-terminal mutation. Interestingly *GATA2* somatic mutations are also seen in these cases. Patients with a high VAF of an N-terminal deletion or a family history of AML should be counseled and potentially undergo germline studies. In these families, AML occurs in childhood or early adulthood and has morphologic and immunophenotypic features similar to cases with acquired biallelic *CEBPA* mutations. AML with germline *CEBPA* mutations also has a relatively good prognosis; however, these patients may experience late relapse, which may be better considered a second primary AML, because the 3' mutation is often different from the original AML.

Diagnostic pearls/pitfalls

– AML with biallelic *CEBPA* mutation has a favorable prognosis compared to other types of AML. It is typified by the presence of 1 N-terminal mutation and 1 C-terminal mutation, requiring sequencing for detection.

– The morphology of AML with biallelic *CEBPA* mutation is nonspecific, often presenting as AML with/without maturation. Multilineage dysplasia may be present but does not change prognosis. Many cases will have aberrant CD7 expression detectable on flow cytometry.

– *GATA2* is often comutated in AML with biallelic *CEBPA* mutation, although most cases have normal karyotype; del(9q) may occur and does not change prognosis. However, little is known about the impact of other karyotypic abnormalities.

– A family history of AML or high VAF (40%-50%) of an N-terminal mutation should prompt evaluation for germline mutation of *CEBPA*, which is a separate WHO diagnosis and has prognostic impact for the patient and family members.

Readings

Ahn JY, Seo K, Weinberg O, Boyd SD, Arber DA. A comparison of two methods for screening *CEBPA* mutations in patients with acute myeloid leukemia. J Mol Diagn. 2009;11(4):319-23. **DOI: 10.2353/jmoldx.2009.080121**

Bacher U, Schnittger S, Macijewski K, et al. Multilineage dysplasia does not influence prognosis in *CEBPA*-mutated AML, supporting the WHO proposal to classify these patients as a unique entity. Blood. 2012;119(20):4719-22. **DOI: 10.1182/blood-2011-12-395574**

Dufour A, Schneider F, Metzeler KH, et al. Acute myeloid leukemia with biallelic *CEBPA* gene mutations and normal karyotype represents a distinct genetic entity associated with a favorable clinical outcome. J Clin Oncol. 2010;28(4):570-7. **DOI: 10.1200/JCO.2008.21.6010**

Green CL, Koo KK, Hills RK, et al. Prognostic significance of *CEBPA* mutations in a large cohort of younger adult patients with acute myeloid leukemia: impact of double *CEBPA* mutations and the interaction with *FLT3* and *NPM1* mutations. J Clin Oncol. 2010;28(16):2739-47. **DOI: 10.1200/JCO.2009.26.2501**

Greif PA, Dufour A, Konstandin NP, et al. *GATA2* zinc finger 1 mutations associated with biallelic *CEBPA* mutations define a unique genetic entity of acute myeloid leukemia. Blood. 2012;120(2):395-403. **DOI: 10.1182/blood-2012-01-403220**

Ng CWS, Kosmo B, Lee PL, et al. *CEBPA* mutational analysis in acute myeloid leukaemia by a laboratory-developed next-generation sequencing assay. J Clin Pathol. 2018;71(6):522-31. **DOI: 10.1136/jclinpath-2017-204825**

Nie Y, Su L, Li W, et al. Novel insights of acute myeloid leukemia with *CEBPA* deregulation: Heterogeneity dissection and re-stratification [published online ahead of print, 2021 Jun 1]. Crit Rev Oncol Hematol. 2021;163:103379. **DOI: 10.1016/j.critrevonc.2021.103379**

Pabst T, Eyholzer M, Fos J, et al. Heterogeneity within AML with *CEBPA* mutations; only *CEBPA* double mutations, but not single *CEBPA* mutations are associated with favourable prognosis. Br J Cancer. 2009;100(8):1343-6. **DOI: 10.1038/sj.bjc.6604977**

Reckzeh K, Cammenga J. Molecular mechanisms underlying deregulation of C/EBPalpha in acute myeloid leukemia. Int J Hematol. 2010;91(4):557-68. **DOI: 10.1007/s12185-010-0573-1**

Taskesen E, Bullinger L, Corbacioglu A, et al. Prognostic impact, concurrent genetic mutations, and gene expression features of AML with *CEBPA* mutations in a cohort of 1182 cytogenetically normal AML patients: further evidence for *CEBPA* double mutant AML as a distinctive disease entity. Blood. 2011;117(8):2469-75. **DOI: 10.1182/blood-2010-09-307280**

Tawana K, Wang J, Tenneville A, et al. Disease evolution and outcomes in familial AML with germline *CEBPA* mutations. Blood. 2015;126(10):1214-23. **DOI: 10.1182/blood-2015-05-647172**

Wouters BJ, Lowenberg B, Erpelinck-Verschueren CAJ, et al. Double *CEBPA* mutations, but not single *CEBPA* mutations, define a subgroup of acute myeloid leukemia with a distinctive gene expression profile that is uniquely associated with a favorable outcome. Blood. 2009;113(13):3088-91. **DOI: 10.1182/blood-2008-09-179895**

Christopher Ryder

23

Acute myeloid leukemia with mutated *RUNX1* & concurrent isolated trisomy 13

History A 70-year-old male presented to the emergency department with fever and weakness. Selected results of the CBC are shown at right. A peripheral smear was reviewed and a bone marrow biopsy obtained.

WBC	$1.2 \times 10^9/L$
HGB	7.8 g/dL
HCT	23.3%
MCV	114 fL
Platelets	$126 \times 10^9/L$

Morphology & flow cytometry The peripheral blood smear demonstrated macrocytic anemia with anisocytosis, neutropenia including toxic-appearing neutrophils, and occasional blasts which had a high nuclear:cytoplasmic ratio and fine chromatin. A bone marrow biopsy was performed, and the aspirate smears showed a predominance of small to medium-sized blasts with minimal cytoplasm and without granulation or Auer rods **f23.1**. Background trilineage hematopoiesis was present but reduced and a subset of erythroid precursors had mild dysplasia with occasional nuclear irregularities. The clot and core sections revealed a hypercellular marrow (50%) with sheets of blasts **f23.2a**. Immunohistochemical stains highlighted 30%-40% blasts that were positive for CD34 **f23.2b** and negative for myeloperoxidase (MPO), lysozyme, CD79a, and CD3.

Flow cytometry **f23.3** showed that the leukemic blasts were positive for CD34, CD117 (partial), CD13, HLA-DR, TdT, and CD7 (partial). They were negative for MPO, CD3 (surface and cytoplasmic), and CD19. The immunophenotypic findings were most suggestive of an acute myeloid leukemia (AML) with minimal differentiation, pending results of cytogenetic and molecular studies.

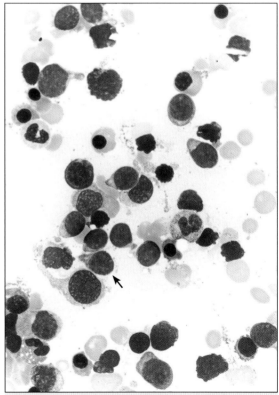

f23.1 Bone marrow aspirate showing small to intermediate-sized blasts (arrow)

    ISBN 978-089189-6814

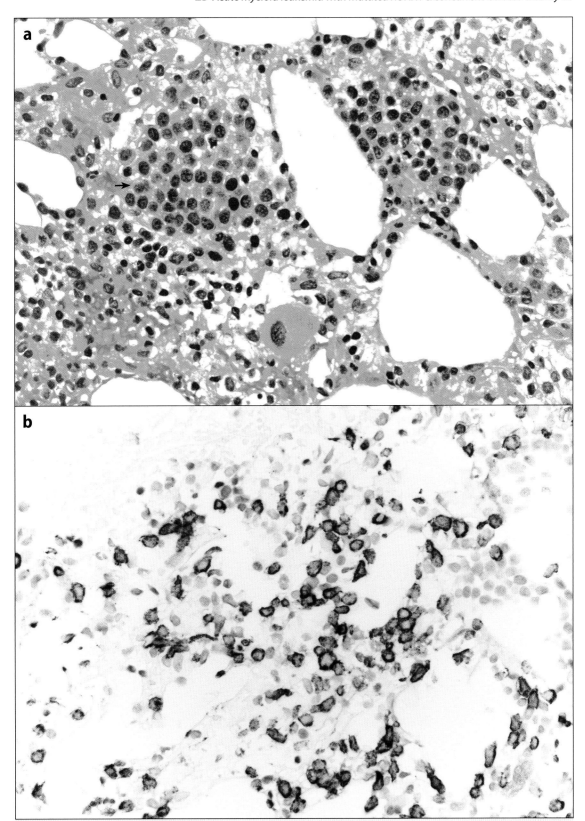

f23.2 Hypercellular clot section showing **a** sheets of small to intermediate-sized blasts (arrow); **b** the blasts are positive for CD34 by immunohistochemical staining

23 *Acute myeloid leukemia with mutated RUNX1 & concurrent isolated trisomy 13*

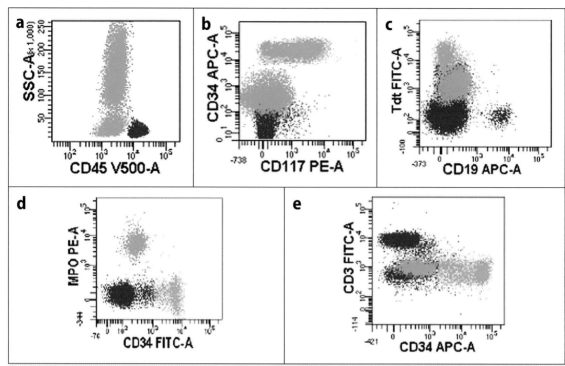

f23.3 Flow cytometry performed on the bone marrow demonstrates **a** a CD45 dim blast population (highlighted in blue), which is positive for **b** CD34 & CD117 (partial) as well as **c** TdT, but negative for CD19, **d** MPO & **e** cytoplasmic CD3; granulocytes are highlighted in green & lymphocytes in red

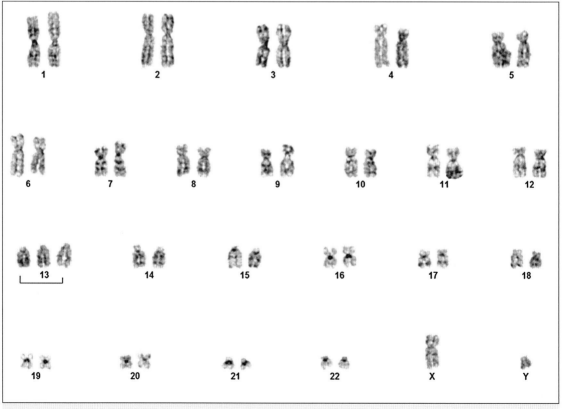

f23.4 Karyotype demonstrating trisomy 13 as the sole cytogenetic abnormality

ISBN 978-089189-6814   ©2021 ASCP

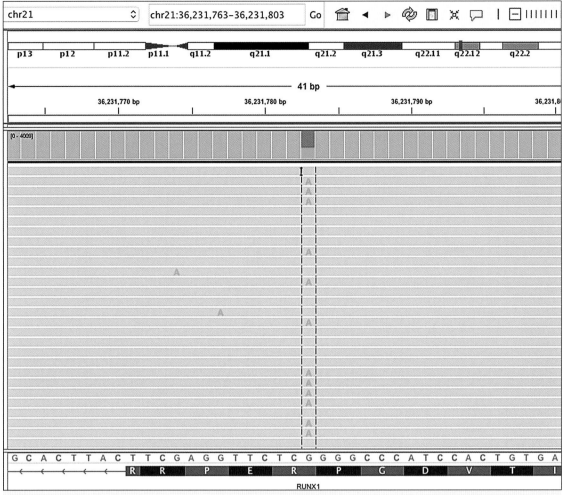

f23.5 Somatic variant analysis using a targeted myeloid NGS panel; annotated reads mapped to the *RUNX1* locus demonstrate p.R174* (c.520C>T), highlighted in green (hg19, Integrative Genomics Viewer browser, showing the reverse strand) [see **fA.8**, p312]

Genetics/molecular results Chromosome analysis identified an abnormal male karyotype with isolated trisomy 13 **f23.4** and FISH studies were negative for AML- or MDS-associated recurrent genetic abnormalities. A myeloid NGS panel revealed several pathogenic variants: *RUNX1* p.R174* (c.520C>T) with a variant allele frequency (VAF) of 41% **f23.5**, *SRSF2* p.P95L (c.284C>T) VAF 30%, and *TET2* p.G223Mfs*28 (c.664_665dupCA) VAF 29%. Based on the morphologic, flow cytometric, and genetic/molecular findings, a final diagnosis of **AML with mutated *RUNX1*** (World Health Organization [WHO] provisional entity) was rendered.

Discussion The transcription factor gene *RUNX1* (runt-related transcription factor 1; formerly *CBFA2/AML1*) on chromosome 21 encodes a master regulator of hematopoiesis whose dysregulation is involved in a number of different hematologic neoplasms. *RUNX1* mutation occurs in 10%-15% of adult AML cases and less frequently in pediatric AML. The *RUNX1* gene is also recurrently rearranged in both B-lymphoblastic leukemia/lymphoma (B-ALL) with t(12;21)(p13.2;q22.1) and AML with t(8;21) (q22;q22.1) (**Case 19**). In addition to AML, inactivating or dominant-negative mutations of *RUNX1* can be seen in MDS, chronic myelomonocytic leukemia, and B-ALL. *RUNX1* mutations are also associated with secondary AML and frequently coincide with the development of MDS/AML in patients with Fanconi anemia and congenital neutropenia.

AML with mutated *RUNX1* is a provisional entity in the 2017 WHO classification of hematologic neoplasms because of its distinct clinicopathologic features. Importantly, this alteration carries negative prognostic significance. To make a diagnosis of AML with mutated *RUNX1*, at least 20% blasts must be present in the peripheral blood and/or bone marrow and other AML-associated recurrent cytogenetic abnormalities, *NPM1* and biallelic *CEBPa* mutations, and criteria for a therapy-related myeloid neoplasm (t-MN) or AML with myelodysplasia-related changes (AML-MRC) must not be present. If a *RUNX1* mutation is detected, especially at a VAF approaching 50%, assessment for a germline mutation should be considered. Congenital *RUNX1* mutations are associated with an autosomal dominant familial platelet disorder with predisposition to hematologic malignancies, which can result in thrombocytopenia, prolonged bleeding, and increased risk of leukemia, although there is significant clinical heterogeneity. Such testing becomes more critical if a family member is being considered as a donor for allogeneic stem cell transplant. The population prevalence of germline *RUNX1* mutation remains to be determined; however, a recent study found that up to 30% of *RUNX1*-mutated AML harbor germline mutations.

Although AML with mutated *RUNX1* does not have a specific blast morphology, cases classified as AML M0 (minimally differentiated) based on the French-American-British (FAB) criteria are enriched for this mutation. In this example case, the blasts had an early stem cell morphology and were negative for MPO and positive for TdT. In such cases, it is critical to exclude lymphoblastic leukemia or mixed phenotype acute leukemia (MPAL) (**Case 53**) by evaluating for appropriate lineage markers. Recurrent genetic abnormalities associated with *RUNX1*-mutated AML include specific trisomies (+8, +13, +21) and frequent mutations in spliceosome and chromatin modifier genes. Correspondingly, molecular testing in this patient identified comutated *SRSF2*, which encodes for a component of the spliceosome complex. *SRSF2* mutations are reportedly specific for secondary AML, and spliceosome mutations are associated with worse prognosis in *RUNX1*-mutated AML. Of note, the patient in this case had a reported history of cytopenias that had not been further evaluated before presentation with AML, so an antecedent MDS could not be excluded.

Trisomy 13 is a rare recurrent event in AML, with isolated +13 accounting for <1% of AML cases. Isolated +13 is enriched in AML M0 and has a high association with *RUNX1* mutation (>75% of cases). However, +13 in the context of a complex karyotype does not seem to correlate with *RUNX1* mutation. The mechanism for leukemogenesis related to +13 may involve upregulation of *FLT3* located at 13q12, because leukemic cells with +13 demonstrate elevated FLT3 expression; it has been postulated that an increased receptor density may facilitate autoactivation of this tyrosine kinase. Interestingly, a study of AML with isolated +13 identified *RUNX1* (75%) and *SRSF2* (81%) as the two most common coexisting genetic changes; recurring comutations in *ASXL1* and *BCOR* were also identified, demonstrating a unique pathobiology for this AML subgroup.

Diagnostic pearls/pitfalls

– Although no specific morphologic finding is associated with AML with mutated *RUNX1*, cases classified as AML M0 based on FAB criteria are enriched for this mutation. The expression of TdT by minimally differentiated blasts necessitates exclusion of acute lymphoblastic leukemia or MPAL using appropriate lymphoid lineage markers (eg, cCD3, CD19, cCD22, CD79a).

– The diagnosis of AML with mutated *RUNX1* requires the exclusion of other recurrent AML-defining genetic changes and must lack criteria for the diagnosis of t-MN or AML-MRC.

– The presence of *RUNX1* mutation with VAF approaching 50% should prompt consideration for germline testing, especially if a relative is being considered as a donor for stem cell transplant. Germline *RUNX1* mutations are associated with a familial platelet disorder with predisposition to hematologic malignancies.

– Isolated trisomy 13 is a rare genetic finding in AML, and if present, suggests the presence of mutated *RUNX1* and poor prognosis. Trisomy 13 in the context of a complex karyotype, however, is not associated with *RUNX1* mutation.

Readings

Dicker F, Haferlach C, Kern W, Haferlach T, Schnittger S. Trisomy 13 is strongly associated with *AML1/RUNX1* mutations and increased FLT3 expression in acute myeloid leukemia. Blood. 2007;110:1308-16. **DOI: 10.1182/blood-2007-02-072595**

Gaidzik VI, Teleanu V, Papaemmanuil E, et al. *RUNX1* mutations in acute myeloid leukemia are associated with distinct clinico-pathologic and genetic features. Leukemia. 2016;30:2160-8. **DOI: 10.1038/leu.2016.126**

Haferlach T, Stengel A, Eckstein S, et al. The new provisional WHO entity '*RUNX1* mutated AML' shows specific genetics but no prognostic influence of dysplasia. Leukemia. 2016;30:2109-12. **DOI: 10.1038/leu.2016.150**

Herold T, Metzeler KH, Vosberg S, et al. Isolated trisomy 13 defines a homogeneous AML subgroup with high frequency of mutations in spliceosome genes and poor prognosis. Blood. 2014;124:1304-11. **DOI: 10.1182/blood-2013-12-540716**

Lindsley RC, Mar BG, Mazzola E, et al. Acute myeloid leukemia ontogeny is defined by distinct somatic mutations. Blood. 2015;125:1367-76. **DOI: 10.1182/blood-2014-11-610543**

Matsuno N, Osato M, Yamashita N, et al. Dual mutations in the *AML1* and *FLT3* genes are associated with leukemogenesis in acute myeloblastic leukemia of the M0 subtype. Leukemia. 2003;17:2492-9. **DOI: 10.1038/sj.leu.2403160**

Schlegelberger B, Heller PG. RUNX1 deficiency (familial platelet disorder with predisposition to myeloid leukemia, FPDMM). Semin Hematol. 2017;54:75-80. **DOI: 10.1053/j.seminhematol.2017.04.006**

Simon L, Spinella J-F, Yao C-Y, et al. High frequency of germline *RUNX1* mutations in patients with *RUNX1*-mutated AML. Blood. 2020;135(21):1882-1886. **DOI: 10.1182/blood.2019003357**

Sood R, Kamikubo Y, Liu P. Role of *RUNX1* in hematological malignancies. Blood. 2017;129:2070-82. **DOI: 10.1182/blood-2017-12-819789**

Christopher Ryder

24

Therapy-related acute myeloid leukemia with t(8;16)(p11.2;p13.3) *KATA-CREBBP*

History A 61-year-old male was experiencing complete remission 1 year after chemoimmunotherapy for high-grade B-cell lymphoma, not otherwise specified. He presented for routine follow-up and was found to have new-onset leukocytosis and thrombocytopenia. CBC is shown at right.

Because of a concern for relapsed lymphoma, a bone marrow biopsy was performed for further evaluation.

WBC	46.1×10^9/L
RBC	4.79×10^{12}/L
HGB	13.9 g/dL
HCT	42.8%
MCV	89 fL
RDW	17.4%
Platelets	40×10^9/L

Morphology & flow cytometry The peripheral blood showed a predominance of large atypical monocytic cells with fine nuclear chromatin and moderately abundant cytoplasm, with some cells demonstrating delicate nuclear clefts consistent with promonocytes **f24.1**. In the bone marrow aspirate smears, blasts and promonocytes were predominant (83%) and, interestingly, some of these cells demonstrated erythrophagocytosis **f24.2**. Occasional small, hypolobated megakaryocytes were also noted in the aspirate **f24.3a**. No significant atypia was identified in residual granulocytic or erythroid precursors. The bone marrow core biopsy was 80%-90% cellular and showed a predominance of immature mononuclear cells; immunohistochemistry for lysozyme (muramidase) highlighted >90% of marrow cells **f24.3b**. Flow cytometric studies identified a large population of monocytic blasts/blast equivalents with high forward and side scatter properties; these cells were negative for CD34 and CD117, positive for HLA-DR, CD33, CD15, CD4, and myeloperoxidase (MPO) and showed heterogeneous CD13, CD14, and CD56 expression **f24.4**. No evidence of a clonal B-cell population was identified. These findings led to a final diagnosis of **therapy-related myeloid neoplasm** (t-MN) presenting as an **acute myeloid leukemia** (AML) **with monocytic differentiation**.

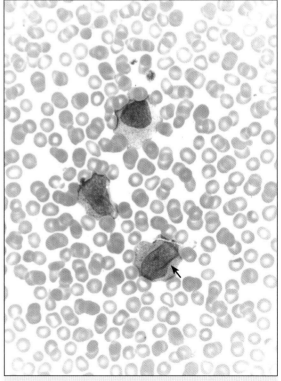

f24.1 Peripheral blood showing blasts with abundant cytoplasm and fine granules; note the delicate nuclear fold (arrow), consistent with a promonocyte

  ISBN 978-089189-6814 ©2021 ASCP

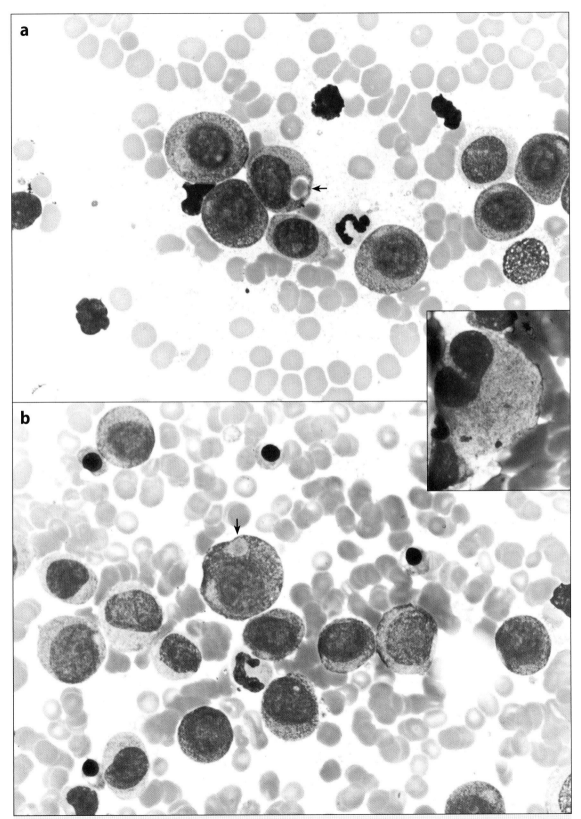

f24.2 Bone marrow showing blasts with more monoblastic morphology than those in peripheral blood, including occasional forms with erythrophagocytosis (denoted by arrows); an example of an atypical megakaryocyte is shown in the inset

24 *Therapy-related acute myeloid leukemia with t(8;16)(p11.2;p13.3) KATA-CREBBP*

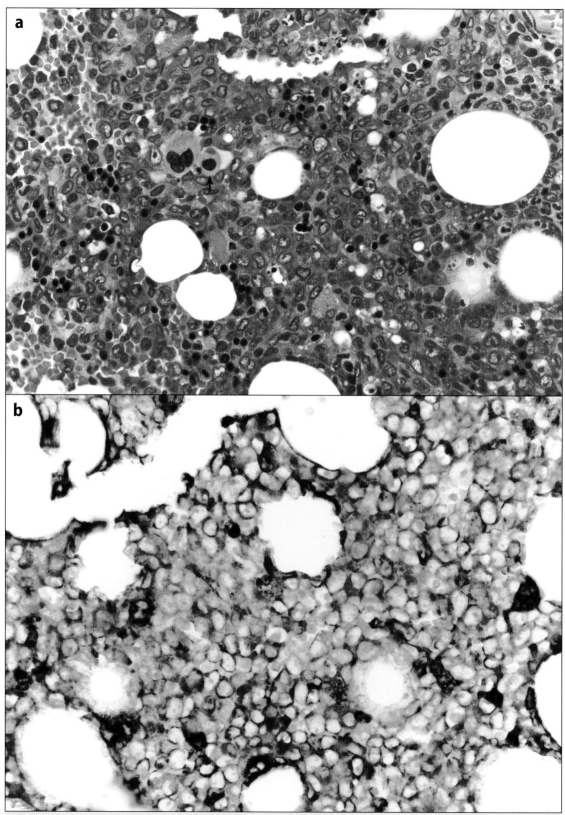

f24.3 a The bone marrow core biopsy demonstrates a predominance of monocytic blasts & occasional small, hypolobated megakaryocytes (arrow); **b** imunostaining for lysozyme highlights the monocytic infiltrate

ISBN 978-089189-6814   ©2021 ASCP

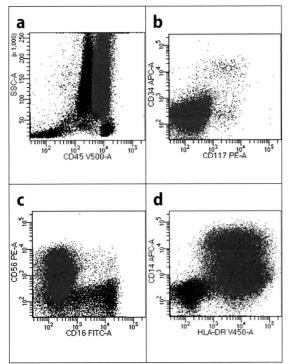

f24.4 Flow cytometry demonstrates **a** a large population of atypical cells (colored in red) with high side scatter that **b** are negative for CD34 & CD117, positive for **c** CD56 & **d** variably positive for CD14, indicating monocytic differentiation

Genetics/molecular results Karyotype revealed the presence of t(8;16)(p11.2;p13.3) in 8 of 20 metaphases as the sole cytogenetic abnormality **f24.5**. FISH studies were negative for any typical recurrent chromosomal abnormality associated with AML. Molecular studies, including NGS, identified only a nonsense mutation in *TET2* (p.Q1532*; c.4594C>T) with a variant allele frequency of 46%.

Discussion The translocation t(8;16)(p11.2;p13.3) is a rare, recurrent cytogenetic abnormality in AML (<1% of cases). Although AML cases with this translocation appear to exhibit unique clinicopathologic features, such cases are not currently a distinct entity recognized by the 2017 World Health Organization classification of hematopoietic neoplasms. Published case series of this rare entity have noted clinical associations with leukemia cutis, coagulopathy, and poor prognosis, although prognosis may depend on the clinical scenario (as described later in this case). In this example case, the patient did not exhibit skin findings but did have an elevated D-dimer and mildly prolonged prothrombin time without apparent bleeding complications. The patient had a relapse <3 months after completion of standard induction therapy.

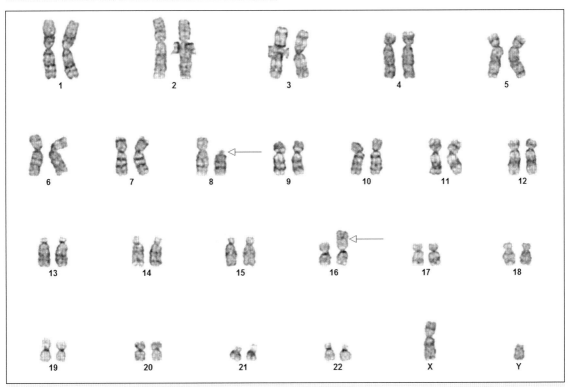

f24.5 Karyotype showing t(8;16)(p11.2p13.3) with arrows denoting the truncated chromosome 8 missing a portion of the p arm & an abnormal chromosome 16 containing the p arm material from chromosome 8

From a morphologic and phenotypic standpoint, AML with t(8;16) tends to have monocytic or myelomonocytic features and frequently shows dual positivity for nonspecific esterase and MPO. Notably, a majority of cases show erythrophagocytosis by blasts. The identification of erythrophagocytosis by leukemic blasts should prompt the consideration of testing for the t(8;16) translocation and/or variant translocations involving the *KAT6A* gene on chromosome 8. The monocytic appearance of blasts and association with coagulopathy may raise clinical suspicion for microgranular acute promyelocytic leukemia (APL; see **Case 20**), but the 2 diseases show distinct immunophenotypes, with t(8;16) AML blasts generally being negative for CD34 and CD117 and positive for HLA-DR, monocytic markers, and CD56, whereas APL blasts are typically positive for CD117 and negative for CD34 and HLA-DR.

The translocation t(8;16)(p11.2;p13.3) results in fusion of the 5' region of *KAT6A (*also known as *MYST3, MOZ)* on chromosome 8 with the 3' end of *CREBBP (*also known as *CBP, KAT3A)* on chromosome 16, both of which encode proteins with histone acetyltransferase activity. The exact role of the resultant fusion protein in leukemogenesis is not well established but the proteins encoded by *KAT6A* and *CREBBP* have known roles in hematopoiesis. Preclinical studies show similarities in function between *KAT6A* and *KMT2A (MLL)*. In line with these observations, t(8;16) AML shows a gene expression profile similar to that of *MLL*-rearranged AML and translocations involving both genes have a tendency to occur in therapy-related myeloid neoplasms having monocytic differentiation and short latency (see **Case 25**). Moreover, *KMT2A (MLL)* has even been reported to be fused with *CREBBP* in AML.

The mutational landscape of t(8;16) AML has not been well-characterized, but various mutations have been reported in a handful of cases including *RUNX1, ASXL1, FLT3,* and *DNMT3A,* among others.. In the example case, the presence of a *TET2* mutation may represent a cooperative leukemogenic event, a bystander mutation, or preexisting age-related clonal hematopoiesis.

AML with t(8;16) has primarily been described in 2 settings: as a t-MN and as a pediatric (or even congenital) AML. In the therapy-related setting, the observed interval from treatment for primary malignancy to t-MN is often short and lacks a preleukemic (myelodyspastic) phase. In adult case series, AML with t(8;16) shows a poor prognosis, likely related to the high rate of t-MN in this cohort. In the pediatric setting, AML with t(8;16) shows an intermediate risk; however, spontaneous remission may ensue in congenital cases (diagnosed <1 month of age). These patients may benefit from a "watch-and-wait" management approach, although only a subset of these cases achieves sustained remission (akin to the natural history of transient abnormal myelopoiesis of Down syndrome [see **Case 28**]). Therefore, close clinical monitoring is necessary in pediatric cases of AML with t(8;16).

Although there is a strong association of erythrophagocytosis with t(8;16) AML, this unique morphologic feature is not specific to leukemias harboring this translocation. Cases of AML with inv(8)(p11q13) and t(16;21)(p11q22) have also been reported to show this phenomenon, as well as rare case reports of AML with other genetic findings, B-lymphoblastic leukemia/lymphoma (B-ALL), and even T-lymphoblastic leukemia/lymphoma (T-ALL).

Diagnostic pearls/pitfalls
– The t(8;16)(p11.2;p13.3) translocation is associated with therapy-related myeloid neoplasm, presenting as AML with monocytic differentiation and erythrophagocytosis by blasts; testing for this gene rearrangement should be considered in cases in which these morphologic features are observed.
– Cases of AML with t(8;16) may occasionally present both clinically and morphologically like APL, with coagulopathy and promonocytic morphology that may mimic a microgranular APL. However, the blast immunophenotype is usually distinct between the 2 diseases, with t(8;16) AML generally being CD117-negative, HLA-DR-positive, and CD34-negative, whereas APL is typically CD117-positive, HLA-DR-negative, and CD34-negative.
– Some pediatric/congenital AML cases with t(8;16) demonstrate spontaneous remission and may benefit from close observation.

ISBN 978-089189-6814 ©2021 ASCP

Readings

Cha WI, Hannah RL, Dawson MA, et al. The transcriptional coactivator Cbp regulates self-renewal and differentiation in adult hematopoietic stem cells. Mol Cell Biol. 2011;31:5046-60. **DOI: 10.1128/MCB.05830-11**

Coenen EA, Zwaan CM, Reinhardt D, et al. Pediatric acute myeloid leukemia with t(8;16)(p11;p13), a distinct clinical and biological entity: a collaborative study by the International-Berlin-Frankfurt-Munster AML-study group. Blood. 2013;122:2704-13. **DOI: 10.1182/blood-2013-02-485524**

Diab A, Zickl L, Abdel-Wahab O, et al. Acute myeloid leukemia with translocation t(8;16) presents with features which mimic acute promyelocytic leukemia and is associated with poor prognosis. Leuk Res. 2013;37:32-6. **DOI: 10.1016/j.leukres.2012.08.025**

Haferlach T, Kohlmann A, Klein HU, et al. AML with translocation t(8;16)(p11;p13) demonstrates unique cytomorphological, cytogenetic, molecular and prognostic features. Leukemia. 2009;23:934-43. **DOI: 10.1038/leu.2008.388**

Sheikh BN, Yang Y, Schreuder J, et al. MOZ (*KAT6A*) is essential for the maintenance of classically defined adult hematopoietic stem cells. Blood. 2016;128:2307-18. **DOI: 10.1182/blood-2015-10-676072**

Sobulo OM, Borrow J, Tomek R, et al. MLL is fused to CBP, a histone acetyltransferase, in therapy-related acute myeloid leukemia with a t(11;16)(q23;p13.3). Proc Natl Acad Sci U S A. 1997;94:8732-7. **DOI: 10.1073/pnas.94.16.8732**

Xie W, Hu S, Xu J, Chen Z, Medeiros LJ, Tang G. Acute myeloid leukemia with t(8;16)(p11.2;p13.3)/*KAT6A-CREBBP* in adults. Ann Hematol. 2019 May;98(5):1149-1157. **DOI: 10.1007/s00277-019-03637-7**

Kwadwo A Oduro & Rose C Beck

25

Therapy-related myeloid neoplasm presenting as a myeloid sarcoma with rearrangement of *KMT2A* (*MLL*)

History A 54-year-old female with a history of breast cancer (invasive ductal carcinoma), diagnosed 4 years prior and treated with surgery and adjuvant chemotherapy (cyclophosphamide, docetaxel and anti-estrogens), presented with knee pain. X-ray was negative but MRI revealed a 2.5-cm tibial lesion. A biopsy of the lesion was nondiagnostic, showing only sclerosis with remodeling changes, and the pain resolved with physical therapy. Initial follow up PET/CT and MRI showed no significant changes. However, followup MRI 1 year later showed growth of the tibial lesion, now measuring 6 cm, as well as new lesions in the femur and fibula. CBC and differential were performed and were normal (selected results are shown at right). A biopsy of the tibial lesion was performed. Based on the results of tibial biopsy, an iliac crest bone marrow biopsy and aspiration were also performed.

Morphology & flow cytometry Histologic sections of the tibial lesion demonstrated a diffuse infiltrate of medium-sized, discohesive cells with a moderate amount of cytoplasm and irregular nuclear contours with dispersed chromatin **f25.1**. There was prominent crush artifact and abundant associated reactive bone. The morphologic findings were consistent with a hematologic neoplasm rather than metastatic breast carcinoma. IHC demonstrated that the neoplasm was positive for CD45, Pax5, c-myc, and bcl-2. The tumor cells were negative for all other B-cell markers (CD20, CD19, CD79a, OCT-2, Bob.1), T-cell markers (CD3, CD2, CD5, CD8), and markers of immaturity (CD34, CD117, TdT, CD10), as well as myeloperoxidase (MPO), cyclin D1, and CD30. Based on the tibial biopsy, an unusual hematopoietic neoplasm was suspected.

WBC	4.5×10^9/L
HGB	12 g/dL
Platelets	221×10^9/L

A bone marrow biopsy revealed a hypercellular marrow completely replaced by tumor cells **f25.2**. The aspirate smear revealed 52% blasts with ovoid to mildly irregular nuclei, fine chromatin, single nucleoli, and variably abundant cytoplasm, morphologically consistent with monoblasts. A cytochemical stain for nonspecific esterase (NSE) was positive in these cells. Flow cytometry **f25.3** confirmed the presence of atypical myeloid cells with an immunophenotype suggestive of monocytic differentiation: positive for CD33, CD15, CD64, HLA-DR, CD4 (dim), CD56 (dim), and negative for CD34, CD117, and MPO. CD14 was also negative. Furthermore, additional IHC revealed that the tumor cells in both the iliac crest biopsy and tibial lesion expressed lysozyme **f25.1d** as well as Pax5.

The overall findings indicated a diagnosis of **myeloid sarcoma and acute myeloid leukemia** (AML) **with monocytic differentiation, therapy-related**.

25 *Therapy-related myeloid neoplasm presenting as a myeloid sarcoma with rearrangement of KMT2A (MLL)*

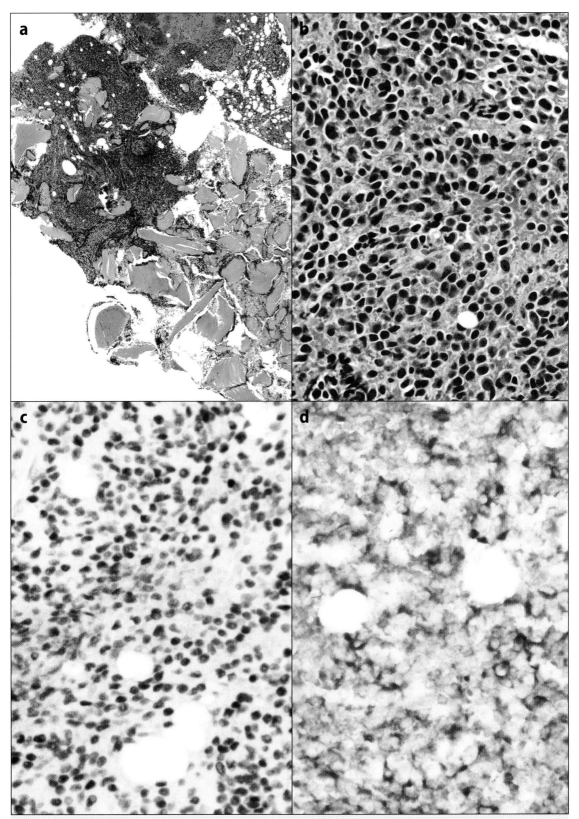

f25.1 Images of the tibial lesion demonstrate **a** a destructive mass of **b** small mononuclear cells that are positive for **c** PAX5 by IHC; **d** a lysozyme stain performed after the initial evaluation is also positive in the infiltrate

25 Therapy-related myeloid neoplasm presenting as a myeloid sarcoma with rearrangement of KMT2A (MLL)

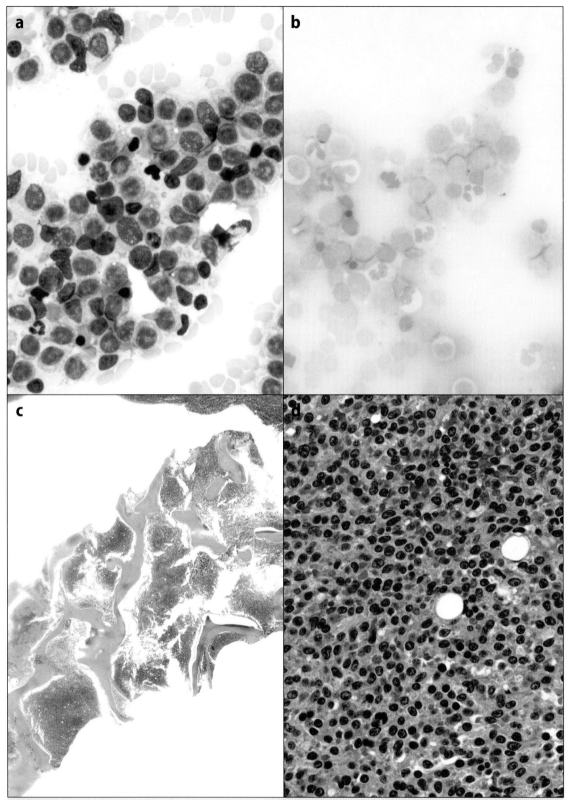

f25.2 **a** Sheets of atypical monocytic cells are present in the bone marrow aspirate smear with blasts that are **b** positive for nonspecific esterase (brown staining); **c** the core biopsy likewise shows **d** sheets of atypical mononuclear cells, similar in histology to those present in the tibial lesion

25 Therapy-related myeloid neoplasm presenting as a myeloid sarcoma with rearrangement of KMT2A (MLL)

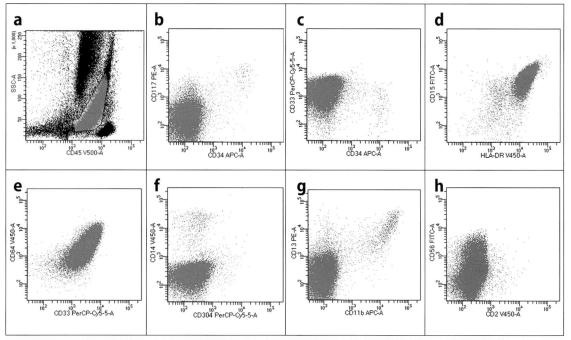

f25.3 Flow cytometry delineates an atypical myeloid population with **a** dim to moderate CD45 expression & high side scatter, at 54% of total events (highlighted in orange). The atypical population is **b** negative for the immature blast markers CD34 & CD117 but **c-e** positive for the monocytic markers CD33, CD15, HLA-DR & CD64. It is also **f-g** negative for CD14, CD304, CD13, and CD11b, although **h** dim aberrant CD56 expression is present

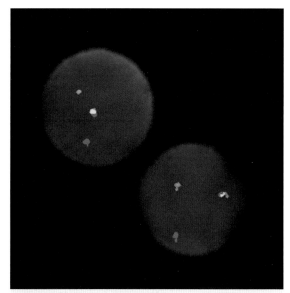

f25.4 Break-apart FISH probes for *KMT2A* (*MLL*) rearrangement demonstrate splitting of 1 yellow into separate orange & green signals, indicating presence of rearrangement

Genetics/molecular results The karyotype showed 46,XX in a total of 7 metaphases and was considered suboptimal because of low cell recovery. FISH using a break-apart probe for *KMT2A* (*MLL*) at 11q23 was positive for a *KMT2A* rearrangement in 74% of the cells **f25.4**; FISH for all other recurrent abnormalities in AML was negative. Additional FISH using dual fusion probes confirmed the presence of t(9;11) *MLLT3-KMT2A* fusion in 53% of cells. A targeted myeloid NGS panel identified only a DNMT3A p.N838Afs*13 (c.2512_2522del11) variant in 29% of reads.

Discussion Most of the time AML presents as "leukemic" disease with circulating blasts and associated cytopenias. However, rarely, AML manifests as a masslike lesion(s), referred to traditionally as a "myeloid sarcoma." Myeloid sarcomas may not necessarily be accompanied by morphologic evidence of peripheral blood or bone marrow involvement, but if left untreated, a leukemic phase will typically ensue. In some cases, myeloid sarcoma may be detected in a patient with a history of AML, as a manifestation of persistent or relapsed disease. Despite its name, it is important that myeloid sarcoma be treated systemically as AML and not as a soft tissue neoplasm, even when a circulating or medullary component is not present.

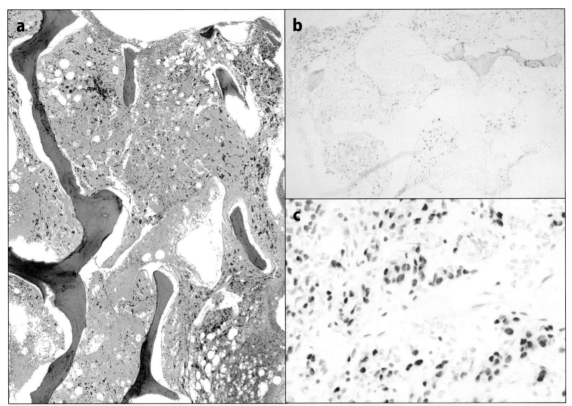

f25.5 Follow-up bone marrow biopsy 14 days after induction of therapy, showing **a** hypocellular bone marrow with **b, c** residual leukemia readily detected by Pax5 IHC

Myeloid sarcoma can be particularly challenging to diagnose in patients without a prior diagnosis of AML. The site of involvement can be variable and is most often in a nonhematopoietic tissue. Thus, neoplasm of hematopoietic origin may not be readily considered in the differential diagnosis and appropriate stains may not be applied until later in the evaluation. Furthermore, AML with monocytic differentiation, including most cases of AML with *KMT2A (MLL)* rearrangement, frequently lack expression of common myeloblast markers such as CD34, CD117, and MPO; these monocytic AMLs have a higher tendency for tissue infiltration compared with other AMLs. In the example case, clinically and radiologically, the patient was thought to have metastatic breast cancer. Even when morphologic findings suggested a hematologic neoplasm, the initial IHC performed on the tibial lesion could not establish a diagnosis.

Evaluation of the tibial lesion was complicated by the observed aberrant strong expression of Pax5, which initially suggested a B-lymphoid neoplasm, although the paradoxical lack of other B-cell markers indicated the need for additional studies. B-cell marker expression by AML has been described for AMLs with

aberrations involving *RUNX1,* such as AML with t(8;21) *RUNX1-RUNX1T1*, which can show expression of Pax5, CD19, or CD79a (see **Case 19**). However, expression of these B-cell markers is typically weak and/or partial, unlike the strong diffuse Pax5 staining present in this case. Interestingly, although initially confusing, the strong Pax5 expression was diagnostically helpful in follow-up biopsies for highlighting residual leukemic blasts, which lacked expression of CD34 or CD117 **f25.5**. Notably, Pax5 expression by itself is insufficient for defining B-cell lineage to evaluate for B/myeloid mixed phenotype acute leukemia (MPAL; **Case 53**). It is interesting to note that *KMT2A (MLL)* rearrangements occur not just in AML but also in acute lymphoblastic leukemia and B/myeloid MPAL, highlighting the lineage promiscuity that can occur in association with this genetic abnormality (see **Case 47** for additional discussion of 11q23 rearrangements in acute leukemia).

According to the 2017 World Health Organization criteria, this patient's disease is best classified as a therapy-related myeloid neoplasm (t-MN) based on the history of prior chemotherapy with cyclophosphamide, an alkylating agent. t-MN occurring after alkylating agents tend to be associated with a complex karyotype and 17p abnormalities as well as a longer latency period (~5-7 years after treatment). In contrast, t-MNs with *KMT2A (MLL)* rearrangements most often occur after topoisomerase or radiation therapy (both not received by this patient), with a shorter latency of 1-3 years. The designation of t-MN is significant for risk stratification, because de novo AML with t(9;11) *MLLT3-KMT2A* is considered an intermediate risk by the National Comprehensive Care Network, whereas t-MN is considered high-risk disease. It is important to note that other *KMT2A (MLL)* rearrangements in AML are considered high risk, underscoring the necessity of determining the specific 11q23 rearrangement in all cases with karyotyping or FISH using dual fusion probes. Identification of the specific *KMT2A (MLL)* rearrangement also provides a molecular target for assessment of residual disease. Specialized techniques for detecting low-level individual *KMT2A (MLL)* fusions include quantitative reverse transcriptase PCR, digital droplet PCR, or NGS; some are commercially available, but their clinical usefulness is still being evaluated.

Diagnostic pearls/pitfalls

– AML can present as a mass lesion, myeloid sarcoma, in unusual locations and should be considered in the differential diagnosis when an undifferentiated neoplastic lesion is difficult to classify.

– Monocytic leukemias often lack expression of common myeloblast markers (CD34, CD117, MPO). High-quality touch prep or aspirate smears are critical for evaluating atypical monocytic populations in bone marrow, whereas NSE cytochemistry, lysozyme immunostain, and flow cytometry can be helpful in identifying monocytic differentiation.

– Aberrant B-cell marker expression can occur in AML and does not warrant a classification of a MPAL. An aberrant immunophenotype can be diagnostically useful for detecting persistent or relapsed disease.

– *KMT2A* rearrangement is one of the classic genetic abnormalities seen in t-MN but also occurs in de novo AML and acute lymphoblastic leukemia. Identifying the specific translocation partner is important for risk stratification in AML and may be useful for disease monitoring.

Readings

Afrin S, Zhang CRC, Meyer C, et al. Targeted next-generation sequencing for detecting *MLL* gene fusions in leukemia. Mol Cancer Res. 2018;16(2):279-85.
DOI: 10.1158/1541-7786.MCR-17-0569

Afrin S, Zhang CRC, Meyer C, et al. Quantitative analysis of MLL fusion transcripts by droplet digital PCR to monitor minimal residual disease in *MLL*-rearranged acute myeloid leukemia [abstract]. Blood. 2018;132(suppl 1):2746.
DOI: 10.1182/blood-2018-99-117761

Hokland P, Ommen HB, Nyvold CG et al 2012. Sensitivity of minimal residual disease in acute myeloid leukaemia in first remission: methodologies in relation to their clinical situation. Br J Haematol. 2012;158(5):569-80.
DOI: 10.1111/j.1365-2141.2012.09203.x

Liu J, Wang Y, Xu LP, et al. Monitoring mixed lineage leukemia expression may help identify patients with mixed lineage leukemia--rearranged acute leukemia who are at high risk of relapse after allogeneic hematopoietic stem cell transplantation. Biol Blood Marrow Transplant. 2014;20(7):929-36.
DOI: 10.1016/j.bbmt.2014.03.008

Meyer C, Burmeister T, Gröger D, et al. The *MLL* recombinome of acute leukemias in 2017. Leukemia. 2018;32(2):273-84.
DOI: 10.1038/leu.2017.213

O'Donnell MR, Tallman MS, Altman JK, et al, 2019. NCCN guidelines version 3.2020: acute myeloid leukemia.
https://www.nccn.org/professionals/physician_gls/pdf/aml.pdf

Swerdlow SH, Campo E, Harris NL, et al. World Health Organization Classification of Tumours of Haematopoietic and Lymphoid Tissues. 4th ed. Lyon, France: IARC Press; 2017.
ISBN: 9789283244943

Rose C Beck

26

Therapy-related acute myeloid leukemia with complex karyotype including amplification of *KMT2A* (*MLL*)

History A 69-year-old female had a history of chronic lymphocytic leukemia, treated with chemotherapy, with subsequent development of myelodysplastic syndrome (MDS) several years later. She was started on azacytidine; after 2 cycles, she presented to her physician with fever, nonproductive cough, and increasing fatigue. She was admitted for neutropenic fever. CBC results are shown at right. A blood smear review was performed.

Morphology & flow cytometry The peripheral blood smear showed granulocytic left shift with hypogranularity as well as 30% blasts, which were medium to large in size and had high nuclear:cytoplasmic ratios. The blast morphology was not suggestive of acute promyelocytic leukemia **f26.1**.

A bone marrow biopsy was performed and the aspirate smear demonstrated 40% blasts with significant erythroid dysplasia, including prominent megaloblastoid change, and megakaryocytic dysplasia **f26.2**. Flow cytometry of the bone marrow demonstrated 32% blasts with a typical myeloid phenotype including positivity for CD34, CD117, CD33, HLA-DR, and CD13 **f26.3**. Based on the morphologic and immunophenotypic findings as well as the patient's history of treated CLL, a diagnosis of **acute myeloid leukemia** (AML), **therapy-related**, was made.

Genetics/molecular results The karyotype **f26.4** was complex and showed: 45,XX, −5, −7, add(11)(q25), −19,+mar1,+mar2[16]/45,idem, add(7)(q11.2), −add(11), −17, +mar3[4].

WBC	2.7×10^9/L
HGB	6.5 g/dL
HCT	19.3%
MCV	99 fL
Platelets	66×10^9/L

Two related clones were identified; both shared monosomy of 5, 7, and 19, as well as 2 marker chromosomes of unknown origin. The larger clone also contained an abnormal chromosome 11 with a large segment of indistinctly banded additional material on the long arm, consistent with amplification of genomic sequence via a homogeneously staining region (HSR). The marker 1 chromosome also contained a similar region, also suggesting the presence of an additional HSR.

FISH studies confirmed the presence of monosomies of 5 and 7. In addition, multiple copies of the *KMT2A* (*MLL*) probe were seen and, on metaphase FISH, corresponded to the HSR observed on chromosome 11, consistent with amplification of the *KMT2A* region at 11q23, without rearrangement **f26.5**.

Limited molecular studies were performed and were negative for mutations in *FLT3*, *NPM1*, or *CEBPA*.

26 *Therapy-related acute myeloid leukemia with complex karyotype including amplification of KMT2A (MLL)*

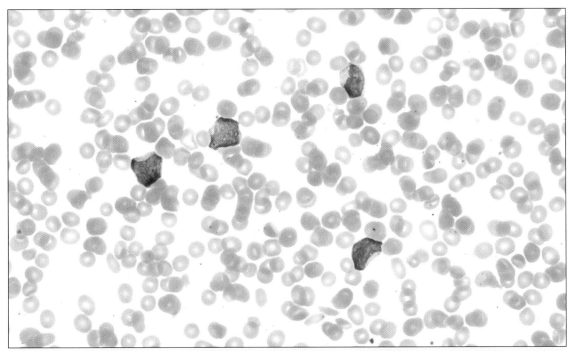

f26.1 Peripheral blood showing blasts with high nuclear:cytoplasmic ratios as well as granulocytic left shift with dysplasia

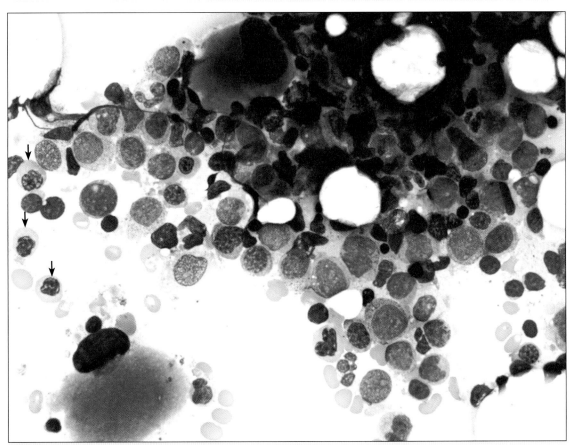

f26.2 Bone marrow aspirate containing increased blasts, erythroid cells with dysplasia & megaloblastoid change (arrows) & hypolobated megakaryocytes

26 *Therapy-related acute myeloid leukemia with complex karyotype including amplification of KMT2A (MLL)*

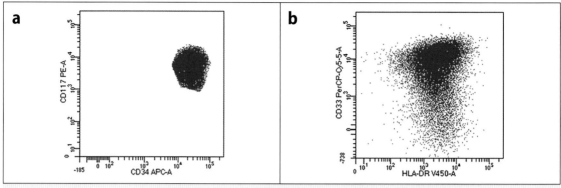

f26.3 Flow cytometry demonstrating 32% **a** CD34-positive, CD117-positive myeloblasts which also express **b** CD33 & HLA-DR

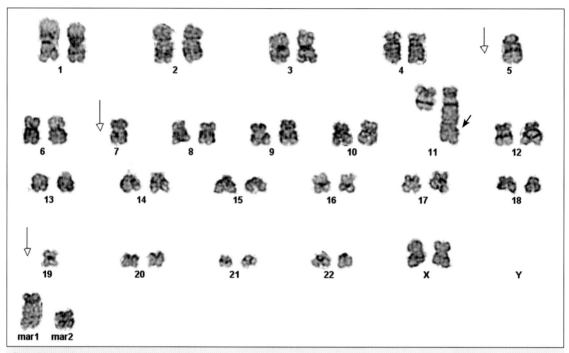

f26.4 The predominant clone in the karyotype demonstrates monosomy 5, 7, and 19 (light arrows), as well as a homogenously staining region (HSR) on 11q (dark arrow) and two marker chromosomes ("mar1" and "mar2")

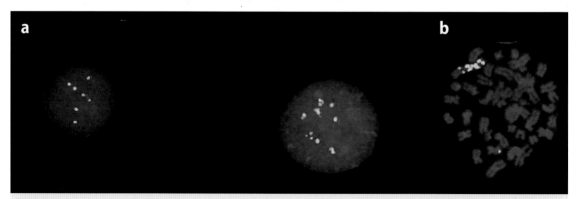

f26.5 **a** Break-apart probe for *KMT2A* at 11q23 (yellow, consisting of 1 orange & 1 green signal in juxtaposition) shows multiple intact signals within each nucleus, consistent with amplification of *KMT2A* without rearrangement; **b** on metaphase FISH, these signals are contained on a single chromosome, corresponding to the homogeneously staining region on chromosome 11 observed on karyotyping

ISBN 978-089189-6814 ©2021 ASCP

Discussion Therapy-related myeloid neoplasm (t-MN) is defined in the 2017 World Health Organization classification hematopoietic neoplasms as cases of AML, myelodysplastic syndrome (MDS), or MDS/myeloproliferative neoplasm that occur after cytotoxic chemotherapy or radiation therapy administered for a prior neoplastic process. The most commonly associated cytotoxic agents include alkylating agents (eg, melphalan, cyclophosphamide, nitrogen compounds, platinum-containing agents) and topoisomerase inhibitors (eg, etoposide, doxorubicin, mitoxantrone). t-MNs arising from alkylating agents or radiation typically occur at least 3 years after treatment, usually present with bone marrow failure and MDS, and are associated with complex karyotypes including unbalanced chromosome abnormalities. In contrast, t-MNs arising from topoisomerase inhibitors typically occur within 1-5 years of treatment and tend to present as AML with balanced translocations, most commonly involving the *KMT2A (MLL)* gene at 11q23, though therapy-related cases of AML with t(8;21)(q22;q22.1), t(15;17)(q24.1;q21.1), or inv(16)(p13.1q22) also occur. Although therapy-related hematopoietic neoplasms are most commonly myeloid, rare cases of acute lymphoblastic leukemia (ALL) have been reported; these cases typically also have chromosomal rearrangements involving 11q23. In general, therapy-related neoplasms portend a poor prognosis and are often refractory to treatment.

Unbalanced abnormalities of chromosomes 5 and 7, as seen in this case, are common in the complex karyotypes seen in t-MN resulting from alkylating agent therapy. Mutations of *TP53* at chromosome 17p are also common (assay not performed in this patient). In this case, the presence of *KMT2A (MLL)* amplification was also detected. *KMT2A* gene amplification, variably defined as >3-5 copies of *KMT2A* identified by FISH, is a rare genetic finding in hematopoietic neoplasms and is most commonly seen in AML or MDS, especially therapy-related cases. Clinically, this unusual genetic finding is associated with coagulopathy, including disseminated intravascular coagulation, and resistance to therapy, with median overall survival of only 1 month in a series of 21 patients with AML or MDS. Interestingly, rare cases of therapy-related B-cell ALL with *KMT2A* amplification have been reported, reiterating the importance of *KMT2A* in the pathogenesis of therapy-related hematopoietic neoplasms. See **Cases 25 & 47** for discussion of *KMT2A* rearrangements in acute leukemias.

Recent case-control studies have associated preexisting age-related clonal hematopoiesis with increased incidence of t-MN in patients who received chemotherapy. Stem cells carrying somatic myeloid mutations, especially in *TP53*, are hypothesized to be chemoresistant and to preferentially expand after cytotoxic therapy, contributing to the development of t-MN.

Unfortunately, in this patient, follow-up bone marrow biopsy performed after four cycles of induction chemotherapy demonstrated 63% blasts, consistent with refractory leukemia, and the patient elected to go to hospice care.

Diagnostic pearls/pitfalls

- Patients who have received cytotoxic therapy or ionizing radiation are at increased risk for secondary hematologic neoplasms, most commonly of the myeloid type, but rarely of the lymphoid type.
- The 2 main subtypes of t-MNs, those occurring after alkylating agents and those occurring after topoisomerase inhibitors, have distinct clinical courses and genetic findings.
- The term "homogeneously staining region (HSR)" refers to an intrachromosomal region with uniform staining by G-banding, indicative of gene amplification.
- AML presenting with prominent background dysplasia may meet criteria for t-MN or AML with myelodysplasia-related changes (in the absence of *NPM1* mutation), and knowledge of clinical history is necessary to make the distinction.

Readings

Chua CC, Fleming S, Wei AH. Clinicopathological aspects of therapy-related acute myeloid leukemia and myelodysplastic syndrome. Best Pract Res Clin Haematol. 2019;32:3-12. **DOI: 10.1016/j.beha.2019.02.007**

Desai P, Roboz GJ. Clonal hematopoiesis and therapy related MDS/AML. Best Pract Res Clin Haematol. 2019;32:13-23. **DOI: 10.1016/j.beha.2019.02.006**

Racke F, Cole C, Walker A, Jones J, Heerema NA. Therapy-related pro-B cell acute lymphoblastic leukemia: report of two patients with MLL amplification. Cancer Genet. 2012;205:653-6. **DOI: 10.1016/j.cancergen.2012.11.001**

Swerdlow SH, Campo E, Harris NL, et al. World Health Organization Classification of Tumours of Haematopoietic and Lymphoid Tissues. 4th ed. Lyon, France: IARC Press; 2017. **ISBN: 9789283244943**

Tang G, DiNardo C, Zhang L, et al. MLL gene amplification in acute myeloid leukemia and myelodysplastic syndromes is associated with characteristic clinicopathological findings and TP53 gene mutation. Hum Pathol. 2015;46:65-73. **DOI: 10.1016/j.humpath.2014.09.008**

Erika M Moore

27

Acute megakaryoblastic leukemia with RAM phenotype & *CFBA2T3-GLIS2*

History A 15-month-old female presented with intermittent fevers for 3 weeks and hesitancy to walk on her right leg. CBC results are shown at right. Morphologic review of the blood smear showed only rare atypical lymphocytes. Magnetic resonance imaging of the right femur showed focal areas of altered marrow signal and heterogeneous enhancement.

Morphology & flow cytometry A bone marrow biopsy specimen was obtained and the aspirate smear demonstrated numerous intermediate-sized to large blasts with fine chromatin, inconspicuous nucleoli, a variable amount of basophilic cytoplasm, and cytoplasmic blebbing, with markedly decreased background hematopoiesis. The core biopsy was 100% cellular with sheets of blasts **f27.1**.

Flow cytometry showed 53% blasts with the following immunophenotype: dim to negative CD45, HLA-DR negative, partial CD34, dim CD117, bright CD56, moderate CD33, dim to negative CD38, and partial CD41, CD61, and CD36 **f27.2**. Myeloperoxidase (MPO) staining was negative. Based on the morphologic and flow cytometric findings, a diagnosis of **acute megakaryoblastic leukemia** was rendered.

Genetics/molecular results Cytogenetics showed an abnormal female karyotype with trisomy 3 in 9 of 20 metaphases **f27.3**. FISH studies demonstrated gain of 3q21 and 3q26, consistent with the identified trisomy 3 **f27.4**. Additional FISH studies were negative for inversion 3, t(3;3), t(8;21), *KMT2A (MLL)*

WBC	4.7×10^9/L
RBC	2.83×10^{12}/L
HGB	7.6 g/dL
HCT	23.2%
MCV	82 fL
RDW	14.9%
Platelets	237×10^9/L

rearrangement, t(15;17), t(6;9), inv(16), *TP53* deletion, trisomy 8, and deletions of 5q/5 and 7/7q. A targeted myeloid NGS panel was negative for myeloid-associated mutations including *FLT3*. Additional testing via the Children's Oncology Group demonstrated a *CBFA2T3-GLIS2* fusion transcript using PCR.

ISBN 978-089189-6814 ©2021 ASCP

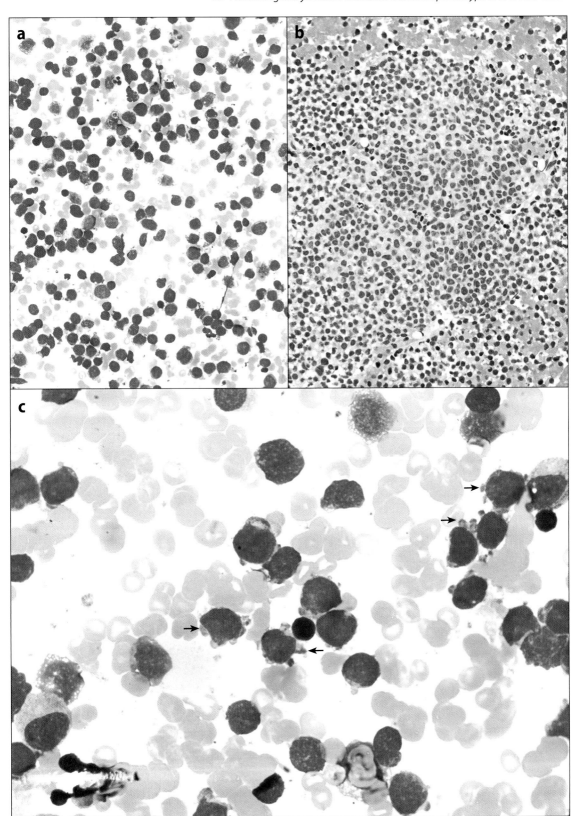

f27.1 **a** Bone marrow aspirate & **b** bone marrow clot section showing sheets of blasts without significant residual hematopoiesis; **c** bone marrow aspirate smear showing intermediate-sized to large blasts with cytoplasmic blebs (arrows)

27 Acute megakaryoblastic leukemia with RAM phenotype & CFBA2T3-GLIS2

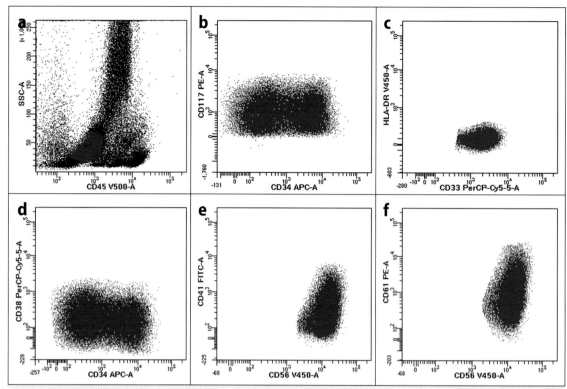

f27.2 Flow cytometry demonstrating megakaryoblasts (highlighted in red), which are **a** dim to negative for CD45, **b** CD34 partial positive, CD117 positive, **c** HLA-DR negative, CD33 positive, **d** CD38 dim to negative, **e-f** CD56 bright positive, and partially positive for CD41 & CD61

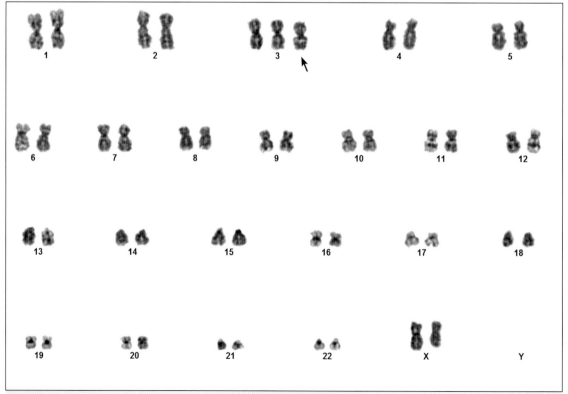

f27.3 Karyotype demonstrating trisomy 3 as the sole cytogenetic abnormality

ISBN 978-089189-6814   ©2021 ASCP

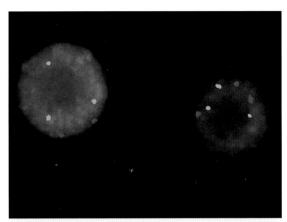

f27.4 FISH for *RPN1* (green) & *MECOM* (orange) demonstrating 3 *RPN1* signals & 3 *MECOM* signals, both of which hybridize to the 3q region, consistent with the trisomy 3 seen on karyotype

Discussion Acute megakaryoblastic leukemia, also known as M7 in the French-American-British classification of acute myeloid leukemia (AML), is a rare subtype of AML comprising <5% of AML cases, occurring in both pediatric and adult patients. By definition, at least half of the blasts present are of megakaryocytic lineage. In the absence of evidence for AML with myelodysplasia-related changes, therapy-related myeloid neoplasm, AML with recurrent genetic abnormality or Down syndrome, acute megakaryoblastic leukemia is classified as AML, not otherwise specified (NOS), in the 2017 World Health Organization (WHO) classification of hematologic neoplasms. Specific WHO subclassifications of AML which frequently present as megakaryoblastic leukemia include AML with the recurrent cytogenetic abnormality t(1;22)(p13.3;q13.1), which occurs predominantly in infants and children <3 years of age, and AML associated with Down syndrome, which usually arises within the first 5 years of life. Despite falling within different AML subclassifications, all cases of acute megakaryoblastic leukemia have similar morphologic features in that the blasts are characteristically intermediate to large in size with basophilic cytoplasm and often have distinct cytoplasmic blebs. However, blast morphology can vary significantly, and some blasts may be small with a high nuclear to cytoplasmic ratio, appearing more like lymphoblasts. Circulating

megakaryocytes, large hypogranular platelets, and megakaryocytic fragments can all be seen in the peripheral blood smear. Micromegakaryocytes are common in the bone marrow and should not be counted as blasts. Acute megakaryoblastic leukemia is often associated with extensive bone marrow fibrosis, presenting challenges to diagnosis, because the fibrosis can lead to a "dry" trap or aspicular aspirate smears, making the blast count difficult to enumerate. In addition, fibrosis can distort the morphologic features in the bone marrow core biopsy and may mimic a metastatic tumor. In such cases, immunophenotyping is essential to establish cell lineage. The blasts typically express at least 1 megakaryocytic marker such as CD41, CD61, CD42b, CD31, or factor VIII, but tend to be negative for more typical blast markers such as CD34 and HLA-DR, as well as TdT and markers of granulocytic differentiation such as MPO and Sudan black B.

By definition, cases of AML, NOS, that are megakaryoblastic do not have a recurrent WHO-defined genetic abnormality. However, there is a distinct association between acute megakaryoblastic leukemia and the *CBFA2T3-GLIS2* fusion transcript, as well as the particular immunophenotype detected in this case. Features of the immunophenotype of this acute megakaryoblastic leukemia have been described as the "RAM phenotype" (named after the initials of a patient with this phenotype), defined by bright CD56 expression, dim to negative CD45 and CD38 expression, and lack of HLA-DR. A study from the Children's Oncology Group (COG) described this phenotype in detail, noting that RAM cases had a higher prevalence of megakaryoblastic lineage and were associated with a high induction failure rate and poor outcome in patients that would otherwise be considered standard risk. In addition, the *CBFA2T3-GLIS2* fusion transcript is associated with both megakaryoblastic lineage and the RAM phenotype. *CBFA2T3* is part of the *RUNX1TI* transcription complex and is important for self-renewal and differentiation of hematopoietic stem cells. *GLIS2* is a zinc finger protein transcription factor present in the kidney and not normally expressed in hematopoietic cells. The precise mechanism by which this fusion causes leukemogenesis is currently unknown, but based on mouse models, is thought to lead to increased stem cell capacity for self-renewal. *CBFA2T3-GLIS2* has been described exclusively in pediatric AML patients having normal karyotype, and it results from a cryptic inversion of chromosome 16, inv(16)(p13.3q24.3), distinct from the recurrent AML abnormality inv(16)(p13.1q22) *CBFB-MYH11*. Slightly more than half of studied patients with the RAM phenotype harbor *CFBA2T3-GLIS2*. This association may in part be attributed to study findings suggesting that the fusion protein can directly regulate the expression of CD56. Although there is clearly a relationship between acute megakaryoblastic leukemia, RAM phenotype, and presence of the *CFBA2T3-GLIS2* fusion, not all AML cases with the RAM phenotype or with *CFBA2T3-GLIS2* are of megakaryoblastic lineage. At the time of writing, assays to detect this fusion are not widely available and testing is generally performed via COG.

Because of the predicted aggressive nature of this rare type of leukemia, the patient in this case underwent allogeneic stem cell transplantation shortly after chemotherapy was initiated. However, extramedullary relapse occurred <2 years later, and the patient died <3 years after diagnosis, despite multiple attempts at salvage therapy.

Diagnostic pearls/pitfalls

– AML with the RAM phenotype (CD56 bright, CD45 dim to negative, CD38 dim to negative, and HLA-DR negative) is associated with a poor prognosis, even in patients who would otherwise be classified as standard risk, and if present, should be emphasized in pathology reports.

– The *CBFA2T3-GLIS2* fusion transcript is cryptic on karyotype analysis but confers an independently poor prognosis. Therefore, cytogenetically normal pediatric cases of acute megakaryoblastic leukemia or nonmegakaryoblastic AML with a RAM phenotype may warrant targeted PCR testing for this rare rearrangement.

– Cytoplasmic staining for CD41 or CD61 is a more specific and sensitive method to detect megakaryocytic lineage, because platelets can adhere to the cell surface of blasts and produce misleading flow cytometry results with surface CD41 or CD61 staining.

– The core biopsy morphology in acute megakaryoblastic leukemia may be misleading and resemble metastatic carcinoma or even a sarcoma. This fact, coupled with the frequent lack of CD34 expression and positive CD56 expression in megakaryocytic blasts, can lead to a misdiagnosis. Careful phenotypic analysis, including the use of megakaryocytic markers, should be undertaken to avoid this pitfall.

Readings

Eidenschink Brodersen L, Alonzo TA, Menssen AJ, et al. A recurrent immunophenotype at diagnosis independently identifies high-risk pediatric acute myeloid leukemia: a report from Children's Oncology Group. Leukemia. 2016;30(10):2077-80. **DOI: 10.1038/leu.2016.119**

Gruber TA, Downing JR. The biology of pediatric acute megakaryoblastic leukemia. Blood. 2015;126(8):943-9. **DOI: 10.1182/blood-2015-05-567859**

Gruber TA, Larson Gedman A, Zhang J, et al. An Inv(16) (p13.3q24.3)-encoded *CBFA2T3-GLIS2* fusion protein defines an aggressive subtype of pediatric acute megakaryoblastic leukemia. Cancer Cell. 2012;22(5):683-97. **DOI: 10.1016/j.ccr.2012.10.007**

Hara Y, Shiba N, Ohki K, et al. Prognostic impact of specific molecular profiles in pediatric acute megakaryoblastic leukemia in non-Down syndrome. Genes Chromosomes Cancer. 2017;56(5):394-404. **DOI: 10.1002/gcc.22444**

Masetti R, Bertuccio SN, Pession A, Locatelli F. *CBFA2T3-GLIS2*-positive acute myeloid leukaemia: a peculiar paediatric entity. Br J. Haematol. 2019;184(3):337–347. PMID: 30592296 **DOI: 10.1111/bjh.15725**

Masetti R, Pigazzi M, Togni M, et al. *CBFA2T3-GLIS2* fusion transcript is a novel common feature in pediatric, cytogenetically normal AML, not restricted to FAB M7 subtype. Blood. 2013;121(17):3469-72. **DOI: 10.1182/blood-2012-11-469825**

Smith JL, Ries RE, Hylkema T, et al. Comprehensive transcriptome profiling of cryptic *CBFA2T3-GLIS2* fusion-positive AML defines novel therapeutic options: a COG and TARGET pediatric AML study. Clin Cancer Res. 2020 Feb 1;26(3):726-737. **DOI: 10.1158/1078-0432.CCR-19-1800**

Swerdlow SH, Campo E, Harris NL, et al. World Health Organization Classification of Tumours of Haematopoietic and Lymphoid Tissues. 4th ed. Lyon, France: IARC Press; 2017. **ISBN: 9789283244943**

Voigt AP, Brodersen LE, Alonzo TA, et al. Phenotype in combination with genotype improves outcome prediction in acute myeloid leukemia: a report from Children's Oncology Group protocol AAML0531. Haematologica. 2017;102(12):2058-68. **DOI: 10.3324/haematol.2017.169029**

Kwadwo Oduro

28

Transient abnormal myelopoiesis of Down syndrome with *GATA1* mutation

History A 3-day-old male, born at 34.5 weeks of gestation, was evaluated in the neonatal intensive care unit for prematurity. Physical examination demonstrated dysmorphism concerning for Down syndrome (DS) including brachycephaly, upslanting eyes, epicanthal folds, small palpebral features, flat facial profile, increased spacing between first and second toes, and a single palmar crease. Physical examination was also notable for absence of hepatosplenomegaly. He was in no acute distress. CBC (selected results shown at right) revealed a leukocytosis but normal hemoglobin and platelet count for age.

Morphology & flow cytometry Review of the peripheral blood smear showed frequent large immature forms consistent with blasts, comprising >50% of the leukocytes. Rare naked megakaryocyte nuclei were also identified **f28.1**.

Flow cytometry of the peripheral blood identified a population of myeloblasts, with the following immunophenotype: positive for CD117, CD7, CD56, CD36, CD38, and CD45 (dim); partially positive for CD34, CD41, and CD61; negative for CD13, CD33, CD14, CD15, HLA-DR, B lymphoid markers (CD19, CD10, CD22), and other T-cell markers (CD2, CD5, CD3). In addition to the blasts having partial expression of the megakaryocytic markers CD41 and CD61 **f28.2**, there was also a population of cells having CD41 and CD61 but having only dim to no CD117; these cells likely represented immature megakaryocyte precursors.

Genetics/molecular results Chromosome analysis performed on blood confirmed constitutional trisomy 21 with male karyotype. *GATA1* mutation testing was performed using an assay combining both next-generation and Sanger sequencing methods, and identified a c.−19−1G>A variant in 50% of sequencing reads.

WBC	40.9×10^9/L
HGB	21.0 g/dL
Platelets	165×10^9/L

Based on the clinical context of a patient with trisomy 21 and the finding of myeloid blasts with megakaryocytic differentiation in the first week of life, a presumptive diagnosis of **transient abnormal myelopoiesis of Down syndrome** was rendered. This was corroborated by the identification of the *GATA1* mutation.

Discussion The presence of >20% blasts in the peripheral blood or bone marrow is generally diagnostic of an acute leukemia. However, in some situations this is not necessarily true. Other cases in this volume have addressed acute myeloid leukemia (AML) that can be diagnosed with <20% blasts, such as AML with t(8;21) *RUNX1-RUNX1T1* and AML with t(15;17) *PML-RARA* (**Cases 19 & 20**, respectively). Conversely, the presence of increased blasts, even approaching leukemia levels, may not indicate a neoplastic condition. The current case illustrates such a scenario.

As the name suggests, transient abnormal myelopoiesis associated with Down syndrome (TAM) occurs exclusively in individuals with DS and is frequently self-limiting. It occurs in 10% of individuals with DS and typically manifests in the first week of life. It is characterized by the presence of circulating blasts which can significantly exceed the 20% threshold for diagnosing AML in other contexts. The myeloproliferation shows megakaryocytic differentiation, typically in the form of megakaryoblasts, which are larger than typical myeloblasts, have basophilic cytoplasm, and often show cytoplasmic blebbing. Even in the absence of these characteristic

   ISBN 978-089189-6814   ©2021 ASCP

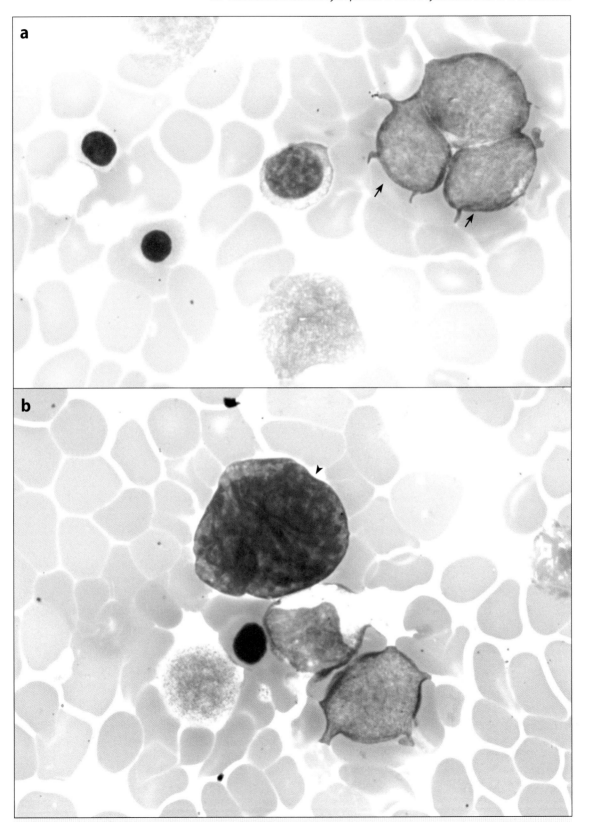

f28.1 Peripheral blood smear showing **a** large blasts with basophilic cytoplasm (arrows), as well as **b** occasional megakaryocyte nuclei (arrowhead)

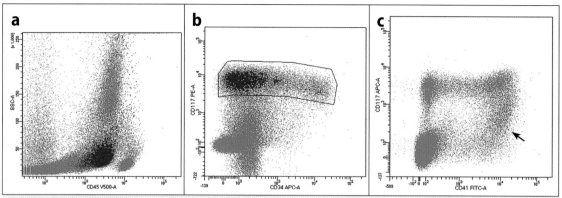

f28.2 Flow cytometry of blood demonstrating an increased **a** CD45 dim blast population (highlighted in red) that is positive for **b** CD117, CD34 (partial) & **c** CD41; in addition, other immature CD41 positive megakaryocytic cells that are dim to negative for CD117are also present (arrow)

morphologic findings, flow cytometry may show blasts expressing markers of megakaryocytic differentiation such as CD41, CD61, and CD42b, as well as other immature cells at different stages of megakaryocyte differentiation, as demonstrated in the current case.

Individuals with DS have an increased risk for acute leukemia, in particular B-lymphoblastic leukemia/lymphoma (B-ALL) and AML. Distinguishing TAM from B-ALL or nonmegakaryocytic AML is relatively straightforward because flow cytometry can readily and reliably distinguish lymphoblasts from myeloblasts and provide a detailed immunophenotypic characterization of myeloblasts, if present. In contrast, it is difficult to conclusively differentiate TAM from acute megakaryoblastic leukemia occurring in DS patients (ie, myeloid leukemia associated with Down syndrome [ML-DS], in the World Health Organization 2017 classification of hematopoietic neoplasms), based on pathologic features alone. These two entities are not distinguishable morphologically. In addition to showing expression of markers of megakaryocyte lineage, the blasts in both TAM and ML-DS tend to have variable CD34 expression, often show aberrant CD7 and CD56 expression, and express myeloid markers such as CD117 and CD33, but are negative for myeloperoxidase, CD15, and CD11a. Expression of CD11b and CD13 may favor ML-DS over TAM, as these markers are expressed in 80%-90% of ML-DS cases vs 10%-20% of TAM cases; however, these trends are not absolute. In clinical practice, circulating blasts with megakaryocytic phenotype appearing in the first week of life is considered TAM until proven otherwise. These patients are monitored without specific treatments unless there are so-called "life-threatening symptoms" (LTS), which occur in about a quarter of cases. LTS include hyperviscosity, absolute blast count $>100 \times 10^9/L$, hepatosplenomegaly causing respiratory symptoms,

heart failure not due to congenital heart defect, renal/hepatic dysfunction, disseminated intravascular coagulation (DIC) with bleeding, and hydrops fetalis. Of note, this particular patient lacked any LTS.

At the molecular level, TAM and ML-DS are both characterized by the presence of mutations in the gene encoding GATA1, a transcription factor crucial for the development and proliferation of erythroid and megakaryocytic precursors. Both disorders demonstrate similar types of mutations in *GATA1*, which are acquired in the prenatal period and result in overexpression of a normally occurring, shortened form of GATA1 (GATA1s) having an N-terminal truncation. *GATA1* mutations are typically assessed by sequencing methods, although immunohistochemistry to evaluate for loss of the full length GATA1 protein has been developed. The *GATA1* c.-19-1G>A variant in this patient is a splice site mutation located in intron 1, upstream of the translation initiation site located in exon 2 of the *GATA1* gene, and was present at an allele frequency of 50%, indicating a somatic mutation, since *GATA1* is hemizygous, being located on the X chromosome (an inherited *GATA1* mutation in this infant with male karyotype would have allelic frequency ~100%). A mutation at this splice site is predicted to result in impaired splicing of the 5' untranslated region and has been associated with N-terminal-truncated GATA1 protein in one report. Some DS individuals may have detectable *GATA1* mutation but do not develop increased blasts, indicating that the combined genetic abnormalities of mutated *GATA1* and trisomy 21 are not by themselves sufficient to cause TAM or ML-DS. Although additional molecular/genetic abnormalities have been identified in some patients with TAM, they are not always functional and their role in TAM pathogenesis is unclear. Interestingly, the resolution of TAM is associated with eradication of detectable *GATA1* mutation as demonstrated using sensitive molecular techniques.

ISBN 978-089189-6814 ©2021 ASCP

Although TAM generally has a good prognosis, ~10% of individuals die of complications of this disorder—most frequently from hepatic failure or DIC—with risk of death influenced by the presence of hepatomegaly alone or in combination with other LTS. About 90% of patients diagnosed with TAM will spontaneously clear circulating blasts in ~3 months. However, some patients have persistent or increasing blast frequency and these may represent bonafide ML-DS cases. Furthermore, ~20% of TAM patients who clear their circulating blasts will subsequently develop ML-DS within the first 4 years of life. Increased risk of subsequent ML-DS has been associated with the presence of additional cytogenetic abnormalities (in addition to trisomy 21), type of *GATA1* mutation in one study (higher risk for variants that are associated with lower expression of GATA1s), and functional mutations in other genes. This includes loss-of-function mutations in genes encoding cohesion components (eg, *CTCF*) and epigenetic regulators (eg, *EZH2, KANSL1*) and gain-of-function mutations in *JAK/STAT* and *RAS* pathway genes.

This patient did not demonstrate LTS at diagnosis or during follow-up and was managed conservatively. His circulating blast frequency steadily dropped from 50% at diagnosis to 35% after 1 week, 10% after 1 month, and finally no circulating blasts were detectable after 2.5 months. Six months after birth, the patient continued to have persistent cytopenia in the form of mild neutropenia (absolute neutrophil count of 0.51×10^9/L), which can happen in about a quarter of TAM patients. However, lack of LTS or hepatomegaly, clearance of circulating blasts, absence of cytogenetic abnormalities besides constitutional trisomy 21, and the presence of a splicing *GATA1* mutation (which is associated with high-level GATA1s expression), all suggest a good outcome for this patient.

Diagnostic pearls/pitfalls

 – Circulating blasts occurring in the first week of life in individuals with DS are more likely to represent TAM as opposed to AML.
 – The blasts in TAM show megakaryoblastic/megakaryocytic differentiation and are often not distinguishable from the megakaryoblasts of ML-DS, based on morphology or immunophenotype, or even presence of *GATA1* mutation.
 – Children with TAM have increased risk of developing ML-DS within the first 4 years of life

Readings

Alford KA, Reinhardt K, Garnett C, et al. Analysis of *GATA1* mutations in Down syndrome transient myeloproliferative disorder and myeloid leukemia. Blood. 2011;118(8):2222-38. **DOI: 10.1182/blood-2011-03-342774**

Boztug H, Schumich A, Pötschger U, et al. Blast cell deficiency of CD11a as a marker of acute megakaryoblastic leukemia and transient myeloproliferative disease in children with and without Down syndrome. Cytometry B Clin Cytom. 2013;84(6):370-8. **DOI: 10.1002/cyto.b.21082**

De Vita S, Mulligan C, McElwaine S, et al. Loss-of-function *JAK3* mutations in TMD and AMKL of Down syndrome. Br J Haematol. 2007;137(4):337-41. **DOI: 10.1111/j.1365-2141.2007.06574.x**

Gamis AS, Alonzo TA, Gerbing RB, et al. Natural history of transient myeloproliferative disorder clinically diagnosed in Down syndrome neonates: a report from the Children's Oncology Group Study A2971. Blood. 2011;118(26):6752-9; quiz 6996. **DOI: 10.1182/blood-2011-04-350017**

Groet J, McElwaine S, Spinelli M, et al. Acquired mutations in *GATA1* in neonates with Down's syndrome with transient myeloid disorder. Lancet. 2003;361(9369):1617-20. **DOI: 10.1016/S0140-6736(03)13266-7**

Kanezaki R, Toki T, Terui K, et al. Down syndrome and *GATA1* mutations in transient abnormal myeloproliferative disorder: mutation classes correlate with progression to myeloid leukemia. Blood. 2010;116(22):4631-8. **DOI: 10.1182/blood-2010-05-282426**

Karandikar NJ, Aquino DB, McKenna RW, et al. Transient myeloproliferative disorder and acute myeloid leukemia in Down syndrome: an immunophenotypic analysis. Am J Clin Pathol. 2001;116(2):204-10. **DOI: 10.1309/XREF-C9T2-6U0A-4EDT**

Labuhn M, Perkins K, Matzk S, et al. Mechanisms of progression of myeloid preleukemia to transformed myeloid leukemia in children with Down syndrome. Cancer Cell. 2019;36(2):123-138 e10. **DOI: 10.1016/j.ccell.2019.06.007**

Lee WY, Weinberg OK, Evans AG, et al. Loss of full-length *GATA1* expression in megakaryocytes is a sensitive and specific immunohistochemical marker for the diagnosis of myeloid proliferative disorder related to Down syndrome. Am J Clin Pathol. 2018;149(4):300-9. **DOI: 10.1093/ajcp/aqy001**

Litz CE, Davies S, Brunning RD, et al. Acute leukemia and the transient myeloproliferative disorder associated with Down syndrome: morphologic, immunophenotypic and cytogenetic manifestations. Leukemia. 1995;9(9):1432-9. **PMID: 7658708**

Massey GV, Zipursky A, Chang MN, et al; Children's Oncology Group (COG). A prospective study of the natural history of transient leukemia (TL) in neonates with Down syndrome (DS): Children's Oncology Group (COG) study POG-9481. Blood. 2006;107(12):4606-13. **DOI: 10.1182/blood-2005-06-2448**

Pine SR, Guo Q, Yin C, et al. *GATA1* as a new target to detect minimal residual disease in both transient leukemia and megakaryoblastic leukemia of Down syndrome. Leuk Res. 2005;29(11):1353-6. **DOI: 10.1016/j.leukres.2005.04.007**

Wang L, Peters JM, Fuda F, et al. Acute megakaryoblastic leukemia associated with trisomy 21 demonstrates a distinct immunophenotype. Cytometry B Clin Cytom. 2015;88(4):244-52. **DOI: 10.1002/cytob.21198**

Yoshida K, Toki T, Okuno Y, et al. The landscape of somatic mutations in Down syndrome-related myeloid disorders. Nat Genet. 2013;45(11):1293-9. **DOI: 10.1038/ng.2759**

Yumura-Yagi K, Hara J, Kurahashi H, et al. Mixed phenotype of blasts in acute megakaryocytic leukaemia and transient abnormal myelopoiesis in Down's syndrome. Br J Haematol. 1992;81(4):520-5. **DOI: 10.1111/j.1365-2141.1992.tb02985.x**

Zucker J, Temm C, Czader M, et al. A child with dyserythropoietic anemia and megakaryocyte dysplasia due to a novel 5'UTR *GATA1s* splice mutation. Pediatr Blood Cancer. 2016;63(5):917-21. **DOI: 10.1002/pbc.25871**

Howard Meyerson

29

Chronic lymphocytic leukemia/ small lymphocytic lymphoma with *TP53* mutation

History A 78-year-old man was noted incidentally to have leukocytosis on a CBC drawn during workup of a kidney stone. The CBC results are shown to the right. The patient was referred to an oncologist and a peripheral blood specimen was sent for morphologic review, flow cytometry, and genetic studies.

Morphology & flow cytometry The peripheral blood smear revealed a lymphocytosis of small, mature-appearing lymphocytes with "soccer ball-like" nuclei and some smudge cells **f29.1**. Flow cytometry analysis revealed an atypical population of lymphocytes constituting 60% of all leukocytes; this population was positive for CD5, CD19, CD20 (dim), CD23, CD43 (dim), CD79b (dim), and CD200, and negative for CD10, CD38, and surface light chain **f29.2**.

Genetics/molecular results FISH was positive for biallelic deletion of 13q14.3 in 62.4% and deletion of 17p13.1 in 76% of cells **f29.3**. FISH was negative for t(11;14) *CCND1-IGH* translocation and deletion of 11q or addition of chromosome 12. Somatic mutation analysis using a targeted NGS panel for lymphoid genes revealed a *TP53* mutation (*TP53* p.N131Y; c.391A>T) with variant allele frequency of 45%. Sequencing of the immunoglobulin heavy chain variable (IGHV) region revealed 92.4% identity with germline indicating a mutated IGHV, with IgVH3-74*01 and IgVH3-74*03 the closest matched germline alleles. Based on the morphologic, immunophenotypic, and genetic results, a diagnosis of **chronic lymphocytic leukemia (CLL)/small lymphocytic lymphoma** was rendered.

Discussion CLL is the most common leukemia in adults in Western countries, typically affecting older individuals and often with an indolent clinical course. When presenting as primarily nodal disease, this entity

WBC	16.5×10^9/L
Differential	
Polymorphonuclear leukocytes	17%
Lymphocytes	69%
Monocytes	12%
Eosinophils	1%
Basophils	1%
RBC	3.58×10^{12}/L
HGB	9.6 g/dL
HCT	30.9%
MCV	86 fL
RDW	15.5%
Platelets	120×10^9/L

is termed small lymphocytic lymphoma. Most cases of CLL are detected incidentally on routine CBC showing an absolute lymphocytosis, with peripheral smear demonstrating a predominance of small mature lymphocytes having clumped chromatin. In this example case, a diagnosis of CLL was made based on the presence of typical morphology and immunophenotype (CD5+, CD23+, CD20dim, CD200+ clonal B cell population), in the presence of an absolute clonal lymphocyte count >5 × 10^9/L, the minimum level required for the diagnosis of CLL. A bone marrow or lymph node biopsy is not necessary to establish the diagnosis. The main differential diagnosis includes leukemic mantle cell lymphoma (MCL), which was excluded in this case based on the absence of the t(11;14)(q13;q32) *CCND1-IGH*. FISH for t(11;14) or immunostaining for cyclin D1 to exclude MCL is recommended in suspected CLL cases, because

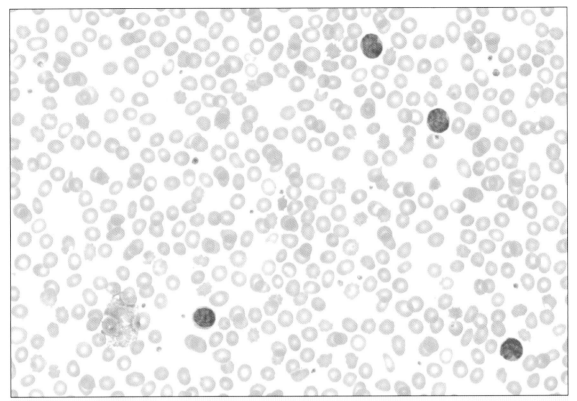

f29.1 Peripheral blood smear demonstrating small lymphocytes with condensed chromatin

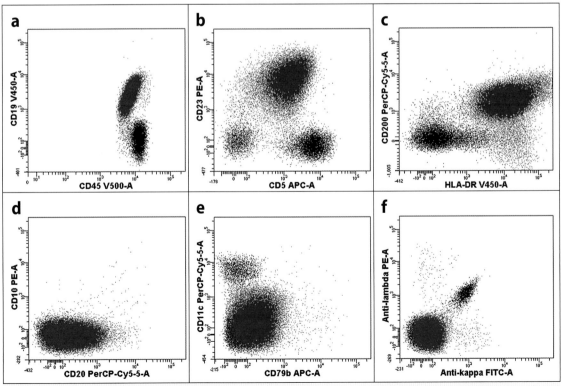

f29.2 Flow cytometry of the peripheral blood smear demonstrating an abnormal **a** CD19+, **b** CD5+, CD23+, **c** CD200+, **d** CD10–, CD20+ (dim), **e** CD79b+ (dim), **f** surface light chain-negative B-cell population (highlighted in red)

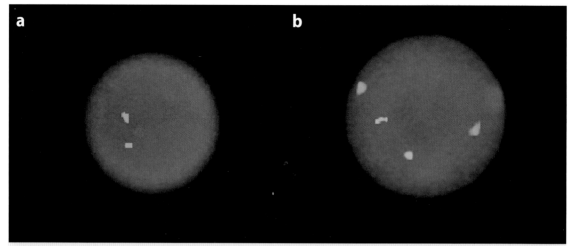

f29.3 a FISH probes *TP53* (17p13, orange) & *ATM* (11q22, green) showing 2 green signals with loss of 1 orange signal, consistent with *TP53* deletion without loss of *ATM*; **b** FISH probes *CEP12* (centromere 12, green), *LAMP1* (13q34, aqua) & *D13S319* (13q14.3, orange) demonstrate loss of both orange signals, consistent with biallelic deletion of 13q14.3 without loss of the entire 13q arm

some MCLs express variable amounts of CD23. Other phenotypic features of MCL that may help to distinguish the process from CLL include moderate to strong expression of CD20 and CD79b, expression of FMC-7, and lack of CD43 and CD200.

Genetic studies are important for determining prognosis and therapy in CLL and have become an essential part of the diagnostic evaluation. Standard genetic studies for CLL include FISH for del(13/13q), del(11q), del(17p), and trisomy 12 as well as for t(11;14); *IGHV* gene mutational analysis and evaluation for somatic mutations, particularly *TP53*, are also recommended. When performed, karyotype assessment requires stimulation of CLL cells with CpG oligonucleotides, because CLL cells rarely divide in culture without stimulation. A complex karyotype (having ≥3 unrelated chromosome abnormalities) is a poor prognostic factor. A summary of typical genetic aberrations found in CLL and their significance is shown in **t29.1**.

This patient had biallelic deletion of 13q14. Deletion of chromosome region 13q14, typically monoallelic, is the most common structural genetic abnormality in CLL. Patients with this abnormality have a favorable prognosis, with a median survival of ~11 years when del(13q14) is present as the sole cytogenetic abnormality. Biallelic 13q14 deletion (where both chromosomes demonstrate the deletion) occurs in ~8%-10% of patients and appears to convey similarly favorable prognosis as monoallelic del(13q14). However, the percentage of 13q14 deleted cells (>60%-80% depending on study) and the size of the

deletion (large size with deletion of the *RB1* gene) appear to adversely affect outcome, although the latter is rarely evaluated unless microarray studies are performed. When present in combination with adverse factors such as del(11q) or del(17p), del(13q14) modestly mitigates these poor prognostic factors.

TP53 mutation and del(17p) often occur together in CLL (as in this case) and adversely affect time to therapy, overall survival (median 32 months), and response to therapy. *TP53* mutations are most often encountered in exons 4-8, in the DNA binding domain, but may also affect other regions of the molecule. These mutations are particularly deleterious because p53 protein triggers cell cycle arrest after DNA damage, allowing for DNA repair. When p53 function is perturbed, replication following DNA damage occurs more readily, allowing for the potentially permanent incorporation of harmful DNA mutations. Even minor *TP53*-mutated subclones in CLL impart an adverse prognostic effect.

Other frequently detected FISH abnormalities in CLL are del(11q) and trisomy 12 (the second most common cytogenetic abnormality in CLL). Trisomy 12 carries an intermediate prognosis, with median survival of ~111 months, similar to patients with CLL having a normal karyotype. Prognosis in CLL patients with trisomy 12, however, is negatively affected by the occurrence of additional chromosomal aberrations such as del(11q) or del(17p) [as is the case with del(13q)]. Trisomy 12 is often associated with atypical CLL morphology, including cells with clefted nuclei

ISBN 978-089189-6814

t29.1 Common FISH abnormalities (with associated genes) & somatic mutations with prognostic significance in CLL

Genes	Function	Frequency	IgVH	Prognosis	Comments
FISH abnormality; involved genetic loci					
del(13q14); MiR 15A,16-1	increased cyclin D2/D3; increased Bcl-2	40%-50%	mutated	favorable	occurs early in disease
trisomy 12	unknown	~15%	unmutated	intermediate	atypical morphology, associated with *NOTCH1* mutations
del(11q22-23); *ATM, BIRC3*	impaired DNA damage response; NF-κB signaling	10%-15%	unmutated	adverse	adenopathy; associated with *ATM, BIRC3 & SF3B1* mutations
del(17p); *TP53*	impaired DNA damage response	5%-10%	unmutated	adverse	occurs later in disease; associated with *TP53* mutations
Somatic mutation					
TP53	impaired DNA damage response	~5%-10%	unmutated	adverse	occurs later in disease
ATM	impaired DNA damage response	~10%	unmutated	adverse	occurs later in disease
NOTCH1	activated Notch signaling	~10%	unmutated	adverse	occurs later in disease & in Richter transformation; associated with trisomy 12
BIRC3	non-canonical NF-κB signaling	~10%-15%	unmutated	adverse	occurs later in disease; associated with del(11q)
SF3B1	splicing factor	~10%-15%	unmutated	adverse	occurs later in disease; associated with high WBC, male sex, del(11q)
MYD88	toll-like receptor/ canonical NF-κB signaling	~3%	mutated	favorable	occurs later in disease; associated with younger age
POT1	telomere protection	~5%	unmutated	adverse	p.Gln376Arg specifically associated with familial CLL
RPS15	ribosomal protein	~5%	unmutated	adverse	associated with del(17p) & *TP53* mutation
FBXW7	Notch signaling	3%-5%	no association	no effect	associated with trisomy 12
NFKBIE	canonical NF-κB signaling	6%	unmutated	adverse	associated with sterotyped IgHV use (subset #1)

CLL, chronic lymphocytic leukemia; IGHV, immunoglobulin heavy chain variable

and increased prolymphocytes in the peripheral blood, as well as *NOTCH1* mutations and unmutated IGHV regions (as described later). The third most common cytogenetic abnormality in CLL, del(11q), is known to be associated with extensive adenopathy and more rapid disease progression, with shortened median survival (~79 months) compared to patients with del(13q) or trisomy 12. Therapeutic approaches incorporating alkylating agents may be beneficial in CLL patients with del(11q).

TP53 mutations and del(17p) are associated with poor response to conventional chemotherapy in CLL. Therefore, current suggested front-line treatment regimens for these cases are the Bruton tyrosine kinase (BTK) inhibitors ibrutinib or acalabrutinib, or the BCL-2 inhibitor venetoclax in combination with anti-CD20 monoclonal antibody. However, therapy with these reagents has led to development of resistance. BTK resistance has been correlated with acquired mutations in the *BTK* gene itself or phospholipase C-γ2,

PLCG2. More recently, resistance to venetoclax has been described to be mediated by a Gly101Val mutation in *BCL2*. As such, NGS panels evaluating lymphoid neoplasms may also evaluate for these aberrations.

The *IGHV* genes are a family of genes encoding a component of the antigen recognition portion of the B-cell receptor (BCR), with each individual BCR using a single *IGHV* gene. Somatic mutations occur in these genes after antigen exposure as part of the honing of the normal B-cell immune response. Approximately 50%-60% of patients with CLL have *IGHV* genes with somatic mutations, defined as <98% homology with germline *IGHV* gene sequences. IGHV-unmutated CLL is associated with poor prognosis and significantly decreased survival compared with CLL having mutated IGHV, and is associated with CD38, CD49d, and ZAP-70 expression as well as adverse genetic mutations, including those in *TP53, ATM, NOTCH1, SF3B1,* and *BIRC3*. Interestingly, preferential *IGHV3-21* gene usage is also associated with poor outcome, irrespective of the mutational status. Approximately 30% of CLL patients carry quasi-similar, if not identical, BCRs, a phenomenon termed BCR stereotypy, which suggests that antigen stimulation may underlie the pathogenesis of CLL. The stereotyped BCRs have been grouped into different subsets, some of which have been shown to affect prognosis.

In this case, the patient's CLL carried a mutated *IGHV* that was not *IGHV3-21*, as well as biallelic deletion of 13q14, both favorable findings. Nonetheless, del(17p) and a *TP53* mutation were present and the relatively high percentage of del(13q)-positive cells make this case a high-risk CLL. Because of the minimally affected blood cell counts and absence of symptoms, the patient is currently being monitored without therapy. He will likely need therapy in the near future based on the adverse genetics, requiring either a BTK or BCL-2 inhibitor as front-line treatment. Long-term outcome is expected to be poor.

Diagnostic pearls/pitfalls

– Genetic analysis including FISH, *IGHV* mutation status, and assessment for *TP53* mutation is recommended for all new diagnoses of CLL, for prognostication purposes.

– Unfavorable chromosomal abnormalities in CLL include del(17p), del(11q), and complex karyotype (≥3 abnormalities).

– Somatic mutations in *TP53, ATM, NOTCH1, SF3B1, BIRC3, RPS15,* and *NFKBIE* are associated with adverse prognosis. Targeted NGS panels for evaluation of lymphoid neoplasms may include these genes.

– Molecular assessment of *IGHV* gene mutation status is important in the diagnostic workup, since unmutated *IgHV* (defined as >98% homology with germline sequences) has an unfavorable prognosis and is associated with expression of CD38, ZAP-70, and CD49d.

– Cases of CLL having del(17p) or *TP53* mutations are typically refractory to standard chemotherapy and benefit from therapy with either BTK or BCL-2 inhibitors.

– Resistance mutations may develop in the *BTK* or *PLCG2* genes after therapy with a BTK inhibitor or in the *BCL2* gene after therapy with a BCL-2 inhibitor.

ISBN 978-089189-6814   ©2021 ASCP

Readings

Blombery P, Anderson MA, Gong JN, et al. Acquisition of the recurrent Gly101Val mutation in *BCL2* confers resistance to venetoclax in patients with progressive chronic lymphocytic leukemia. Cancer Discovery. 2019;9(3):342-53. **DOI: 10.1158/2159-8290.CD-18-1119**

Bosch F, Dalla-Favera R. Chronic lymphocytic leukaemia: from genetics to treatment. Nat Rev Clin Oncol. 2019;16(11):684-701. **DOI: 10.1038/s41571-019-0239-8**

Cavallari M, Cavazzini F, Bardi A, et al. Biological significance and prognostic/predictive impact of complex karyotype in chronic lymphocytic leukemia. Oncotarget. 2018;9(76):34398-412. **DOI: 10.18632/oncotarget.26146**

Crespo M, Bosch F, Villamor N, et al. ZAP-70 expression as a surrogate for immunoglobulin-variable-region mutations in chronic lymphocytic leukemia. N Engl J Med. 2003;348(18):1764-75. **DOI: 10.1056/NEJMoa023143**

Dal Bo M, Rossi FM, Rossi D, et al. 13q14 deletion size and number of deleted cells both influence prognosis in chronic lymphocytic leukemia. Genes Chromosomes Cancer. 50(8):633-43, 2011. **DOI: 10.1002/gcc.20885**

Damle RN, Wasil T, Fais F, et al. Ig V gene mutation status and CD38 expression as novel prognostic indicators in chronic lymphocytic leukemia. Blood. 1999;94(6):1840-7. **PMID: 10477712**

Diop F, Moia R, Favini C, Spaccarotella E, et al. Biological and clinical implications of *BIRC3* mutations in chronic lymphocytic leukemia. Haematologica. 2020;105(2):448-56. **DOI: 10.3324/haematol.2019.219550.**

Döhner H, Stilgenbauer S, Benner A, et al. Genomic aberrations and survival in chronic lymphocytic leukemia. N Engl J Med. 2000;343(26):1910-6. **DOI: 10.1056/NEJM200012283432602**

Gattei V, Bulian P, Del Principe MI, et al. Relevance of CD49d protein expression as overall survival and progressive disease prognosticator in chronic lymphocytic leukemia. Blood. 2008;111(2):865-73. **DOI: 10.1182/blood-2007-05-092486**

Hotinski AK, Best OG, Kuss BJ. The future of laboratory testing in chronic lymphocytic leukaemia. Pathology. 2021 Apr;53(3):377-384. **DOI: 10.1016/j.pathol.2021.01.006**

Hu B, Patel KP, Chen HC, et al. Routine sequencing in CLL has prognostic implications and provides new insight into pathogenesis and targeted treatments. Br J Haematol. 2019;185(5):852-64. **DOI: 10.1111/bjh.15877**

Hu B, Patel KP, Chen HC, et al. Association of gene mutations with time-to-first treatment in 384 treatment-naive chronic lymphocytic leukaemia patients. Br J Haematol. 2019;187(3):307-18. **DOI: 10.1111/bjh.16042**

Lee J, Wang YL. Prognostic and predictive molecular biomarkers in chronic lymphocytic leukemia. J Mol Diagn. 2020 Sep;22(9):1114-1125. **DOI: 10.1016/j.jmoldx.2020.06.004.**

Ljungström V, Cortese D, Young E, et al. Whole-exome sequencing in relapsing chronic lymphocytic leukemia: clinical impact of recurrent RPS15 mutations. Blood. 2016;127(8):1007-16. **DOI: 10.1182/blood-2015-10-674572**

Stamatopoulos K, Belessi C, Moreno C, et al. Over 20% of patients with chronic lymphocytic leukemia carry stereotyped receptors: pathogenetic implications and clinical correlations. Blood. 2007;109(1):259-70. **DOI: 10.1182/blood-2006-03-012948**

Van Dyke DL, Shanafelt TD, Call TG, et al. A comprehensive evaluation of the prognostic significance of 13q deletions in patients with B-chronic lymphocytic leukaemia. Br J Haematol. 2010;148(4):544-50. **DOI: 10.1111/j.1365-2141.2009.07982.x**

Woyach JA, Furman RR, Liu TM, et al. Resistance mechanisms for the Bruton's tyrosine kinase inhibitor ibrutinib. N Engl J Med. 2014;370(24):2286-94. **DOI: 10.1056/NEJMoa1400029**

Zenz T, Eichhorst B, Busch R, et al. *TP53* mutation and survival in chronic lymphocytic leukemia. J Clin Oncol. 2010;28(29):4473-9. **DOI: 10.1200/JCO.2009.27.8762**

Howard Meyerson

30
B-cell prolymphocytic leukemia with gain of *c-MYC*

History An 83-year-old man with a 2-year history of "atypical CLL" presented for management of his lymphocytosis. The CBC results are shown at right. A bone marrow biopsy was performed with flow cytometry and genetic studies.

Morphology & flow cytometry The accompanying peripheral blood smear revealed a predominance of lymphocytes that were medium-sized with a moderate amount of cytoplasm and round to oval nuclei having single prominent nucleoli **f30.1a**. These cells were enumerated at 73% of white cells. The bone marrow aspirate smear demonstrated normal trilineage maturation and 44% lymphocytes morphologically similar to those seen in the blood **f30.1b**. The clot section and trephine core biopsy revealed multiple aggregates of small to medium-sized lymphocytes **f30.2**. Flow cytometry showed 49% atypical lymphocytes that were positive for CD5 (moderate), CD19, CD20 (moderate), CD38 (dim), CD43, CD79b (moderate), and κ light chain, and negative for CD10, CD11c, CD23, CD43, and CD200 **f30.3**. Immunohistochemistry for cyclin D1 and SOX11, performed on the core biopsy, were both negative.

Genetics/molecular results Chromosome analysis performed on the bone marrow revealed a complex karyotype **f30.4**:

47,X,–Y,+1,del(1)(p13),+3,t(3;18)(p26;q21.2),der(14)t(1;14)(q21;q32).

FISH was positive for deletion of *IGH* (14q32) in 52.8% of cells but negative for del(11q), trisomy 12, del(13q)/–13, and del(17p). Because of the prolymphocytic morphology of the cells in the peripheral blood, FISH for *c-MYC* was performed

WBC	22.9×10^9/L
Differential	
Polymorphonuclear leukocytes	12%
Bands	1%
Lymphocytes	81%
Monocytes	5%
Eosinophils	1%
RBC	4.48×10^{12}/L
HGB	13.9 g/dL
HCT	42.1%
MCV	94 fL
RDW	13.8%
Platelets	155×10^9/L

using an *IGH-MYC* dual fusion probe set. FISH was positive for gain (4 copies) of *MYC* (8q24) in 47.6% of metaphase cells. A t(8;14) *IGH-MYC* fusion was not detected **f30.5**. Somatic mutation analysis using a targeted NGS panel for 30 lymphoid-related genes revealed *TRAF3* p.K429 c.1285A>T with a variant allele frequency of 45%. Based on the morphology, flow cytometry, and genetics/molecular results, a diagnosis of **B-cell prolymphocytic leukemia** (B-PLL) was made.

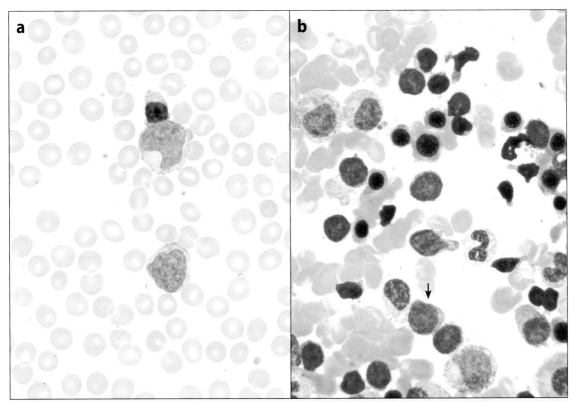

f30.1 **a** Peripheral blood & **b** bone marrow demonstrating intermediate-sized lymphocytes with prominent nucleoli & a moderate amount of cytoplasm (arrow)

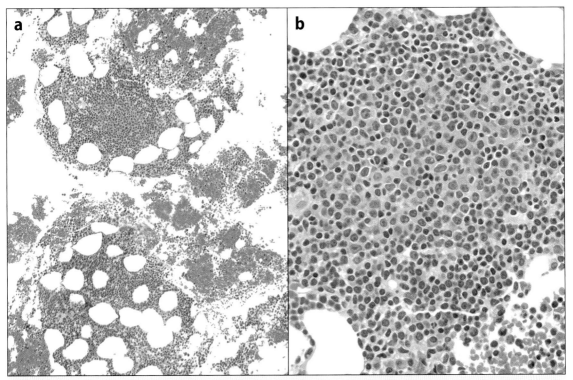

f30.2 Bone marrow clot section demonstrating **a** multiple lymphoid aggregates composed of **b** mixed small to intermediate-sized lymphocytes

30 B-cell prolymphocytic leukemia with gain of c-MYC

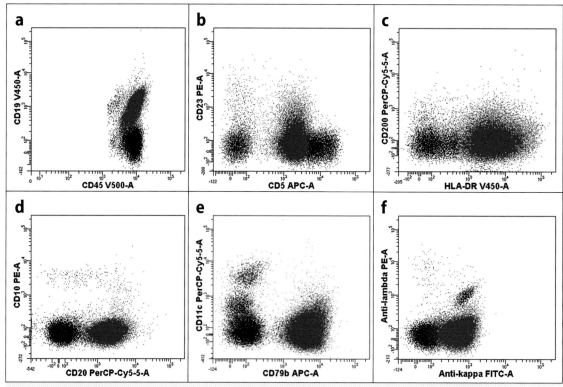

f30.3 Flow cytometry performed on the bone marrow aspirate demonstrates **a** a CD19+, **b** CD5+ (moderate), CD23–, **c** CD200–, **d** CD10–, CD20+ (moderate), **e** CD11c–, CD79b+ (moderate), **f** κ-restricted B-cell population (highlighted in red)

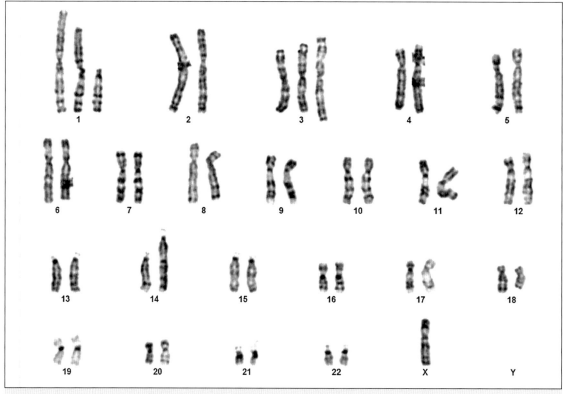

f30.4 Chromosome analysis demonstrating complex karyotype including gains of chromosomes 1 & 3

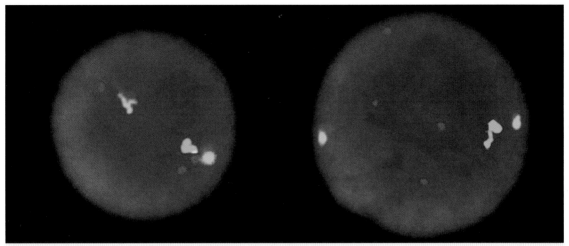

f30.5 FISH probes for *MYC* (8p11, orange), *IGH* (14q32, green) and CEP8 (centromere 8, aqua) demonstrate gain of 2 orange signals consistent with extra copies of the *MYC* region (with a normal number of signals for the chromosome 8 centromere) & loss of 1 green signal, diagnostic of an *IGH* deletion but not for *IGH-MYC* translocation

Discussion B-PLL is a rare B-cell lymphoproliferative disorder of the elderly, with average age at diagnosis ~70 years. Patients usually present with very high white blood cell counts (>100 × 10⁹/L), splenomegaly (often massive), cytopenias, and B symptoms. The disease is considered aggressive, with median survival of 3-5 years; however, a subset of patients may demonstrate a more indolent course. Anemia, lymphocytosis >100 × 10⁹/L, and age >70 years have been associated with more aggressive disease. The diagnosis is based primarily on peripheral blood morphology, with >55% prolymphocytes (of total lymphocytes) in the peripheral blood smear. Prolymphocytes are typically medium in size, with more open chromatin and abundant cytoplasm, as well as a prominent nucleolus, as compared to lymphocytes found in chronic lymphocytic leukemia (CLL). Circulating mantle cell lymphoma (MCL) must be excluded because leukemic MCL may demonstrate similar morphology and immunophenotype (see **Case 32**). Approximately a quarter of cases meeting morphologic criteria will harbor a *CCND1* rearrangement and should therefore be classified as leukemic or blastoid MCL rather than B-PLL.

No specific immunophenotype characterizes B-PLL. The leukemia cells are positive for CD5 in more than half of patients and typically lack CD10. Cases with CD5 expression may resemble MCL on immunophenotyping, with moderate to strong expression of CD19, CD20, and surface light chain, expression of FMC-7, and lack of CD23 and CD200. However, both cyclin D1 and SOX11 should be negative in B-PLL. B-PLL may represent the end stage of a low-grade B-cell lymphoproliferative

disorder such as CLL or splenic marginal zone lymphoma (SMZL), with the acquisition of virulent genetic aberrations resulting in cells with prolymphocytic morphology. This hypothesis may explain the varied and nonspecific phenotype found among B-PLL cases. Nonetheless, there is some debate about whether CLL truly progresses to B-PLL.

In addition to leukemic MCL, based on morphology, the differential diagnosis of B-PLL also includes CLL with increased prolymphocytes and hairy cell leukemia variant (HCL-v). The atypical cells in HCL-v are nucleolated similar to prolymphocytes, which can cause diagnostic confusion; however, the two disorders can usually be distinguished based on immunophenotype and genetic findings. In addition, HCL-v cells tend to be smaller, with smaller nucleoli, often with cytoplasmic projections. Cases of HCL-v typically do not express CD5 or CD10, but instead display moderate expression of CD11c and CD103, markers not seen in B-PLL. At the molecular level, mutations of *MAP2K1* are seen in 30%-40% of HCL-v cases but are not observed in B-PLL. The circulating cells of CLL often include a variable amount of prolymphocytes, making distinction between B-PLL and CLL difficult. Careful evaluation of cells in the thin areas of the peripheral smear usually reveals a substantially smaller percentage of prolymphocytes in CLL. Some CLL cases have cells that are on a continuum from small lymphocytes to slightly enlarged cells having small indistinct nucleoli to prolymphocytes, making the enumeration of prolymphocytes problematic. In these cases, the flow cytometric features can be helpful since the typical CLL phenotype (CD5+, CD23+, CD200+, dim CD20, dim to negative surface light chain) is usually lacking in B-PLL. Genetics may also be useful as *c-MYC* abnormalities are indicative of B-PLL (as described herein) rather than CLL. The common FISH abnormalities found in CLL, del(13q), del(17p) and trisomy 12, may also occur in cases of B-PLL, although del(11q) is quite infrequent in B-PLL.

No unifying genetic abnormality defines B-PLL. However, several features are notable. Compared to other low-grade B-cell lymphoproliferative disorders, B-PLL frequently demonstrates a complex karyotype (at least three unrelated cytogenetic abnormalities), abnormalities of *c-MYC*, deletion of 17p (*TP53*), and *BCOR* mutations (see **t30.1** for genetic features of B-PLL). *C-MYC* aberrations, including mutually exclusive gains and translocations [most commonly t(8;14) *IGH-MYC*], are present in three-quarters of cases and are correlated with expression of CD38. Other nonspecific, unbalanced translocations are very common, occurring in almost all cases of B-PLL that lack *c-MYC* translocation. Although mutation studies are limited, somatic mutations in the *TP53* gene are the most frequently encountered abnormality in B-PLL and often coexist with del(17p). *TP53* mutations and *c-MYC* aberrations occur together in ~20%-25% of cases and may confer a particularly poor prognosis. *BCOR* mutations have been observed in ~25% of cases and are also associated with *c-MYC* translocation. Interestingly *BCOR* mutations are not seen in Burkitt lymphoma but translocation of *c-MYC* is invariably present in that disease. B-PLL, similar to CLL and SMZL, demonstrates immunoglobulin heavy chain variable (IGHV) stereotypy with preferential use of IGHV3 and IGHV4 subgroups (~90% of cases). *IGHV* is frequently mutated.

This patient demonstrated a complex karyotype including trisomy 3 and an unbalanced translocation, as well as del(14q32) *IGH* and gain of *c-MYC* . Of note, gains of *c-MYC* in cases of B-PLL have been associated with a highly complex karyotype (at least 5 cytogenetic abnormalities) and trisomy 3 as seen here. Interestingly, somatic mutation analysis in this case revealed an inactivating mutation of *TRAF3*, which is a negative regulator of the noncanonical NF-κB pathway. Inactivating mutations of *TRAF3* are expected to lead to enhanced NF-κB signaling (see also **Case 36**). Mutations of *TRAF3* have been described in various B-lymphoproliferative disorders, including CLL, SMZL, and lymphoplasmacytic lymphoma. Approximately 10% of low-grade B-cell lymphoproliferative disorders with del(14q32) will also have a *TRAF3* mutation, as seen in

t30.1 Genetic abnormalities found in B-cell prolymphocytic leukemia

Abnormality	Frequency
complex karyotype	~75%
unbalanced translocation	~70%
translocation of *c-MYC*	~60%
gain of *c-MYC*	~15%
del(17p)	~40%
del(13q)	~30%
del(11q)	rare
trisomy 12	~25%
trisomy 3	~25%
trisomy 18	~30%
TP53 mutation	~40%
BCOR mutation	~25%
MYD88 mutation	~25%
SF3B1 mutation	~20%
restricted *IGHV* gene use	IGHV3 (~60%); IGHV4 (~30%)
Table adapted from Chapiro, et al	

this case. *TRAF3* inactivation in these cases is postulated to be biallelic, owing to the fact that *TRAF3* resides with the 14q32 region and has been shown to be deleted when evaluated. The resulting changes are expected to then lead to constitutive NF-κB activation.

The patient is currently being followed without therapy. The decision not to treat was based on the lack of poor clinical prognostic factors, including absence of anemia and relatively low lymphocyte count, as well as lack of the highly adverse genetic finding of coexisting *c-MYC* and *TP53* aberrations.

Diagnostic pearls/pitfalls
– Other B-cell lymphoproliferative disorders that closely resemble B-PLL include leukemic or blastoid MCL, CLL with increased prolymphocytes, and HCL-v. Diagnosis of B-PLL can usually be made based on a combination of morphology, immunophenotype, and genetic testing. In particular, cases with prolymphocytic morphology but with t(11;14) *IGH-CCND1* should be classified as MCL.
– The most common genetic aberrations found in B-PLL are abnormalities of *c-MYC*, a complex karyotype, and deletion and/or mutation of *TP53*.
– Patients with B-PLL having both a *c-MYC* and *TP53* aberration have a particularly poor prognosis.
– *BCOR* mutations are found in 25% of B-PLL cases and are relatively unique to B-PLL among low-grade B-cell lymphoproliferative disorders.

Readings

Chapiro E, Pramil E, Diop M, et al. Genetic characterization of B-cell prolymphocytic leukemia: a prognostic model involving *MYC* and *TP53*. Blood. 2019;134(21):1821-31. **DOI: 10.1182/blood.2019001187**

Collignon A, Wanquet A, Maitre E, et al. Prolymphocytic leukemia: new insights in diagnosis and in treatment. Curr Oncol Rep. 2017;19(4):29. **DOI: 10.1007/s11912-017-0581-x**

Cross M, Dearden C. B and T cell prolymphocytic leukaemia. Best Pract Res Clin Haematol. 2019;32(3):217-28. **DOI: 10.1016/j.beha.2019.06.001**

Dearden C. How I treat prolymphocytic leukemia. Blood. 2012;120(3):538-51. **DOI: 10.1182/blood-2012-01-380139**

Del Giudice I, Davis Z, Matutes E, et al. IgVH genes mutation and usage, ZAP-70 and CD38 expression provide new insights on B-cell prolymphocytic leukemia (B-PLL). Leukemia. 2006;20(7):1231-7. **DOI: 10.1038/sj.leu.2404238**

Flatley E, Chen AI, Zhao X, et al. Aberrations of *MYC* are a common event in B-cell prolymphocytic leukemia. Am J Clin Pathol. 2014;142(3):347-54. **DOI: 10.1309/AJCPUBHM8U7ZFLOB**

Hercher C, Robain M, Davi F, et al; Groupe Français d'Hématologie Cellulaire. A multicentric study of 41 cases of B-prolymphocytic leukemia: two evolutive forms. Leuk Lymphoma. 2001;42(5):981-7. **DOI: 10.3109/10428190109097717**

Huh YO, Lin KI, Vega F, et al. *MYC* translocation in chronic lymphocytic leukaemia is associated with increased prolymphocytes and a poor prognosis. Br J Haematol. 2008;142(1):36-44. **DOI: 10.1111/j.1365-2141.2008.07152.x**

Lens D, Coignet LJ, Brito-Babapulle V, et al. B cell prolymphocytic leukaemia (B-PLL) with complex karyotype and concurrent abnormalities of the *p53* and *c-MYC* gene. Leukemia. 1999;13(6):873-6. **DOI: 10.1038/sj.leu.2401416**

Nagel I, Bug S, Tönnies H, et al. Biallelic inactivation of *TRAF3* in a subset of B-cell lymphomas with interstitial del(14)(q24.1q32.33). Leukemia. 2009;23(11):2153-5. **DOI: 10.1038/leu.2009.149**

Sandes AF, de Lourdes Chauffaille M, Oliveira CR, et al. CD200 has an important role in the differential diagnosis of mature B-cell neoplasms by multiparameter flow cytometry. Cytometry B Clin Cytom. 2014;86(2):98-105. **DOI: 10.1002/cyto.b.21128**

Schlette E, Bueso-Ramos C, Giles F, et al. Mature B-cell leukemias with more than 55% prolymphocytes: a heterogeneous group that includes an unusual variant of mantle cell lymphoma. Am J Clin Pathol. 2001;115(4):571-81. **DOI: 10.1309/PPK0-TJUK-1UAR-3194**

Shvidel L, Shtalrid M, Bassous L, et al. B-cell prolymphocytic leukemia: a survey of 35 patients emphasizing heterogeneity, prognostic factors and evidence for a group with an indolent course. Leuk Lymphoma. 1999;33(1-2):169-79. **DOI: 10.3109/10428199909093739**

van der Velden VH, Hoogeveen PG, de Ridder D, et al. B-cell prolymphocytic leukemia: a specific subgroup of mantle cell lymphoma. Blood. 2014;124(3):412-9. **DOI: 10.1182/blood-2013-10-533869**

31

Howard Meyerson

Hairy cell leukemia with *BRAF* V600E

History A 56-year-old female presented with fatigue, abdominal discomfort with bloating, and pancytopenia. Imaging studies revealed mild splenomegaly with no other abnormalities. CBC results are shown at right. A bone marrow biopsy with genetic studies was performed.

Morphology & flow cytometry The peripheral blood smear was unremarkable. The bone marrow aspirate was aspicular and hypocellular. Hematopoietic progenitors were normal with a relative decrease in granulocytic elements. However, a population of atypical, slightly enlarged lymphocytes was identified, constituting 20% of marrow cells. These cells had ovoid to kidney-shaped nuclei with moderate delicate grey cytoplasm, and some had fine cytoplasmic projections **f31.1**. The trephine biopsy was 40% cellular with a subtle interstitial infiltrate of cells having monocytoid nuclei and ample pale cytoplasm, imparting a "fried-egg" appearance to the marrow. IHC revealed the atypical lymphocytes to be positive for CD20 as well as *BRAF* V600E, as detected by a specific anti-*BRAF* V600E antibody **f31.2**. Flow cytometry demonstrated a clonal population of B cells that was CD5-negative, CD10-negative, CD11c-positive (bright), CD19-positive, CD20-positive (bright), CD22-positive (bright), CD25-positive (moderate), CD38-negative, CD103-positive, CD123-positive, and κ-positive **f31.3**. Based on the morphologic and immunophenotypic findings, a diagnosis of **hairy cell leukemia** (HCL) was rendered.

Genetics/molecular results Cytogenetic analysis showed a normal 46,XX female karyotype in all 20 metaphases. FISH studies were not performed. A *BRAF* p.V600E c.1799T>A mutation was detected with allele-specific PCR using DNA isolated from the bone marrow clot section.

WBC	2.4×10^9/L
Differential	
Polymorphonuclear leukocytes	28%
Bands	3%
Lymphocytes	63%
Monocytes	4%
Eosinophils	2%
RBC	3.39×10^{12}/L
HGB	11.2 g/dL
HCT	32.2%
MCV	95 fL
RDW	13.1%
Platelets	64×10^9/L

ISBN 978-089189-6814

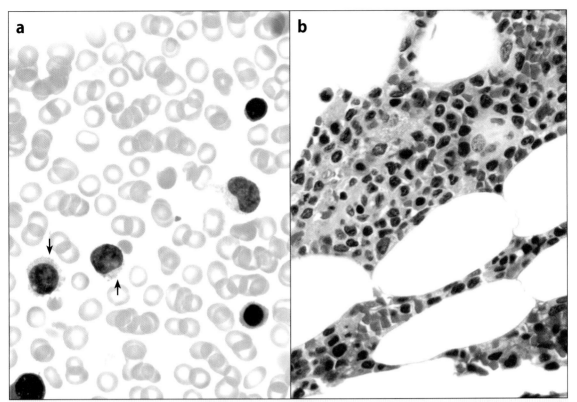

f31.1 **a** Bone marrow aspirate demonstrating atypical lymphoid cells with delicate cytoplasmic projections (arrows); **b** bone marrow core showing interstitial infiltrate of lymphoid cells with abundant cytoplasm

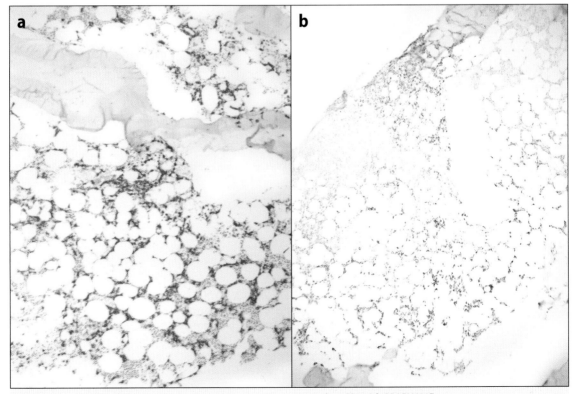

f31.2 Immunostains performed on the core biopsy demonstrating positivity for **a** CD20 & **b** *BRAF* V600E

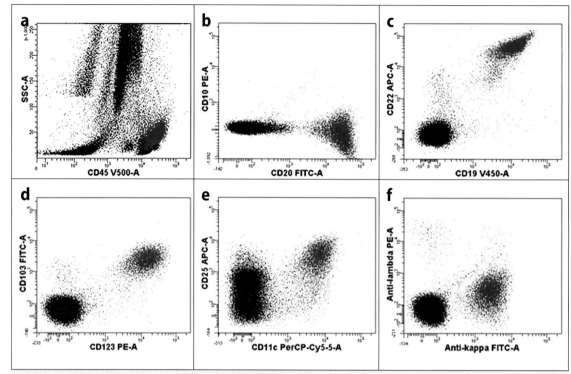

f31.3 Flow cytometry dot plots from bone marrow aspirate: **a** A CD45 bright, **b** CD20+, CD10–, **c** CD19+, CD22+ (bright), **d** CD103+, CD123+, **e** CD25+ (moderate), CD11c+, **f** κ restricted B-cell population is identified (shown in red), consistent with hairy cell leukemia

Discussion HCL typically presents in middle-aged adults with a male predominance (M:F = 4:1). Patients usually have pancytopenia with splenomegaly and a "dry tap" upon bone marrow aspiration (due to the extensive fibrosis associated with HCL), with a diffuse infiltrate of atypical lymphocytes present in core biopsy sections, as seen in this case. Patients often present with marked monocytopenia and neutropenia, which may lead to infectious complications. The differential diagnosis for HCL generally includes other B-cell disorders associated with villous lymphocytes, in particular splenic marginal zone lymphoma (SMZL) and hairy cell leukemia variant (HCL-v), as well as aplastic anemia in rare instances. Usually, these different processes can be readily distinguished by a combination of morphology, immunophenotype, and genetic studies (**t31.1** and as discussed later in this case).

Morphologically, HCL cells have a monocytoid, oval to slightly indented nucleus with a moderate amount of pale, blue-grey cytoplasm having characteristic thin, delicate extensions, as seen in **f31.1**. Only rare HCL cells may be present in the blood smear, and the hairy extensions may not always be evident, especially in the bone marrow aspirate smear. The cytoplasm of HCL

cells often appears fuzzy at its border (given that the cells are mature B cells, a more thoughtful name for this entity may have been *fuzzy cell lymphoma*). In contrast, the cells of SMZL usually have round to oval nuclei and may demonstrate a moderate amount of cytoplasm with bipolar, "torpedo"-like cytoplasmic tufts; fine "hairy" projections are usually lacking in SMZL cells. HCL-v cells generally demonstrate round to oval nuclei with a small discrete nucleolus, a feature distinct from cells of HCL. A moderate amount of cytoplasm is usually present in HCL-v cells, often with a few delicate, wispy protrusions. In addition, HCL-v is often associated with an elevated white blood cell count, a feature typically lacking in classic HCL.

Occasionally HCL may be mistaken for aplastic anemia when the marrow is extensively involved. Few hematopoietic cells may be present on the aspirate and the wide spacing of the hairy cell nuclei on the core biopsy, together with a lack of normal hematopoietic elements, may give the erroneous impression that the HCL cells represent normal stromal cells. A CD20 stain on the core biopsy helps resolve this issue.

HCL cells have a unique immunophenotype and are almost always positive for CD11c, CD25, CD103, and

t31.1 Key differences between B-cell disorders associated with villous lymphocytes

	Hairy cell leukemia	Hairy cell leukemia variant	Splenic marginal zone lymphoma
Morphology on Wright-stained smears & immunophenotype			
nucleus	oval, indented with finer chromatin & without obvious nucleolus	round to oval with single distinct nucleolus & variable chromatin	round with clumped chromatin & small to absent nucleoli
cytoplasm	fine projections, often circumferential	occasional fine cytoplasmic projections	usually tufted projections that are polar or "torpedo"-like
immunophenotype	CD11c+ (bright) CD25+ CD103+ CD123+ annexin 1+	CD11c+ (bright) CD25– CD103+/– CD123dim/– annexin 1–	CD11c–/+ CD25– CD103– CD123dim/– annexin 1–
Incidence of molecular & cytogenetic findings			
BRAF V600E	~100%	0%	0%
MAP2K1 mutation	0%	30%-40%	0%
KLF2 mutation	~15%	0%	~25%-40%
NOTCH2 mutation	rare	0%	20%-25%
TP53 mutation	rare	~15%	rare
U2AF1 mutation	0%	~15%	0%
MLL3 (KMT2C) mutation	~15%	~25%	rare
CCDN3 mutation	0%	13%	7%
CDKN1B (p27) mutation	~15%	rare	rare
IGVH gene usage	*IGHV*3-30 ~7% *IGHV*3-33 ~7% *IGHV*4-39 ~7%	*IGHV*-34 ~50%	*IGHV*1-2 ~30% *IGHV*4-34 ~10%-15% *IGHV*3-23 ~8%
del(7q)	occasional	unknown	~40%

CD123 **t31.1**. CD11c expression is moderate to strong and CD25 expression is also robust. In addition, the cells demonstrate strong expression of the B-cell antigens CD20, CD22, and CD79b. CD38 is typically negative. Annexin-1 expression, usually assessed by IHC, is felt to be specific for HCL. Cyclin D1 is also weakly positive in HCL cells but they lack a *CCND1* translocation. HCL cells may also express CD10 and rare cases have been shown to be CD5 positive; therefore, expression of CD10 or CD5 does not exclude a diagnosis of HCL.

SMZL cells typically lack CD103 and CD123 and may have low to absent CD25 expression. CD11c is generally low or absent in SMZL, although occasional cases may express CD11c at high levels. HCL-v cells usually have strong expression of CD11c as well as partial expression of CD103, whereas CD123 is generally low or absent. HCL-v cells are universally negative for CD25, a key feature in distinguishing HCL-v from classic HCL. More recently, markers shown to be differentially expressed between HCL and HCL-v include CD43, CD81, and CD200, with CD43 and CD200 having stronger expression and CD81 having weaker expression in HCL, as compared to HCL-v.

It is critical to discriminate HCL from SMZL and HCL-v, because therapy differs for these neoplasms. Of particular importance is distinguishing HCL-v from HCL, because HCL-v is associated with a more aggressive disease course and poor response to the purine analogs typically used to treat HCL. Positive response of HCL to therapy correlates with the presence of the *BRAF* V600E mutation, which is observed in nearly 100% of HCL cases and absent in HCL-v.

BRAF V600E in exon 15 is almost universally present in HCL, with very rare patients having *BRAF* mutations located in exon 11. A *BRAF* V600E-specific monoclonal antibody can be used to detect disease in cases with low tumor burden or in which mutation analysis is not possible. The *BRAF* gene encodes a serine/threonine kinase that plays an important role in the RAS/RAF/MEK/ERK mitotic signaling pathway. The *BRAF* V600E protein product is constitutively active, leading to uncontrolled phosphorylation of MEK and subsequently ERK; ERK then phosphorylates multiple targets which drive cellular activation and proliferation. Among B-cell neoplasms, *BRAF* V600E is not specific to HCL and rarely occurs in chronic lymphocytic leukemia, SMZL, splenic diffuse red pulp lymphoma, and B-cell prolymphocytic leukemia. The clinical impact of *BRAF* mutations in these other B-cell lymphoproliferative disorders is unclear at present.

In addition to *BRAF*, other genes that are recurrently mutated in HCL include *CDKN1B*, *KLF2*, and *KMT2C* (*MLL3*), among others (frequencies shown in **t31.1**). Mutations in *CDKN1B* and *KMT2C (MLL3)* are inactivating, whereas the pathogenic nature of *KLF2* mutations is uncertain. The effect of these mutations on disease course is unclear but one study found that *CDKN1B* mutations did not affect prognosis. *KLF2* is more commonly mutated in SMZL, occurring in ~25%-40% of cases, and mutations are structurally distinct from those in HCL; *KLF2* alterations in HCL are characterized by amino acid substitutions whereas in SMZL the *KLF2* mutations affect splicing or lead to frameshifts (see also **Case 36**). As mentioned, HCL-v is characterized by the absence of *BRAF* V600E, instead having mutations in *MAP2K1* in 30%-40% of cases. Thus, molecular profiling may help to distinguish these three disorders in difficult cases. HCL-v is also notable for heavily biased use of the *IGHV*4-34 immunoglobulin receptor gene, present in ~50% of cases. If sequencing of

IGHV is available, this analysis may be of value in cases in which the distinction between HCL and HCL-v is otherwise difficult.

In this case, the presence of *BRAF* V600E confirmed the diagnosis of classic HCL, and the patient was started on a purine analog, which led to complete remission and appropriate recovery of peripheral blood counts one year later.

Diagnostic pearls/pitfalls

- HCL can be distinguished from HCL-v by mutation profiling. HCL is characterized by near universal presence of *BRAF* V600E, whereas HCL-v always lacks *BRAF* V600E and has preferential usage of IGVH4-34 immunoglobulin receptor in 50% of cases, as well as mutated *MAP2K1* in 30%-40% of cases.
- As opposed to HCL, HCL-v does not respond to purine analogs, and correspondingly, response to purine analogs correlates to the presence of *BRAF* V600E. Thus, *BRAF* mutation analysis should be performed in all suspect cases of HCL.
- A phenotype that is positive for CD11c (bright), CD25 (moderate-bright), CD123, and CD103 is virtually diagnostic for HCL, whereas HCL-v lacks CD25.
- A *BRAF* V600E specific monoclonal antibody is available that can be used to detect disease in cases with low tumor burden or where sequencing is not possible.

Readings

Andersen CL, Gruszka-Westwood A, Østergaard M, et al. A narrow deletion of 7q is common to HCL, and SMZL, but not CLL. Eur J Haematol. 2004.72(6):390-402. **DOI: 10.1111/j.1600-0609.2004.00243.x**

Bikos V, Darzentas N, Hadzidimitriou A, et al. Over 30% of patients with splenic marginal zone lymphoma express the same immunoglobulin heavy variable gene: ontogenetic implications. Leukemia. 2012;26(7):1638-46. **DOI: 10.1038/leu.2012.3**

Dietrich S, Hüllein J, Lee SC, et al. Recurrent *CDKN1B* (p27) mutations in hairy cell leukemia. 2015;126(8):1005-8. **DOI: 10.1182/blood-2015-04-643361**

Durham BH, Getta B, Dietrich S, et al. Genomic analysis of hairy cell leukemia identifies novel recurrent genetic alterations. Blood. 2017;130(14):1644-8. **DOI: 10.1182/blood-2017-01-765107**

Falini B, Martelli MP, Tiacci E. *BRAF* V600E mutation in hairy cell leukemia: from bench to bedside. Blood. 2016;128(15):1918-27. **DOI: 10.1182/blood-2016-07-418434**

Jebaraj BM, Kienle D, Bühler A, et al. *BRAF* mutations in chronic lymphocytic leukemia. Leuk Lymphoma. 2013;54(6):1177-82. **DOI: 10.3109/10428194.2012.742525.**

Langabeer SE, Quinn F, O'Brien D, et al. Incidence of the *BRAF* V600E mutation in chronic lymphocytic leukaemia and prolymphocytic leukaemia. Leuk Res. 2012;36(4):483-4. **DOI: 10.1016/j.leukres.2011.12.015**

ISBN 978-089189-6814 ©2021 ASCP

Pettirossi V, Santi A, Imperi E, et al. *BRAF* inhibitors reverse the unique molecular signature and phenotype of hairy cell leukemia and exert potent antileukemic activity. Blood. 2015;125(8):1207-16. **DOI: 10.1182/blood-2014-10-603100**

Roider T, Falini B, Dietrich S. Recent advances in understanding and managing hairy cell leukemia. F1000Res. 2018;7:F1000 Faculty Rev-509. **DOI: DOI.org/10.12688/f1000research.13265.1**

Salem DA, Scott D, McCoy CS, et al. Differential Expression of CD43, CD81, and CD200 in Classic Versus Variant Hairy Cell Leukemia. Cytometry B Clin Cytom. 2019;96(4):275-82. **DOI: 10.1002/cyto.b.21785**

Sellar RS, Fend F, Akarca AU, et al. *BRAF*(V600E) mutations are found in Richter syndrome and may allow targeted therapy in a subset of patients. Br J Haematol. 2015;170(2):282-5. **DOI: 10.1111/bjh.13291**

Shao H, Calvo KR, Grönborg M, et al. Distinguishing hairy cell leukemia variant from hairy cell leukemia: development and validation of diagnostic criteria. Leuk Res. 2013;37(4):401-9. **DOI: 10.1016/j.leukres.2012.11.021**

Tiacci E, Pettirossi V, Schiavoni G, et al. Genomics of hairy cell leukemia. J Clin Oncol. 2017;35(9):1002-10. **DOI: 10.1200/JCO.2016.71.1556.**

Tiacci E, Trifonov V, Schiavoni G, et al. *BRAF* mutations in hairy-cell leukemia. N Engl J Med. 2011;364(24):2305-15. **DOI: 10.1056/NEJMoa1014209**

Troussard X, Cornet E. Hairy cell leukemia 2018: Update on diagnosis, risk-stratification, and treatment. Am J Hematol. 2017;92(12):1382-90. **DOI: 10.1002/ajh.24936**

Turakhia S, Lanigan C, Hamadeh F, et al. Immunohistochemistry for *BRAF* V600E in the differential diagnosis of hairy cell leukemia vs other splenic B-cell lymphomas. Am J Clin Pathol. 2015;144(1):87-93. **DOI: 10.1309/AJCP5WVXJ2KTLODO**

Waterfall J, Arons E, Walker R, et al. High prevalence of *MAP2K1* mutations in variant and IGHV4-34–expressing hairy-cell leukemias. Nature Genetics 2014;46:8-10. **DOI: 10.1038/ng.2828**

Watkins AJ, Huang Y, Ye H, et al. Splenic marginal zone lymphoma: characterization of 7q deletion and its value in diagnosis. J Pathol. 2010;220(4):461-74. **DOI: 10.1002/path.2665**

Weston-Bell NJ, Tapper W, Gibson J, et al. 2016. Exome sequencing in classic hairy cell leukaemia reveals widespread variation in acquired somatic mutations between individual tumours apart from the signature *BRAF* V(600)E lesion. PLoS One. 11(2):e0149162. **DOI: 10.1371/journal.pone.0149162**

Xi L, Arons E, Navarro W, et al. Both variant and IGHV4-34-expressing hairy cell leukemia lack the *BRAF* V600E mutation. Blood. 2012;119(14):3330-2. **DOI: 10.1182/blood-2011-09-379339**

Erika M Moore

32

Mantle cell lymphoma with t(11;14)(q13;q32) *CCND1-IGH* & mutations in *NOTCH2 & ATM*

History A 52-year-old male presented with mild, persistent pancytopenia. CBC results are shown at right. A bone marrow biopsy with peripheral smear review was performed for further evaluation.

Morphology & flow cytometry A peripheral blood smear demonstrated pancytopenia with rare atypical lymphoid cells having irregular nuclear contours. The bone marrow aspirate showed increased and atypical lymphocytes that were small to intermediate in size with condensed chromatin. The core biopsy was hypercellular (80% cellular) with multiple large interstitial lymphoid aggregates **f32.1**.

Flow cytometry demonstrated a dim κ-restricted B-cell population that was positive for CD5, CD19, CD20, and CD79b, and negative for CD10, CD23, CD25, CD11c, and CD43 **f32.2**.

Immunohistochemical stains performed on the core biopsy demonstrated that the lymphoid aggregates were positive for CD20, CD5, PAX5, cyclin D1, and SOX11 **f32.3**. A Ki-67 stain demonstrated approximately 10%-20% positive cells.

Based on the morphologic and immunophenotypic findings, a diagnosis of **mantle cell lymphoma** was rendered.

WBC	3.2×10^9/L
RBC	4.49×10^{12}/L
HGB	12.4 g/dL
HCT	38.5%
MCV	86 fL
RDW	15.1%
Platelets	76×10^9/L

Genetics/molecular results FISH was positive for a rearrangement between *IGH* and *CCND1* **f32.4**. A targeted NGS panel for lymphoid-related genes demonstrated the following mutations:

NOTCH2 p.R2400* (c. 7198C>T) in 13% of 330 reads **f32.5**
ATM p.D2725V (c. 8174A>T) in 8% of 1511 reads

ISBN 978-089189-6814 ©2021 ASCP

32 Mantle cell lymphoma with t(11;14)(q13;q32) CCND1-IGH & mutations in NOTCH2 & ATM

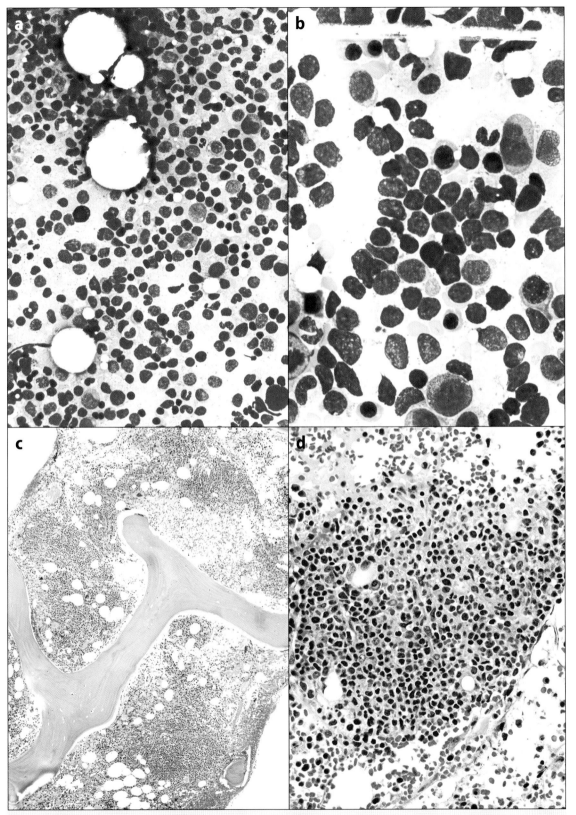

f32.1 a-b The bone marrow aspirate smear demonstrates predominance of small mature lymphocytes with irregular nuclear contours, which form **c-d** loosely paratrabecular and interstitial nodular lymphoid infiltrates in the core biopsy

32 *Mantle cell lymphoma with t(11;14)(q13;q32) CCND1-IGH & mutations in NOTCH2 & ATM*

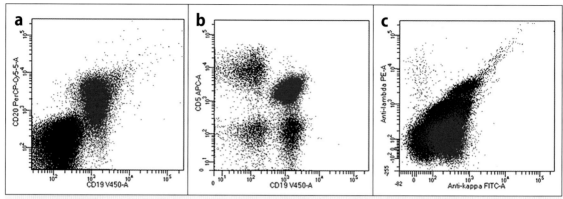

f32.2 Flow cytometric studies (gated on CD45 bright events) demonstrate a **a** CD19+, CD20+, **b** CD5+ B-cell population with dim κ light chain restriction (shown in red)

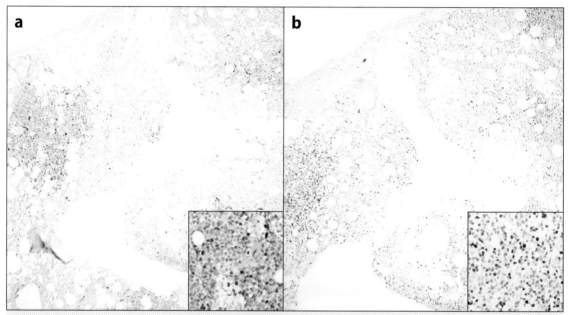

f32.3 Immunohistochemistry performed on the core biopsy is positive for **a** cyclin D1 & **b** SOX11, with higher power insets

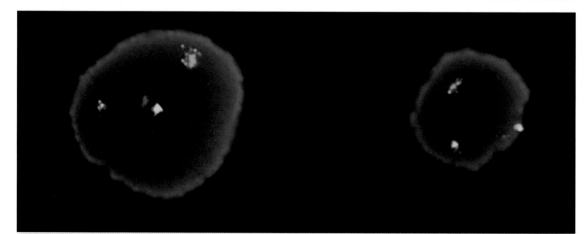

f32.4 Dual fusion FISH probes for *IGH* (14q32, green) & *CCND1* (11q13, orange) demonstrate 1 orange signal, 1 green signal & 2 yellow signals, diagnostic of *IGH-CCND1* fusion

ISBN 978-089189-6814

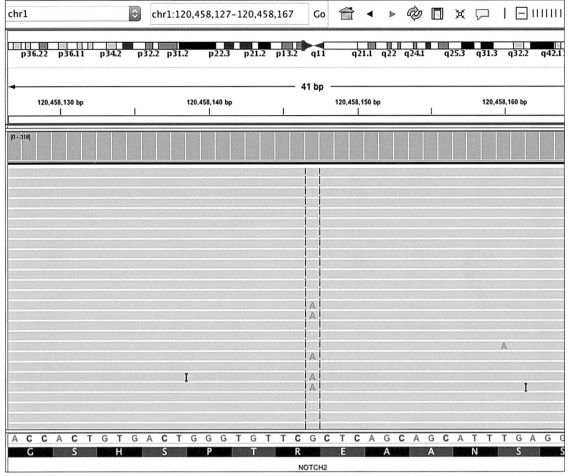

f32.5 Somatic variant analysis using a targeted lymphoid NGS panel showing 1 of 2 mutations detected; annotated reads mapped to the *NOTCH2* locus demonstrate p.R2400* (c. 7198C>T) in 13% of reads, highlighted in green (showing the reverse strand; hg19, Integrative Genomics Viewer browser) [see **fA.8**, p312]

Discussion Mantle cell lymphoma (MCL) is a B-cell lymphoma typically composed of monotonous, small to intermediate-sized lymphocytes with irregular nuclear contours and condensed chromatin. It usually occurs in older patients, is more common in men, and is often seen in lymph nodes but can also be present in the bone marrow, spleen, or extranodal sites. Although not positive in every case, aberrantly strong CD5 expression is characteristic of MCL. Therefore, one of the main differential diagnostic considerations is chronic lymphocytic leukemia/small lymphocytic lymphoma (CLL/SLL), because CLL/SLL is also a CD5-positive B-cell lymphoproliferative disorder composed of small lymphocytes. Using flow cytometric studies, MCL is typically differentiated from CLL/SLL by moderate to bright CD20, moderate to bright surface light chain, expression of FMC7, and lack of CD23 and CD200 **t32.1**. Most MCLs will also express nuclear cyclin D1

(by immunohistochemistry) because of the characteristic *IGH-CCND1* translocation, t(11;14)(q13;q32), present in over 95% of cases. A small subset of MCLs (<5%) do not have *IGH-CCND1* and are therefore negative for cyclin D1 expression, but these cases usually express the transcription factor SOX11, which is also positive in the vast majority of MCL cases and therefore a useful marker for those that are cyclin D1-negative. LEF1 is another useful immunostain for differentiating between MCL and CLL/SLL, because it is relatively specific for CLL/SLL and should be negative in MCL **t32.1**.

The primary oncogenic event in the vast majority of MCL cases is t(11;14)(q13;q32), a rearrangement between *CCND1* on 11q13 and the immunoglobulin heavy chain gene (*IGH*) promoter on 14q32; this fusion results in overexpression of cyclin D1 and subsequent cell cycle deregulation. Although this is the initiating event, additional abnormalities are required to develop

t32.1 Comparison between mantle cell lymphoma (MCL) & chronic lymphocytic leukemia/small lymphocytic lymphoma (CLL/SLL)

Feature	MCL	CLL/SLL
morphology	small, irregular nuclear contours, condensed chromatin	small, round, condensed "soccer ball" chromatin
sites of involvement	lymph nodes, frequent extranodal involvement, spleen, bone marrow, peripheral blood	peripheral blood, bone marrow, spleen, lymph nodes; extranodal involvement less common
immunophenotype	CD5+, cyclin D1+, CD23–, FMC7+, CD200–, SOX11+, LEF1–	CD5+, CD20 dim/–, cyclin D1–, CD23+, FMC7–, CD200+, surface light chain dim/–, LEF1+, SOX11–
clinically important chromosomal abnormalities	t(11;14)(q13;q32) *IGH/CCND1* is recurrent	del(13q), trisomy 12, del(11q), del(17p) used for prognostication

MCL and numerous secondary genetic aberrations have been reported. Alterations that affect pathways including apoptosis, chromatin modification, DNA damage response, and the cell cycle have all been described, as well as abnormalities that result in activation of several known oncogenic/signaling pathways including NOTCH, JAK/STAT3, WNT signaling, mTOR and NF-κB, among others. Some of the most commonly mutated genes in MCL are *ATM*, *CCND1*, *MLL2*, *TP53*, and *NOTCH*. Although the prognostic significance of these additional mutations (other than *TP53*) is not entirely certain, one study found that *NOTCH*, *TP53*, and *CCND1* mutations, among others, are much more frequent in blastoid and pleomorphic MCL than in classic MCL. A few other studies have indicated potential for therapeutic targeting of specific mutations such as *NOTCH* or for molecular pathway-related therapies such as those targeting the DNA damage response in cases with *ATM* and *TP53* mutations, for example.

Although most small B-cell lymphomas are relatively indolent, MCL has an aggressive clinical course with a historical median survival of 3-5 years. Although in recent years more aggressive chemotherapy regimens, often followed by autologous stem cell transplantation, have led to improved median survival times, MCL still remains largely uncurable. Both the Ki-67 proliferation index and *TP53* mutation status are important prognostic indicators in MCL. A Ki-67 index >30% is associated with a worse prognosis while Ki-67 <10% is correlated with a better clinical course. Similarly, several studies have shown that MCLs with *TP53* mutations do not respond well to conventional chemotherapeutic

regimens or transplantation and have a poorer overall survival. National Comprehensive Cancer Network guidelines advocate *TP53* mutation analysis in all new cases of MCL.

There are several morphologic variants of MCL that have clinical significance. The 2 morphologic variants associated with more aggressive behavior than typical MCL are termed *blastoid* and *pleomorphic*. Blastoid MCL resembles a lymphoblastic leukemia with monotonous-appearing intermediate-sized cells with fine chromatin and usually a very high mitotic rate. Pleomorphic MCL often consists of many large cells with more vesicular chromatin and prominent nucleoli and can mimic a diffuse large B-cell lymphoma. Both variants are associated with poor overall survival. Conversely, the leukemic, non-nodal-type of MCL, which is defined by peripheral blood, bone marrow, and splenic involvement but without significant lymphadenopathy, is associated with more indolent disease. These variants of MCL may have a somewhat atypical immunophenotype. Leukemic non-nodal cases tend to be SOX11-negative and may be CD5-negative or CD200-positive. Pleomorphic and blastoid variants can lack CD5 and express LEF1. Although the aberrant immunophenotype or unusual morphology in these variant cases may cause confusion, all these variants typically express cyclin D1, allowing for their identification as MCL.

In this patient, the absence of *TP53* mutation predicted response to conventional chemotherapy, which he received shortly after diagnosis.

Diagnostic pearls/pitfalls

- Most but not all cases of MCL carry the t(11;14) *CCND1-IGH* fusion, which results in overexpression of cyclin D1 protein.

- Almost all MCLs are positive by immunohistochemistry for cyclin D1, SOX11, or both. SOX11 is a useful stain to identify cyclin D1-negative MCL though it is often negative in the leukemic non-nodal type of MCL. Using a combination of both stains should allow for recognition of nearly all cases of MCL.

- Although there are distinct immunophenotypic differences between CLL/SLL and MCL, typical patterns are not always present and all cases of suspected CLL should be assessed for cyclin D1 overexpression, either via immunohistochemistry or FISH testing for *CCND1-IGH*, because these 2 disorders differ significantly in their prognoses and therapeutic courses.

- It is good practice to perform a cyclin D1 immunostain on all suspected diffuse large B-cell lymphomas, particularly those that are CD5-positive, to exclude the pleomorphic variant of mantle cell lymphoma.

- *TP53* mutation analysis should be performed in all new cases of MCL, because these mutations confer a worse prognosis and suggest poor response to conventional chemotherapy.

Readings

Beà S, Valdés-Mas R, Navarro A, Salaverria I, et al. Landscape of somatic mutations and clonal evolution in mantle cell lymphoma. Proc Natl Acad Sci U S A. 2013;110(45):18250-5. **DOI: 10.1073/pnas.1314608110**

Determann 0, Hoster E, Ott G, et al. Ki-67 predicts outcome in advanced-stage mantle cell lymphoma patients treated with anti-CD20 immunochemotherapy: results from randomized trials of the European MCL Network and the German Low Grade Lymphoma Study Group. Blood. 2008;111(4):2385-7. **DOI: 10.1182/blood-2007-10-117010**

Greiner TC, Dasgupta C, Ho VV, et al. Mutation and genomic deletion status of ataxia telangiectasia mutated (*ATM*) and p53 confer specific gene expression profiles in mantle cell lymphoma. Proc Natl Acad Sci U S A. 2006;103(7):2352-7. **DOI: 10.1073/pnas.0510441103**

Halldórsdóttir AM, Lundin A, Murray F, et al. Impact of *TP53* mutation and 17p deletion in mantle cell lymphoma. Leukemia. 2011;25:1904-8. **DOI: 10.1038/leu.2011.162**

Jain P, Zhang S, Kanagal-Shamanna R, et al. Genomic profiles and clinical outcomes of de novo blastoid/pleomorphic MCL are distinct from those of transformed MCL. Blood Adv. 2020;4(6):1038-50. **DOI: 10.1182/bloodadvances.2019001396**

Nordström L, Sernbo S, Eden P, et al. *SOX11* and *TP53* add prognostic information to MIPI in a homogenously treated cohort of mantle cell lymphoma—a Nordic Lymphoma Group study. Br J Haematol. 2014;166:98-108. **DOI: 10.1111/bjh.12854**

Sarkozy C, Ribrag V. Novel agents for mantle cell lymphoma: molecular rational and clinical data. Expert Opin Investig Drugs. 2020;29(6):555-66. **DOI: 10.1080/13543784.2020.1760245**

Silkenstedt E, Arenas F, Colom-Sanmartí B, et al. Notch1 signaling in *NOTCH1*-mutated mantle cell lymphoma depends on delta-like ligand 4 and is a potential target for specific antibody therapy. J Exp Clin Cancer Res. 2019;38(1):446. **DOI: 10.1186/s13046-019-1458-7**

Swerdlow SH, Campo E, Harris NL, et al. World Health Organization Classification of Tumours of Haematopoietic and Lymphoid Tissues. 4th ed. Lyon, France: IARC Press; 2017. **ISBN: 9789283244943**

Zhang J, Jima D, Moffitt AB, Qingquan L, et al. The genomic landscape of mantle cell lymphoma is related to the epigenetically determined chromatin state of normal B cells. Blood. 2014;123(19):2988-96. **DOI: 10.1182/blood-2013-07-517177**

Jingwei Li, Valentina Nardi & Annette S Kim

33

Follicular lymphoma with del(1p36)

History An 89-year-old man presented with a 2-month history of progressively enlarging left submandibular adenopathy and was found on subsequent imaging to have multiple cervical, supraclavicular, and axillary lymph nodes enlarged up to 2.0 cm. He denied any "B" symptoms (fever, drenching night sweats, or loss of >10% of body weight over 6 months). CBC results are shown at right. The differential was normal. An initial fine-needle aspiration biopsy was nondiagnostic and the patient subsequently underwent excisional biopsy of the left submandibular lymph node.

Morphology & flow cytometry The gross report indicated a 3.5 cm lymph node that on histologic examination was almost entirely replaced by a proliferation of large, crowded, and expanded follicles composed of numerous centroblasts (>15/high-power field) in a background of centrocytes (small cleaved lymphocytes, **f33.1**, **f33.2**). There were few scattered mitoses within follicles, which lacked polarization and mantle zones.

Immunohistochemistry showed that the neoplastic follicular cells were positive for CD20, BCL2, BCL6, and MUM1 but negative for CD10 **f33.3**. CD21 and CD23 demonstrated extensive expanded and disrupted follicular dendritic cell meshworks **f33.4**. The neoplastic B cells expressed IgM but not IgG, IgD, or IgA. The Ki-67 proliferation index was 70%-80% within the follicles.

Flow cytometric analysis demonstrated a population of B cells (47% of gated events) that was positive for B lymphoid markers CD19 and CD20, exhibited monotypic surface and cytoplasmic κ immunoglobulin light chain expression, and was negative for CD5, CD10, CD23, CD200, and other T-cell markers **f33.5**.

WBC	10.54×10^9/L
HGB	15.2 g/dL
HCT	38.5%
MCV	89.6 fL
Platelets	211×10^9/L

Genetics/molecular results Cytogenetic analysis showed a complex karyotype of 48,XY,del(1)(p36.1p36.3), add(2)(p23), inv(3)(q12q27), der(6;17)(p10;q10), +9,dup(18)(q21q23),+22,+mar[cp7] in the majority of metaphases **f33.6**. FISH analysis was negative for t(14;18) *IGH-BCL2*. Based on the morphologic, immunophenotypic, flow cytometric, and cytogenetic findings, a diagnosis was rendered of a **B-cell lymphoma, most consistent with follicular lymphoma (grade 3A of 3)**.

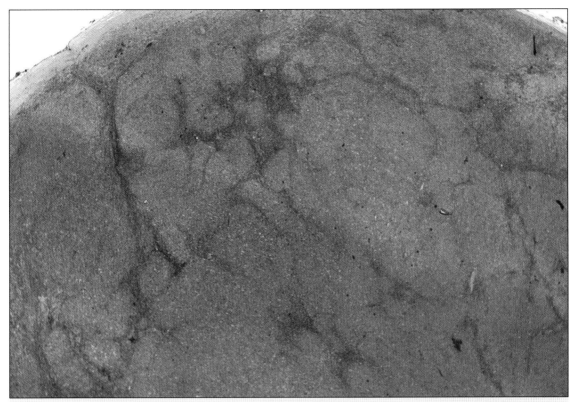

f33.1 H&E stain demonstrating expanded follicles entirely replacing the lymph node

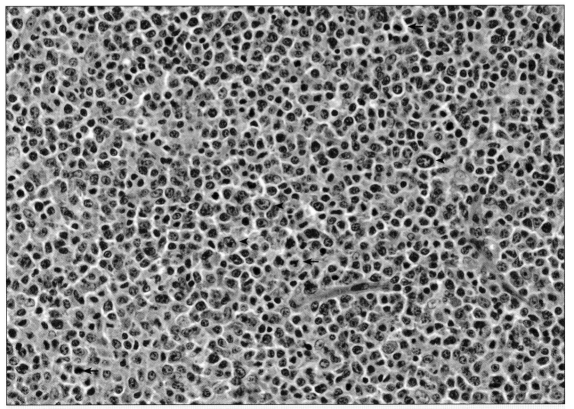

f33.2 H&E stain of the lymph node demonstrating centrocytes & larger centroblasts (arrowheads) & mitotic figures (arrows)

33 *Follicular lymphoma with del(1p36)*

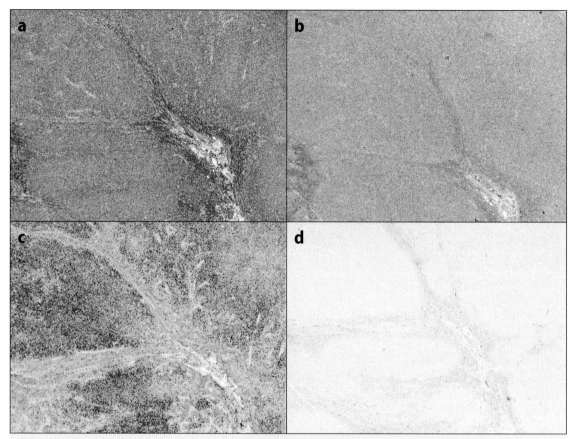

f33.3 IHC demonstrating that the tumor cells are positive for **a** BCL2, **b** BCL6 & **c** MUM1 but **d** negative for CD10

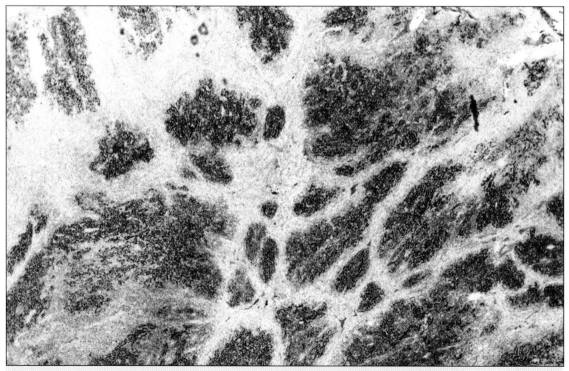

f33.4 CD21 immunohistochemical stain demonstrating expanded & disrupted follicular dendritic cell meshworks

ISBN 978-089189-6814

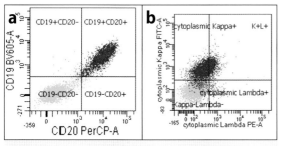

f33.5 Flow cytometric analysis of the lymph node demonstrating a population (highlighted in red) of **a** CD19+, CD20+ B cells which **b** express cytoplasmic κ light chain restriction; background T cells are shown in blue

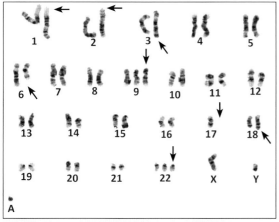

f33.6 Karyotype showing deletion of 1p36.1p36.3; additional chromosomal aberrations include additional material of unknown origin at 2p23, inversion of 3q12q27, derivative chromosome of (6;17)(p10;q10), gain of chromosomes 9 & 22, duplication of 18q21q23 & a marker chromosome

Discussion Follicular lymphoma (FL) is a B-cell neoplasm of follicle center cell origin composed of variable proliferations of numerous neoplastic follicles. The resulting lymph node architecture ranges from a partially follicular pattern to complete effacement by neoplastic follicles, or even a predominantly diffuse pattern with loss of follicular organization. FL cytologic grades (1-2, 3A, or 3B) are based on the number of large centroblasts in a background of centrocytes within the neoplastic follicles. Progression in cytologic grade is common during the natural history of the disease, from a few centroblasts in low-grade FL to numerous centroblasts in high-grade FL, with subsequent transformation in some cases to diffuse large B-cell lymphoma composed of sheets of large centroblasts.

In about 80%-90% of the cases, FL is genetically characterized by the t(14;18)(q32;q21) balanced chromosomal translocation between the *IGH* and *BCL2* genes. This primary event is not sufficient for manifestation of the disease, and acquisition of secondary genetic alterations is necessary for disease progression. *BCL2* translocation to immunoglobulin light chain genes has also been reported in a minority of cases, namely t(2;18)(p11;q21) and t(18;22)(q21;q11), which result in fusion of *BCL2* with κ or λ light chain genes, respectively. Secondary genetic events include mutations in epigenetic genes, in particular genes encoding histone modifiers such as *KMT2D* (*MLL2*), *CREBBP*, *EZH2*, and *EP300*. Other highly recurrently mutated genes include those involved in B-cell signaling pathways, such as *TNFRSF14*, *CARD11*, and *MAP2K1*, as well as the immunomodulator *IRF8*.

Lymphomas having a follicular growth pattern but lacking *BCL2* rearrangement and protein expression occur in both children and adults and often present diagnostic challenges. Large B-cell lymphoma with *IRF4* gene rearrangement occurs mostly in children and young adults and is characterized by strong expression of MUM1 (IRF4) in the neoplastic cells, which typically have a follicular and/or diffuse growth pattern (see **Case 40**). These cases have high-grade morphology and a high proliferation index, but usually have localized disease that responds well to treatment. Large B cell lymphoma with *IRF4* rearrangement must be distinguished from pediatric-type FL (PTFL; see **Case 34**), which also occurs mostly in younger patients, with a similar predilection for the head and neck region. PTFL is associated with a follicular growth pattern and often blastoid morphology with a paradoxically excellent prognosis. PTFL may be difficult to differentiate from either reactive lymphadenopathy or grade 3 FL (especially in adults); the latter distinction is especially important because localized cases of PTFL often do not need treatment beyond surgical excision. PTFL is associated with recurrent aberrations of the *TNFRSF14* locus at 1p36.32, either by copy neutral loss of heterozygosity (CN-LOH) or mutation, as well as recurrent mutations in *MAP2K1*. Interestingly, recurrent deletion of the *TNFRSF14* locus can be found in many adult cases of FL that lack t(14;18); these are associated with predominantly diffuse growth pattern and low-grade histology, often with coexpression of CD10 and CD23 and localized inguinal location. The term *diffuse FL variant* has been proposed for these cases, which often still contain small or microfollicles within diffuse regions. In contrast to the diffuse FL variant, it is well-recognized that many high-grade FLs in adults can be BCL2-negative and lose CD10 expression, especially as they become more diffuse. These cases may also express MUM1 in a diffuse growth pattern; they have relatively poor

t33.1 Lymphomas with follicular growth pattern that are typically negative for t(14;18) *IGH-BCL2*

Entity	Age group	Typical anatomic site	Morphology	Genetic findings	Notable immunophenotype
large B cell lymphoma with IRF4 rearrangement	usually children, young adults; rarely adults	head & neck	intermediate-sized to large cells with open chromatin; follicular or follicular & diffuse pattern	*IRF4* rearrangement; *BCL6* locus breakpoints in some cases	positive: CD20, PAX5, BCL6, MUM1 & in some cases BCL2 Negative: PRDM1(BLIMP1), CD10 in ~30%
pediatric-type FL	children & young adults with a marked male predominance (M:F = 10:1), rarely adults	head & neck; inguinal & femoral lymph nodes less frequent	partial effacement of nodal architecture by intermediate-sized cells; follicular proliferation with expansile follicles having "starry sky" appearance	del(1p36), *TNFRSF14* deletion or mutations, *MAP2K1* mutations in some cases	positive: CD20, PAX5, CD10 & BCL6 negative: BCL2, MUM1
"diffuse variant" of FL	middle-aged adults	inguinal region	diffuse involvement of lymph node by a mixture of centrocytes and centroblasts; scattered "micro" or residual follicles	del(1p36)	positive: CD20, PAX5, CD23, CD10, BCL6 variable: BCL2
primary cutaneous FL	middle-aged adults with a slight male predominance (male:female = 1.5:1)	head & trunk	neoplastic follicular center cells in a follicular or diffuse pattern infiltrating subcutis but sparing dermis	del(14q32.33) & rarely deletion or promoter hypermethylation of *CDKN2A* & *CDKN2B*	positive: CD20, CD79a, CD10 (may be absent), BCL6 negative: BCL2, MUM1

prognosis, and if necessary, can be distinguished from large B-cell lymphoma with *IRF4* gene rearrangement using FISH probes for *IRF4*. Finally, primary cutaneous follicular center lymphoma is also typically negative for *BCL2* rearrangement and protein expression. In this example case, chromosome analysis demonstrated deletion of 1p36 and lack of t(14;18); however, the morphologic and immunophenotypic findings did not suggest the diffuse FL variant.

TNFRSF14 encodes a member of the tumor necrosis factor receptor superfamily. It is thought that the FL disease progression in patients with either mutation or deletion of this gene is because of loss of its tumor suppressor role. For instance, it is known that stimulation of TNFRSF14 in lymphoma cells via LIGHT ligand enhances Fas-induced apoptosis and improves tumor

immunogenicity. Adult FL with deletion 1p36, while bearing aberrations of *TNFRSF14* in common with PTFL, displays a complex mutational profile with recurrent co-occurrence of *STAT6* and *CREBBP* and other epigenetic gene mutations, but not of *MAP2K1*, distinguishing it from the genomically more quiet PTFL.

In conclusion, the 1p36 locus may be affected by a variety of alterations in FL, including copy number variation, acquired CN-LOH, and mutations, and alterations in *TNFRSF14* are among the most common genetic lesions seen in FLs, although not specific for this entity. Alterations at 1p36 can occur in FLs with or without t(14;18) *IGH-BCL2*. However, it should be noted that FISH probes for 1p36 are not widespread for clinical use at this time, making these aberrations difficult to detect in the absence of karyotypic studies.

Diagnostic pearls/pitfalls

– FLs may display a wide range of architectural variation, from a partially follicular pattern to a predominantly diffuse pattern with loss of follicular organization.

– Excisional biopsy is recommended for initial diagnosis of FL because adequate sampling of the lymph node tissue is necessary for accurate grading and to differentiate the focally follicular/predominantly diffuse variant of FL from diffuse large B-cell lymphoma.

– The hallmark t(14;18)(q32;q21) chromosomal translocation between the *IGH* and *BCL2* genes is present in most but not all cases of FL. Distinct variants that typically do not have this translocation are listed in **t33.1**.

– The diffuse variant of FL as well as PTFL frequently demonstrate deletion of 1p36 and absence of t(14;18).

– Aberrations of the *TNFRSF14* locus at 1p36.32 are common in both pediatric and adult types of FL, with or without accompanying t(14;18) *IGH-BCL2*.

Readings

Asmann Y, Maurer M, Wang C, et al. Genetic diversity of newly diagnosed follicular lymphoma. Blood Cancer J. 2014;4:e256. **DOI: 10.1038/bcj.2014.80**

Choi SM, Betz BL, Perry AM et al. Follicular lymphoma diagnostic caveats and updates. Arch Pathol Lab Med. 2018;142(11):1330-40. **DOI: 10.5858/arpa.2018-0217-RA**

Jaffe ES, Narris NL, Swerdlow SH, et al. Follicular lymphoma. In: Swerdlow SH, Campo E, Harris NL, et al. World Health Organization Classification of Tumours of Haematopoietic and Lymphoid Tissues. 4th ed. Lyon, France: IARC Press; 2017:266-277. **ISBN: 9789283244943**

Karube K, Guo Y, Suzumiya J, et al. CD10-MUM1+ follicular lymphoma lacks *BCL2* gene translocation and shows characteristic biologic and clinical features. Blood. 2007;109(7):3076-9. **DOI: 10.1182/blood-2006-09-045989**

Katzenberger T, Kalla J, Leich E, et al. A distinctive subtype of t(14;18)-negative nodal follicular non-Hodgkin lymphoma characterized by a predominantly diffuse growth pattern and deletions in the chromosomal region 1p36. Blood. 2009;113:1053-61. **DOI: 10.1182/blood-2008-07-168682**

Kim AS, Wu CJ, Lovitch SB. Molecular genetic aspects of non-Hodgkin lymphomas. In: Greer JP, Arber DA, Appelbalm FR, et al, eds. Wintrobe's Clinical Hematology. 14th ed. Philadelphia, PA: Wolters Kluwer Health; 2018; chap 88:1843-79. **ISBN: 978-1496347428**

Koster A, Tromp H, Raemaekers J, et al. The prognostic significance of the intra-follicular tumor cell proliferative rate in follicular lymphoma. Haematologica. 2007;92(2):184-90. **DOI: 10.3324/haematol.10384**

Launay E, Pangault C, Bertrand P, et al. High rate of *TNFRSF14* gene alterations related to 1p36 region in de novo follicular lymphoma and impact on prognosis. Leukemia. 2012;26(3):559-62. **DOI: 10.1038/leu.2011.266.**

Mamessier E, Song J, Eberle F, et al. Early lesions of follicular lymphoma: a genetic perspective. Haematologica. 2014;99(3):481-8. **DOI: 10.3324/haematol.2013.094474**

Salaverria I, Philipp C, Oschlies I, et al; Molecular Mechanisms in Malignant Lymphomas Network Project of the Deutsche Krebshilfe; German High-Grade Lymphoma Study Group; Berlin-Frankfurt-Munster-NHL Trial Group. Translocations activating *IRF4* identify a subtype of germinal center-derived B-cell lymphoma affecting predominantly children and young adults. Blood. 2011;118(1):139-47. **DOI: 10.1182/blood-2011-01-330795**

Schmidt J, Gong S, Marafioti T, et al. Genome-wide analysis of pediatric-type follicular lymphoma reveals low genetic complexity and recurrent alterations of *TNFRSF14* gene. Blood. 2016;128(8):1101-11. **DOI: 10.1182/blood-2016-03-703819**

Shanmugam V, Kim AS. Lymphomas. In: Tafe JL, Arcila ME, eds. Genomic Medicine: A Practical Guide. New York, NY: Springer. 2020; chap 16:253-315. **ISBN: 978-3030229214**

Siddiqi I, Friedman J, Barry-Holson K, et al. Characterization of a variant of t(14;18) negative nodal diffuse follicular lymphoma with CD23 expression, 1p36/*TNFRSF14* abnormalities, and *STAT6* mutations. Mod Pathol. 2016;29(6):570-81. **DOI: 10.1038/modpathol.2016.51**

Swerdlow S, Campo E, Pileri S, et al. The 2016 revision of the World Health Organization classification of lymphoid neoplasms. Blood. 2016;127(20):2375-90. **DOI: 10.1182/blood-2016-01-643569**

Zamò A, Pischimarov J, Horn H, et al. The exomic landscape of t(14;18)-negative diffuse follicular lymphoma with 1p36 deletion. Br J Haematol. 2018;180(3):391-4. **DOI: 10.1111/bjh.15041**

Howard Meyerson

34

Pediatric-type nodal follicular lymphoma with *MAP2K1* mutation

History A 69-year-old male was referred to an otolaryngologist for evaluation of a left neck mass. The patient noted left neck swelling for approximately 2 weeks after resolution of an infection of the left eye. On examination, the mass was firm. He had no pain, dysphagia, or "B" symptoms (fever, drenching night sweats, or loss of >10 percent of body weight over 6 months). CBC results are shown at right. The differential was normal.

CT of the neck demonstrated an enlarged, left, level 2 lymph node measuring 2.4 × 1.8 cm, with a few prominent other level 2 and 3 lymph nodes. An excisional biopsy was performed with flow cytometry and genetic studies.

Morphology & flow cytometry Sections from the biopsy demonstrated a lymph node with a nodular growth pattern of uniform-appearing, large follicles throughout the cortex and medulla, surrounded by attenuated mantle zones and separated only by a thin layer of small lymphocytes. The nodules lacked polarity and consisted predominantly of medium-sized lymphocytes with prominent nuclei (centroblast morphology) with numerous interspersed tingible body macrophages imparting a starry sky appearance focally **f34.1**. Immunohistochemistry (IHC) revealed cells with a germinal center phenotype (CD10 positive, BCL-6 positive, MUM1 negative) but with weak to absent expression of BCL2 **f34.2**. The proliferation fraction assessed by Ki-67 staining was ~95% **f34.2**. On flow cytometry, a clonal population of dim κ-restricted to surface immunoglobulin-negative B cells with weak expression of CD19 and CD79b and moderate expression of CD20 was detected **f34.3**. These findings indicated a lymphoma of germinal center origin with a follicular pattern but high-grade morphology.

WBC	5.2 × 10⁹/L
RBC	4.72 × 10¹²/L
HGB	14.9 g/dL
HCT	43.9%
MCV	93 fL
RDW	12.5%
Platelets	246 × 10⁹/L

Genetics/molecular results FISH studies for *MYC*, *BCL2*, and *BCL6* gene rearrangements and *IGH/MYC* fusion were performed on the formalin-fixed, paraffin-embedded tissue sections and were negative. A targeted lymphoid NGS panel was also performed on cells from the flow cytometry specimen and identified a *MAP2K1* p.K57N (c.171G>C) mutation in 26% of reads **f34.4**. Based on the overall morphologic, immunophenotypic, and genetic/molecular findings, a final diagnosis of **pediatric-type nodal follicular lymphoma** was rendered.

Discussion Follicular lymphomas (FLs) are a group of lymphoid neoplasms that arise from germinal center B cells. These lymphomas typically grow in a nodular pattern, recapitulating the normal follicular architecture of the lymph node. Most FLs occur in adults >30 years of age and are clinically indolent but incurable lesions, often disseminated throughout the body at the time of detection. Bone marrow involvement occurs in roughly 75% of cases of adult FL at diagnosis. Morphologically, FL usually shows a proliferation of uniform, back-to-back lymphoid nodules with attenuated to absent mantle zones, loss of the normal germinal center light zone/dark zone polarity, and absence of tingible body macrophages. Cytologically, the neoplastic cells are composed of a mixture of small irregular (or "cleaved") cells (centrocytes) and large cells (centroblasts). Cell size

ISBN 978-089189-6814

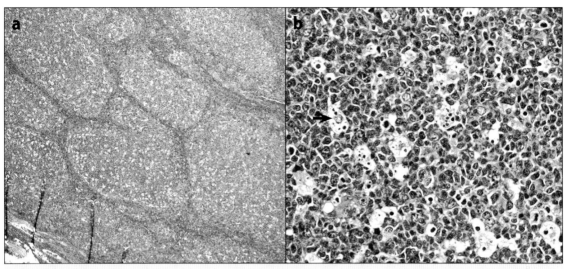

f34.1 Lymph node demonstrating **a** large, monotonous-appearing follicles composed of **b** centroblasts with numerous tingible body macrophages (arrow)

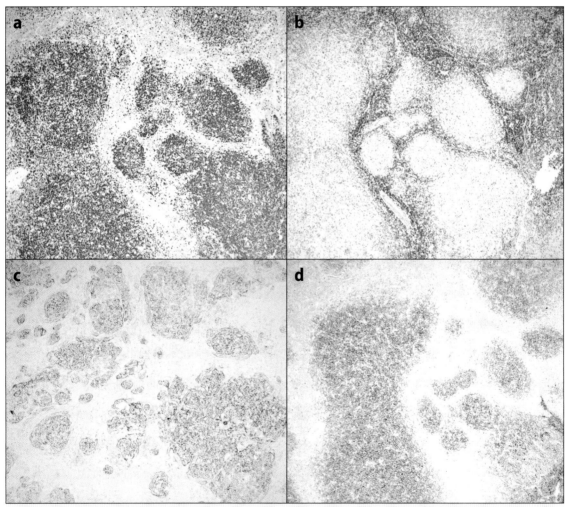

f34.2 Immunohistochemical stains demonstrating many follicles, which are **a** positive for CD10 & **b** negative for BCL2; the follicles have irregular outlines but **c** preserved CD21-positive follicular dendritic cell meshworks & **d** a high Ki-67 proliferation fraction

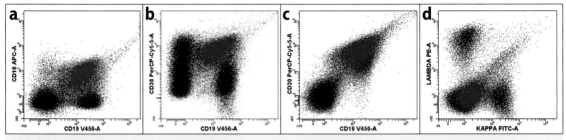

f34.3 Flow cytometry performed on the lymph node demonstrates an abnormal B-cell population, highlighted in red, which is **a** CD19 dim, CD10 positive, **b** CD38 positive, and **c** CD20 positive, with **d** partial dim κ light chain expression

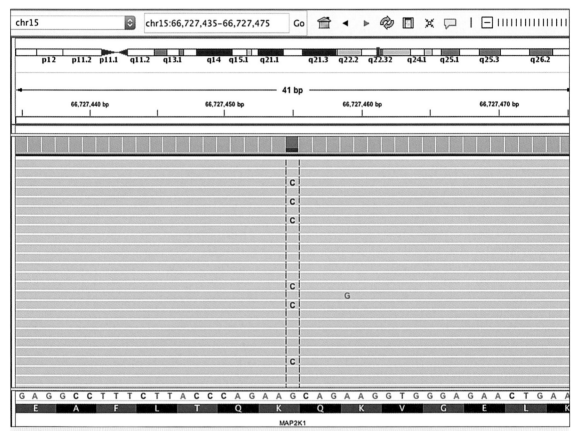

f34.4 Somatic variant analysis using a targeted lymphoid NGS panel; annotated reads mapped to the *MAP2K1* locus demonstrate p.K57N (c.171G>C) in 26% of reads (highlighted in blue; hg19, Integrative Genomics Viewer browser) [see **fA.8**, p312]

may be difficult to ascertain, especially in poorly fixed specimens, and can usually be determined by comparing the lymphoma cell nuclei with that of a normal histiocyte or endothelial cell, which are benchmarks for "large" cells. Most often FLs are composed of small cells, with <15 large cells per high-power field (hpf); these are considered grade 1-2 lesions. Low-grade lesions typically have a low proliferation index, usually <30% as determined with Ki-67 staining. When large cells become more numerous (at least 15/hpf), the lesions are considered grade 3. Grade 3 is further subdivided into grade 3A and 3B types depending on whether the large

cells completely replace the germinal center (3B). Grade 3 cases, particular grade 3B, act more aggressively, with clinical behavior similar to that of diffuse large B-cell lymphoma. The cells in most cases of FL are positive for BCL-2 protein and characterized by the presence of t(14;18)(q32q21) *IGH-BCL2*, which results in uncontrolled expression of BCL-2. Because BCL-2 is antiapoptotic, cells harboring this genetic aberration fail to undergo apoptosis, continue to survive the germinal center environment, and slowly accumulate in the lymph node.

t34.1 Clinical & pathologic features of pediatric-type vs adult-type follicular lymphoma

	Pediatric-type follicular lymphoma	**Adult-type follicular lymphoma**
age	predominantly <18 y, may occur in adults	predominantly adults, rare <18 y
sex	male:female ~10:1	male = female
sites	primarily head, neck & tonsils	no predilection
clinical	localized, curable	disseminated, incurable
histology	mostly intermediate-sized blastoid cells and/or grade 3, tingible body macrophages present	mostly grade 1-2, lack of tingible body macrophages
BCL-2 IHC	negative	positive (90%)
t(14;18) *IGH-BCL2*	absent	present (80%-90%)
deletion 1p36	~40%	40%-50%
BCL6 (3q27) alterations	absent	5%-15%
MAP2K1 mutation	10%-40%	rare
TNFRS14 mutation	30%-50%	30%-50%
IRF8 mutation	p.K66R in 15%-50%	C-terminal insertion/deletion or missense in 15%-20%
KMT2D mutation	0-15%	50%-80%
CREBBP mutation	<5%	50%-70%
EZH2 mutation	rare	15%-30%

The findings delineated above characterize the typical adult-type follicular lymphoma (AFL). Other, less common subtypes of FL have been described. Pediatric-type FL (PTFL), in particular, occurs primarily in children and young adults <30 years of age, although infrequently in older individuals, as illustrated by this case. PTFL has distinct clinical and pathological characteristics that differentiate it from AFL **t34.1**. It is usually localized, most often occurring in the head and neck region or tonsils and with a marked male predominance (10:1). Rarer cases have also been described occurring elsewhere, such as the testis. As opposed to AFL, PTFL is felt to be curable, potentially with excision alone, although some form of systemic therapy is also usually used. Pathologically, PTFL cases most often demonstrate grade 3B histology, although with retention of tingible body macrophages, a finding generally not seen with AFL. Importantly, PTFL cells lack BCL-2 expression and *BCL2* gene rearrangement. As such, a diagnosis of PTFL should be considered in any follicular lesion that is BCL-2-negative on IHC and lacks *BCL2* gene rearrangement. By definition, PTFLs also lack rearrangement of *BCL6*, *c-MYC*, and *IRF4* genes.

Molecular studies have identified recurrent mutations in *MAP2K1* (10%-40%), *TNFRS14* (30%-50%), and *IRF8* (15%-50%) in PTFL, although PTFL has a low overall mutational burden compared to AFL, with ~1-5 mutations per case. Less commonly, other MAP kinase pathway genes may be mutated, suggesting that activation of this signaling cascade is important for PTFL pathogenesis. *MAP2K1* mutations are not common in AFL. AFLs commonly contain *TNFRS14* mutations, limiting the usefulness of this mutation for distinguishing between these disorders. Likewise, loss of chromosome region 1p36 (the *TNFRS14* locus) is seen in a large portion of cases in both AFL and TPFL (see **Case 33**). *IRF8* gene mutations have also been described in AFL but the quality of the mutation differs from that in PTFL and is potentially helpful for discriminating these neoplasms. In particular, *IRF8* p.K66R is characteristically found in PTFL and is predicted to affect DNA binding, whereas the *IRF8* mutations in AFL are frequently located in the C-terminal domain with unclear biologic effects. AFLs often contain mutations in chromatin and histone remodeling genes such as *KTM2D* and *CREBBP*, which are less commonly encountered in PTFL **t34.1**.

The main entities in the differential diagnosis in this example case, aside from AFL, included reactive follicular hyperplasia (RFH) and large B-cell lymphoma with *IRF4* rearrangement. AFL was excluded partly based on the absence of BCL-2 staining and the lack of *BCL2* and *BCL6* gene rearrangements. However, ~10% of AFLs lack BCL-2 protein expression and/or *BCL2* rearrangement, limiting the use of these parameters as the sole means to distinguish AFL from PTFL. In ~50% of "BCL-2 negative" AFLs, lack of BCL-2 expression is a result of an inability to detect somatically mutated BCL-2 protein by a commonly used BCL-2 monoclonal antibody which recognizes residues 41-54 of BCL-2. Genetic studies in these cases will identify *BCL2* rearrangement and the use of alternative anti-BCL-2 antibodies enables detection of the protein. In a small minority of AFLs, BCL-2 is truly not overexpressed and *BCL2* rearrangement is not present. Instead, many of these cases harbor rearrangement of *BCL6* located at chromosome region 3q27. AFLs with *BCL6* rearrangements usually have grade 3B morphology, may lack CD10 expression, and often have associated diffuse large B-cell areas. Interestingly, *BCL6* and *BCL2* rearrangements appear mutually exclusive, and *BCL6* rearrangements are not seen in PTFL. Finally, a third subset of AFL without BCL2 expression will lack both *BCL2* and *BCL6* rearrangements and often demonstrates a complex karyotype.

RFH can be distinguished from PTFL in most cases based on morphology and absence of a clonal B-cell population. In RFH, the follicles are mostly distributed in the nodal cortex, whereas neoplastic follicles in PTFL will involve all regions of the lymph node including the medulla. In addition, reactive follicles maintain normal dark/zone light zone polarity and distinct mantle zones, features usually lost in PTFL. BCL-2 is not expressed in reactive follicles and this may be a source of confusion when evaluating for PTFL. However, the B cells in reactive follicles are polyclonal, a finding best demonstrated by flow cytometry. In rare cases, however, clonal B cells can be detected using flow cytometry and/or molecular methods in lymph nodes with features of RFH. This may lead to a diagnostic dilemma, and diagnosis of PTFL in these cases relies heavily on atypical morphology. Interestingly RFH with clonal B cells has a clinical picture similar to that of PTFL, occurring in children and young adults with a marked male predominance and predilection for lymph nodes of the head and neck as well as tonsils, raising the possibility that these cases are on a biologic continuum with PTFL. Molecular studies have not been undertaken in these cases to determine whether there are somatic mutations similar to those of PTFL.

Large B-cell lymphoma (LBCL) with *IRF4* rearrangement (**Case 40**) is a provisional entity recently included in the 2017 World Health Organization classification of hematopoietic neoplasms. This lymphoma, like PTFL, is associated with young age, head/neck and tonsil localization, and good prognosis. It grows either in a nodular fashion with FL grade 3 morphology or as a diffuse proliferation of large cells, or a mixture of both. Using IHC, these lymphomas are positive for BCL-6 and strongly express MUM1 (IRF4), whereas ~50% of cases lack expression of CD10 and BCL-2. The presence of *IRF4* gene rearrangement confirms the diagnosis. *IRF4* resides at chromosome band 6p25 and gene fusions may occur either with the immunoglobulin heavy chain or the λ or κ light chain loci. Therefore, *IRF4* rearrangement is best detected with FISH using a break-apart probe. Although occasional cases of PTFL will express MUM1 by IHC, this was not observed in the example case, excluding a diagnosis of LBCL with *IRF4* rearrangement. In PTFL cases having MUM1 protein expression, FISH for *IRF4* rearrangement should be performed. Recent studies have shown that LBCL with *IRF4* rearrangement has frequent mutations in *IRF4* and NF-κB pathway genes (*CARD11, CD79B,* and *MYD88*) as well as *CCND3*. *MAP2K1* mutations may also occasionally be present (~10% of cases).

This patient's disease was fully staged with PET/CT and bone marrow biopsy which revealed no additional evidence of disease or organomegaly. He ultimately received treatment with rituximab only.

Diagnostic pearls/pitfalls

– PTFL is characterized by male predominance, localized disease to the head, neck, and tonsils, good prognosis and young age, although occasionally it can occur in older individuals.

– By definition PTFL lacks BCL-2 protein expression and *BCL2, BCL6, c-MYC,* and *IRF4* gene rearrangements and may be confused with BCL-2-negative AFL. If present, a *MAP2K1* mutation can help distinguish between these two types of FL, as can the type of *IRF8* mutation (see **t34.1**).

– BCL-2 protein expression may not be detected in 5%-10% of AFLs with *BCL2* rearrangement with the most commonly used anti-BCL-2 monoclonal antibody, because of point mutations in the *BCL2* gene. Use of alternative anti-BCL-2 monoclonal antibodies will identify the protein.

– PTFL may be confused with reactive follicular hyperplasia, and occasional cases of reactive follicular hyperplasia have clonal B cells detected by flow cytometry. A diagnosis of PTFL requires abnormal morphology as well as demonstration of B-cell clonality.

Readings

Adam P, Baumann R, Schmidt J, et al. The BCL2 E17 and SP66 antibodies discriminate 2 immunophenotypically and genetically distinct subgroups of conventionally BCL2-"negative" grade 1/2 follicular lymphomas. Hum Pathol. 2013;44(9):1817-26. **DOI: 10.1016/j.humpath.2013.02.004**

Agrawal R, Wang J. Pediatric follicular lymphoma: a rare clinicopathologic entity. Arch Pathol Lab Med. 2009;133(1):142-6. **DOI: 10.1043/1543-2165-133.1.142**

Araf S, Fitzgibbon J. Pediatric-type FL: simply different. Blood 2016;128(8):1030-31. **DOI: 10.1182/blood-2016-07-725002**

Bödör C, Grossmann V, Popov N, et al. *EZH2* mutations are frequent and represent an early event in follicular lymphoma. Blood. 2013;122(18):3165-8. **DOI: 10.1182/blood-2013-04-496893**

Bosga-Bouwer AG, van Imhoff GW, Boonstra R, et al. Follicular lymphoma grade 3B includes 3 cytogenetically defined subgroups with primary t(14;18), 3q27, or other translocations: t(14;18) and 3q27 are mutually exclusive. Blood. 2003;101(3):1149-54. **DOI: 10.1182/blood.V101.3.1149**

Ferry JA. Recent advances in follicular lymphoma: pediatric, extranodal, and follicular lymphoma in situ. Surg Pathol Clin. 2010;3(4):877-906. **DOI: 10.1016/j.path.2010.08.002**

Jardin F, Gaulard P, Buchonnet G, et al. Follicular lymphoma without t(14;18) and with *BCL-6* rearrangement: a lymphoma subtype with distinct pathological, molecular and clinical characteristics. Leukemia. 2002;16(11):2309-17. **DOI: 10.1038/sj.leu.2402707**

Koo M, Ohgami RS. Pediatric-type follicular lymphoma and pediatric nodal marginal zone lymphoma: recent clinical, morphologic, immunophenotypic, and genetic insights. Adv Anat Pathol. 2017;24(3):128-35. **DOI: 10.1097/PAP.0000000000000144**

Krysiak K, Gomez F, White BS, et al. Recurrent somatic mutations affecting B-cell receptor signaling pathway genes in follicular lymphoma. Blood. 2017;129(4):473-83. **DOI: 10.1182/blood-2016-07-729954**

Kussick SJ, Kalnoski M, Braziel RM, Wood BL. Prominent clonal B-cell populations identified by flow cytometry in histologically reactive lymphoid proliferations. Am J Clin Pathol. 2004;121(4):464-72. **DOI: 10.1309/4EJ8-T3R2-ERKQ-61WH**

Li H, Kaminski MS, Li Y, et al. Mutations in linker histone genes *HIST1H1* B, C, D, and E; *OCT2* (POU2F2); *IRF8*; and *ARID1A* underlying the pathogenesis of follicular lymphoma. Blood. 2014;123(10):1487-98. **DOI: 10.1182/blood-2013-05-500264**

Louissaint A Jr, Ackerman AM, Dias-Santagata D, et al. Pediatric-type nodal follicular lymphoma: an indolent clonal proliferation in children and adults with high proliferation index and no *BCL2* rearrangement. Blood. 2012;120(12):2395-404. **DOI: 10.1182/blood-2012-05-429514**

Louissaint A Jr, Schafernak KT, Geyer JT, et al. Pediatric-type nodal follicular lymphoma: a biologically distinct lymphoma with frequent *MAPK* pathway mutations. Blood. 2016;128(8):1093-100. **DOI: 10.1182/blood-2015-12-682591**

Lovisa F, Binatti A, Coppe A, et al. A high definition picture of key genes and pathways mutated in pediatric follicular lymphoma. Haematologica. 2019;104(9):e406-9. **DOI: 10.3324/haematol.2018.211631**

Martin-Guerrero I, Salaverria I, Burkhardt B, et al. Recurrent loss of heterozygosity in 1p36 associated with *TNFRSF14* mutations in *IRF4* translocation negative pediatric follicular lymphomas. Haematologica. 2013;98(8):1237-41. **DOI: 10.3324/haematol.2012.073916**

Nann D, Ramis-Zaldivar JE, Müller I, et al. Follicular lymphoma t(14;18)-negative is genetically a heterogeneous disease. Blood Adv. 2020 Nov 24;4(22):5652-5665. **DOI: 10.1182/bloodadvances.2020002944.**

Oschlies I, Salaverria I, Mahn F, et al. Pediatric follicular lymphoma: a clinico-pathological study of a population-based series of patients treated within the Non-Hodgkin's Lymphoma—Berlin-Frankfurt-Münster (NHL-BFM) multicenter trials. Haematologica. 2010;95(2):253-9. **DOI: 10.3324/haematol.2009.013177**

Ozawa MG, Bhaduri A, Chisholm KM, et al. A study of the mutational landscape of pediatric-type follicular lymphoma and pediatric nodal marginal zone lymphoma. Mod Pathol. 2016;29(10):1212-20. **DOI: 10.1038/modpathol.2016.102**

Ramis-Zaldivar JE, Gonzalez-Farré B, Balagué O, et al. Distinct molecular profile of *IRF4*-rearranged large B-cell lymphoma. Blood. 2020;135(4):274-86. **DOI: 10.1182/blood.2019002699**

Schmidt J, Gong S, Marafioti T, et al. Genome-wide analysis of pediatric-type follicular lymphoma reveals low genetic complexity and recurrent alterations of *TNFRSF14* gene. Blood. 2016;128(8):1101-11. **DOI: 10.1182/blood-2016-03-703819**

Schmidt J, Ramis-Zaldivar JE, Nadeu F, et al. Mutations of *MAP2K1* are frequent in pediatric-type follicular lymphoma and result in *ERK* pathway activation. Blood. 2017;130(3):323-7. **DOI: 10.1182/blood-2017-03-776278**

Swerdlow SH, Campo E, Pileri SA, et al. The 2016 revision of the World Health Organization classification of lymphoid neoplasms. Blood. 2016;127(20):2375-90. **DOI: 10.1182/blood-2016-01-643569**

Christopher Ryder

35

Lymphoplasmacytic lymphoma with mutations in *MYD88* & *CXCR4*

History A 69-year-old man with a history of chronic kidney disease, aortic stenosis, and anemia presented at an outpatient cardiology visit with weakness. He was found to be pancytopenic (selected CBC results are shown at right). Subsequently, a bone marrow biopsy was performed for further evaluation. Additional laboratory workup revealed a monoclonal IgM λ paraprotein at 1.7 g/dL and an elevated serum viscosity at 2.06 cP (normal range 1.50-1.80 cP).

Morphology & flow cytometry Review of the peripheral blood smear revealed pancytopenia with mild rouleaux formation and rare plasmacytoid lymphocytes. The bone marrow aspirate showed a lymphoplasmacytic infiltrate with a range of morphologic features, including small mature lymphocytes with clumped nuclear chromatin and scant cytoplasm, lymphoplasmacytoid cells, and plasma cells **f35.1**. The bone marrow core biopsy demonstrated mild hypercellularity with extensive marrow replacement by an interstitial lymphoplasmacytic infiltrate and few areas of residual trilineage hematopoiesis **f35.2**. Immunohistochemistry for CD20 and CD138 demonstrated 50%-60% B cells and 15%-20% plasma cells, respectively, and the plasma cells showed λ restriction **f35.3**. Flow cytometry identified a λ-restricted B-cell population that was negative for CD5 and CD10, as well as a plasma cell population that was positive for CD45, CD19, and λ light chain and negative for CD56 **f35.4**. Few background polytypic B cells and plasma cells were also identified. The overall findings supported a diagnosis of a **B-cell lymphoma with plasmacytic differentiation**, with **lymphoplasmacytic lymphoma** being favored.

WBC	1.4× 10⁹/L
HGB	5.0 g/dL
Platelets	59 × 10⁹/L

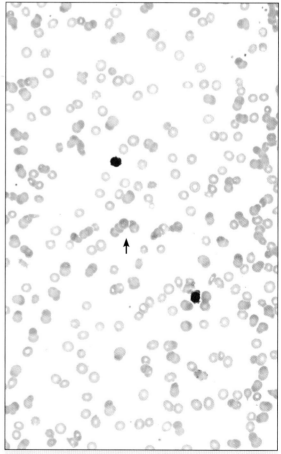

f35.1 Peripheral blood smear demonstrating pancytopenia & rouleaux formation in the red blood cells (arrow)

ISBN 978-089189-6814

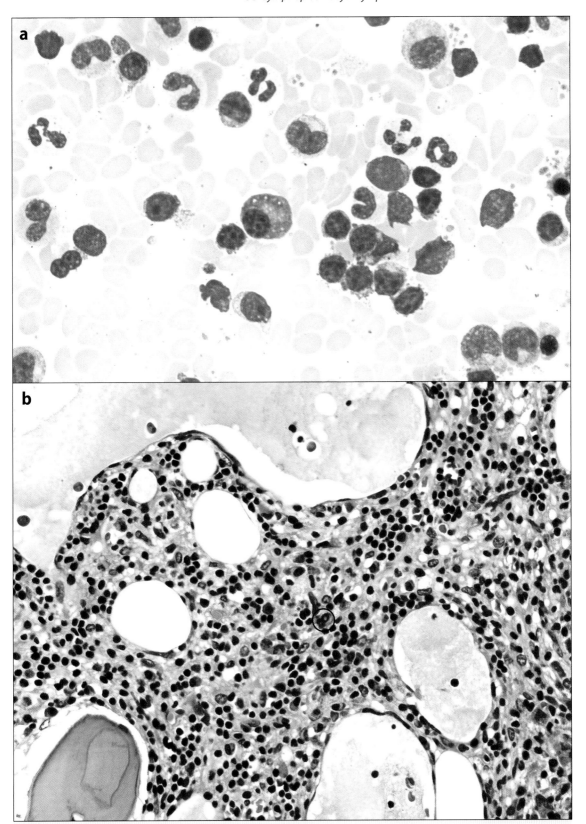

f35.2 a Bone marrow aspirate demonstrating a spectrum of lymphoplasmacytic morphology; **b** bone marrow core biopsy demonstrating a prominent lymphoplasmacytic infiltrate with a rare Dutcher body (circled)

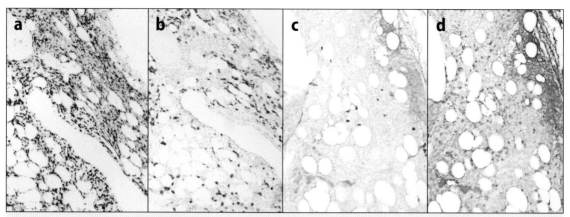

f35.3 Immunohistochemistry performed on the bone marrow core biopsy for **a** CD20, **b** CD138, **c** κ & **d** λ demonstrating an infiltrate of CD20-positive B cells admixed with λ-predominant plasma cells

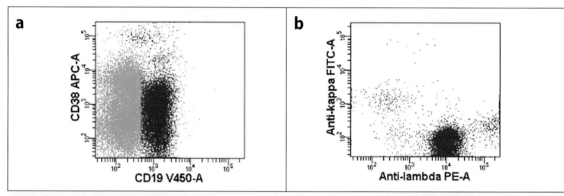

f35.4 Flow cytometric studies demonstrate (**a**) a CD19 positive B-cell population (red) and a CD19 positive, CD38 bright plasma cell population (blue), both of which demonstrate (**b**) intracellular λ light chain restriction; few background polytypic B cells & plasma cells are present in this specimen; T & NK cells are shown in green for comparison

Genetics/molecular results Chromosome analysis revealed a normal male karyotype. A targeted NGS panel for lymphoid-related genes identified *MYD88* p.L265P (c.794T>C, variant allele frequency [VAF] 25% **f35.5**) and *CXCR4* p.R334* (c.1021C>T, VAF 12%). These findings confirmed the diagnosis of **lymphoplasmacytic lymphoma** (LPL).

Discussion The diagnosis of specific B-cell lymphomas with plasmacytic differentiation is often a challenge for hematopathologists. Although nearly all small B-cell lymphomas can present with plasmacytic features, this finding is most commonly seen in marginal zone lymphomas and LPL. The latter is a low-grade B-cell neoplasm that demonstrates a spectrum of morphology in bone marrow, including small lymphocytes with clumped chromatin and scant cytoplasm, plasmacytoid lymphocytes with more abundant cytoplasm and eccentric nuclei, and true plasma cells, although not all of these types of cells may be present in every case. This morphologic heterogeneity recapitulates the

spectrum of B-cell maturation toward plasma cells. Peripheral blood lymphocytosis is variably present in LPL, may display a similar spectrum of morphology, and tends to be less prominent than in other marrow-based lymphoproliferative disorders such as chronic lymphocytic leukemia (CLL).

Most cases of LPL predominantly involve the bone marrow, with only a small minority of cases demonstrating extramedullary disease in addition to or without significant marrow involvement. The pattern of marrow infiltration may be nodular, diffuse, or interstitial, with the lymphoid component generally predominating. In lymph nodes, LPL often appears as a monotonous lymphoplasmacytic infiltrate that preserves the nodal architecture, although more advanced lesions may cause nodal effacement. Dilated sinuses and few residual, often regressed, reactive lymphoid follicles are characteristic. Follicular colonization by lymphoma cells may also be present. Other typical features include Dutcher bodies, increased mast cells, and hemosiderin pigment. The

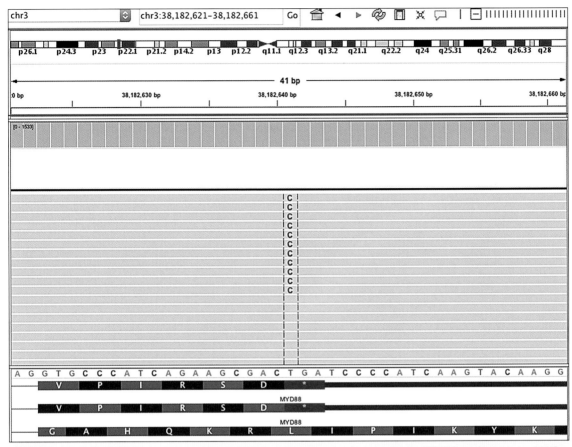

f35.5 Somatic variant analysis using a targeted lymphoid NGS panel; annotated reads mapped to the *MYD88* locus demonstrate p.L265P (c.794T>C), highlighted in blue (hg19, Integrative Genomics Viewer browser) [see **fA.8**, p312]

presence of proliferation centers and/or prominent marginal zone lymphocyte morphology should prompt consideration of small lymphocytic lymphoma or marginal zone lymphoma, respectively.

When evaluating lymphomas with plasmacytic differentiation in bone marrow, the possibility of a coexisting lymphoproliferative disorder and a separate plasma cell neoplasm (PCN) such as myeloma must be excluded. Suspicion for 2 distinct processes should be especially high when the light chain usage is discordant between the B-cell and plasma cell components, albeit with the caveat that very rare cases of biclonal LPL have been reported. Even when the 2 populations share the same light chain restriction, the distinct immunophenotype of the plasma cell component of LPL vs that of the plasma cells of PCN helps discriminate between the 2 entities. The neoplastic plasma cells of PCN are characteristically negative for CD19 and generally show dimmer CD38 and absent CD45 expression compared to normal plasma cells. In contrast, the plasma cell component is positive

for CD19 in the vast majority of low-grade B-cell lymphomas with plasmacytic differentiation, including LPL. In addition, CD56, cyclin D1, and CD117 may be aberrantly expressed at varying rates by PCNs but rarely by the plasma cells of LPL, and surface light chain is more likely to be observed in plasma cells of LPL **t35.1**. The lymphoid component of LPL typically shows a nonspecific phenotype that is most often negative for CD5 and CD10. However, at least partial expression of CD5 has been reported in as many as 43% of cases. Because CD23 expression is also relatively frequent (35%-50% of cases) in the lymphoid cells of LPL, morphologic correlation is helpful to avoid a misdiagnosis of CLL.

Several clinical syndromes are attributed to LPL. Although often used synonymously with LPL, Waldenström macroglobulinemia (WM) is actually a clinical diagnosis defined by the combination of LPL with a detectable monoclonal IgM paraprotein in serum. Most LPL cases meet the criteria for WM. The serum hyperviscosity resulting from elevated levels of

t35.1 Typical immunophenotypic findings in small B-cell lymphoma (BCL) with plasmacytic differentiation vs plasma cell myeloma (PCM)

Disease component	CD19	CD20	CD45	sIg	CD56	CD117	Cyclin D1
Lymphocytes of BCL	+	+	+	+	–	–	–*
Plasma cells of BCL	+	–/+	+ (dim)	–/+	–	–	–
Plasma cells of PCM	–	–/+	–	–	+ (~80%)	+ (~30%)	+ (~25%)

+, positive; –, negative; –/+, minority of cases positive; sIg, surface immunoglobulin receptor
*Rare cases of cyclin D1-positive mantle cell lymphoma may have plasmacytic differentiation

pentameric IgM may cause end-organ damage including cerebral infarction. Importantly, central nervous system (CNS) symptoms caused by hyperviscosity must be distinguished from rare CNS involvement by LPL known as Bing-Neel syndrome, because these 2 conditions require different treatment approaches.

An IgM paraprotein of <3 g/dL, together with <10% marrow lymphoplasmacytic infiltration and no disease-associated cytopenias, symptoms, or extramedullary disease, define IgM monoclonal gammopathy of undetermined significance (MGUS). Because of its unique biology, the 2017 World Health Organization classification of hematopoietic neoplasms lists this precursor lesion as a distinct entity from non-IgM MGUS, including a slightly higher rate of progression as well as a tendency to evolve into lymphoma or primary amyloidosis rather than plasma cell myeloma.

Over the past decade, studies have shown that >90% of LPL cases harbor the *MYD88* L265P mutation. The MYD88 adapter protein mediates signaling for interleukin and toll-like receptors, resulting in activation of the transcription factor NF-κB in B cells; mutated MYD88 drives constitutive NF-κB proliferative and survival signaling. It is important to note that the *MYD88* L265P mutation is not exclusive to LPL. It occurs rarely in other low-grade B-cell lymphomas (including up to 10% of splenic marginal zone lymphomas) as well as in 15%-20% of diffuse large B-cell lymphomas (DLBCLs), particularly CNS and testicular DLBCLs, where it is found in ~2/3 of cases. Consistent with the concept of IgM MGUS being a precursor lesion to LPL, roughly half of IgM MGUS cases harbor *MYD88* L265P as well. In contrast, *MYD88* mutation is absent in the rare IgM plasma cell myelomas; it is also absent in γ heavy chain disease, which may morphologically resemble LPL. *MYD88* L265P has therefore become a powerful molecular marker to confirm a diagnosis of LPL in cases of small B-cell lymphoma with plasmacytic

differentiation. Importantly, for cases in which LPL is not a diagnostic consideration based on morphology, the presence of *MYD88* mutation by itself should not be taken as definitive evidence of LPL. The small proportion of LPL cases with wild-type *MYD88* appear to have worse clinical outcomes than cases with *MYD88* L265P.

The G protein-coupled receptor *CXCR4* is the second most commonly mutated gene in LPL, occurring in 25%-40% of cases. It arises almost exclusively in *MYD88*-mutated cases and is frequently subclonal in nature. Both nonsense and frameshift mutations in the C-terminus lead to a truncated form of CXCR4 that resists normal recycling/downregulation and facilitates constitutive ERK and AKT pathway activation. Of note, somatic *CXCR4* mutations identified in LPL are identical to germline mutations found in WHIM (warts, hypogammaglobulinemia, infections, myelokathexis) syndrome. The presence of mutated *CXCR4* in LPL is reportedly associated with higher disease activity and less robust response to Bruton tyrosine kinase (BTK) inhibitors (ie, ibrutinib), though some studies have found no significant differences. True resistance to ibrutininb in LPL may develop because of a *BTK* mutation, which shows an association with *CXCR4* mutation.

Additional recurrent genetic abnormalities in LPL include mutation of *ARID1A* (up to 17%) and *KMT2D* (*MLL2*; up to 24%), deletion 6q (~50%), and trisomy 4 (~20%). Less frequent mutations in chromatin modifying genes (of which *KMT2D* is one) and genes of the NF-κB and DNA damage response pathways have been reported. These genetic changes lack specificity or robust prognostic information for LPL.

In summary, LPL is a low-grade B-cell lymphoma composed of a morphologic spectrum of lymphoplasmacytic cells and plasma cells, typically expressing a monoclonal IgM monoclonal protein and showing concordant light chain restriction by both lymphocytes and plasma cells. Although LPL was historically a diagnosis of exclusion, at present, the identification of *MYD88* L265P mutation in a small B-cell lymphoma with plasmacytic differentiation and appropriate clinical presentation is essentially diagnostic for LPL. Detection of a concurrent mutation in *CXCR4* offers confirmatory evidence of LPL, because it occurs almost exclusively in LPL among B-cell lymphomas and frequently in combination with *MYD88* L265P.

Diagnostic pearls/pitfalls

– Definitive diagnosis of small B-cell lymphomas with plasmacytic differentiation can be challenging; with the appropriate clinical presentation and histologic features, the presence of *MYD88* L265P mutation strongly argues in favor of a diagnosis of LPL, though a minor proportion of marginal zone lymphomas (mostly splenic) also harbor this mutation.

– *MYD88* L265P mutations are not specific to LPL and are also prevalent in IgM MGUS, a precursor lesion with a low rate of progression to overt lymphoma, as well as a subset of DLBCL.

– Mutation in *CXCR4* co-occurs with *MYD88* L265P in LPL and occurs very rarely in other B-cell lymphomas; although it has been associated with poor response to BTK inhibitors, current guidelines do not recommend altering therapy in cases harboring *CXCR4* mutation.

– The immunophenotype of plasma cells in LPL and other low-grade B-cell lymphomas is distinct from that seen in multiple myeloma **t35.1** and can be used to exclude the presence of coexisting myeloma.

– WM is specifically a clinical syndrome defined by the presence of both LPL and a detectable IgM monoclonal protein, often with resultant characteristic symptoms related to serum hyperviscosity.

Readings

Alley CL, Wang E, Dunphy CH, et al. Diagnostic and clinical considerations in concomitant bone marrow involvement by plasma cell myeloma and chronic lymphocytic leukemia/monoclonal B-cell lymphocytosis: a series of 15 cases and review of literature. Arch Pathol Lab Med. 2013;137:503-17. **DOI: 10.5858/arpa.2011-0696-OA**

Digiuseppe JA. Flow cytometric immunophenotyping of plasmacytic neoplasms. Am J Clin Pathol. 2007;127:172-4. **DOI: 10.1309/T50T3M7WNXYFXCLW**

Dimopoulos MA, Kastritis E. How I treat Waldenström macroglobulinemia. Blood. 2019;134:2022-35. **DOI: 10.1182/blood.2019000725**

Gustine JN, Xu L, Tsakmaklis N, et al. CXCR4 (S338X) clonality is an important determinant of ibrutinib outcomes in patients with Waldenström macroglobulinemia. Blood Adv. 2019;3:2800-3. **DOI: 10.1182/bloodadvances.2019000635**

Hunter ZR, Branagan AR, Manning R, et al. CD5, CD10, and CD23 expression in Waldenström macroglobulinemia. Clin Lymphoma. 2005;5:246-9. **DOI: 10.3816/clm.2005.n.008**

Hunter ZR, Xu L, Tsakmaklis N, et al. Insights into the genomic landscape of MYD88 wild-type Waldenström macroglobulinemia. Blood Adv. 2018;2:2937-46. **DOI: 10.1182/bloodadvances.2018022962**

Kriangkum J, Taylor BJ, Treon SP, et al. Molecular characterization of Waldenstrom's macroglobulinemia reveals frequent occurrence of two B-cell clones having distinct IgH VDJ sequences. Clin Cancer Res. 2007;13:2005-13. **DOI: 10.1158/1078-0432. CCR-06-2788**

Kumar S, Kimlinger T, Morice W. Immunophenotyping in multiple myeloma and related plasma cell disorders. Best Pract Res Clin Haematol. 2010;23:433-51. **DOI: 10.1016/j.beha.2010.09.002**

Martinez-Lopez A, Curiel-Olmo S, Mollejo M, et al. *MYD88* (L265P) somatic mutation in marginal zone B-cell lymphoma. Am J Surg Pathol. 2015;39:644-51. **DOI: 10.1097/PAS.0000000000000411**

Morice WG, Chen D, Kurtin PJ, Hanson CA, Mcphail ED. Novel immunophenotypic features of marrow lymphoplasmacytic lymphoma and correlation with Waldenström macroglobulinemia. Mod Pathol. 2009;22:807-16. **DOI: 10.1038/modpathol.2009.34**

Schmidt J, Federmann B, Schindler N, et al. *MYD88* L265P and *CXCR4* mutations in lymphoplasmacytic lymphoma identify cases with high disease activity. Br J Haematol. 2015;169:795-803. **DOI: 10.1111/bjh.13361**

Schulz R, David D, Farkas DH, Crisan D. Molecular analysis in a patient with Waldenström macroglobulinemia reveals a rare case of biclonality. Mol Diagn. 1996;1:159-66. **DOI: 10.1054/MODI00100159**

Seegmiller AC, Xu Y, Mckenna RW, Karandikar NJ. Immunophenotypic differentiation between neoplastic plasma cells in mature B-cell lymphoma vs plasma cell myeloma. Am J Clin Pathol. 2007;127:176-81. **DOI: 10.1309/5EL22BH45PHUPM8P**

Swerdlow SH, Kuzu I, Dogan A, et al. The many faces of small B cell lymphomas with plasmacytic differentiation and the contribution of *MYD88* testing. Virchows Arch. 2016;468:259-75. **DOI: 10.1007/s00428-015-1858-9**

Treon SP, Cao Y, Xu L, et al. Somatic mutations in *MYD88* and *CXCR4* are determinants of clinical presentation and overall survival in Waldenström macroglobulinemia. Blood. 2014;123:2791-6. **DOI: 10.1182/blood-2014-01-550905**

Treon SP, Xu L, Yang G, et al. MYD88 L265P somatic mutation in Waldenström macroglobulinemia. N Engl J Med. 2012;367:826-33. **DOI: 10.1056/NEJMoa1200710**

Varettoni M, Arcaini L, Zibellini S, et al. Prevalence and clinical significance of the *MYD88* (L265P) somatic mutation in Waldenström macroglobulinemia and related lymphoid neoplasms. Blood. 2013;121:2522-8. **DOI: 10.1182/blood-2012-09-457101**

Wang W, Ding Y, Campbell A, et al. Biclonal presentation of lymphoplasmacytic lymphoma/Waldenström macroglobulinaemia. Pathology. 2019;51:340-3. **DOI: 10.1016/j.pathol.2018.10.022**

Xu L, Tsakmaklis N, Yang G, et al. Acquired mutations associated with ibrutinib resistance in Waldenström macroglobulinemia. Blood. 2017;129:2519-25. **DOI: 10.1182/blood-2017-01-761726**

Howard Meyerson

36

Splenic marginal zone lymphoma with del(7q) & mutations in *CARD11 & CXCR4*

History A 65-year-old male was referred to a hematologist for long-standing thrombocytopenia, initially felt to be autoimmune in nature. CBC results are shown at right. Serologic studies revealed no evidence of platelet-associated antibodies or antibodies to hepatitis C. A monoclonal IgG λ at 0.2 g/dL was identified with serum protein electrophoresis.

Ultrasonography of the spleen demonstrated marked splenomegaly (21 cm) confirmed with CT scan. Only minimal adenopathy was noted. Because of these findings, a bone marrow biopsy with peripheral smear review was performed, with flow cytometry and genetic studies.

Morphology & flow cytometry A peripheral blood smear revealed a lymphocytosis of small to intermediate-sized lymphocytes with a moderate amount of cytoplasm and round to oval nuclei with clumped chromatin **f36.1a**. The bone marrow aspirate smear was aspicular and hemodilute but contained lymphocytes similar to those seen on the peripheral smear **f36.1b**. The trephine core biopsy revealed near complete replacement of the bone marrow by small lymphocytes **f36.2**. Flow cytometry demonstrated an atypical population of lymphocytes, constituting 76% of all cells, which were positive for CD5, CD19, CD20 (moderate), CD79b (moderate), CD20, and λ light chain, and negative for CD10, CD23, CD38, and CD43 **f36.3**. Immunohistochemistry for cyclin D1 and SOX11 performed on the core biopsy specimen was negative.

WBC	5.2×10^9/L
Differential	
Polymorphonuclear leukocytes	25%
Bands	3%
Lymphocytes	67%
Monocytes	5%
RBC	4.06×10^{12}/L
HGB	12.9 g/dL
HCT	39.1%
MCV	96 fL
RDW	14.1%
Platelets	64×10^9/L

Genetics/molecular results Culture failure precluded chromosome analysis. FISH was negative for del(13/13q) del(11q), del(17p), trisomy 12 and t(11;14) *CCND1-IGH*. FISH to detect loss of chromosome 7 or a deletion of its long (q) arm revealed an abnormal signal pattern with 2 chromosome 7 centromere signals and one 7q signal in 46% of nuclei, consistent with del(7q) **f36.4**. Somatic mutation analysis assessed with NGS using a targeted panel of 30 lymphoid-related genes revealed *CARD11* p.D17G (c.50A>G) with 49% variant allele frequency (VAF) and *CXCR4* p.S338* (c.1013C>G) with 40% VAF. A *MYD88* mutation was not detected. Based on the clinical, morphologic, immunophenotypic, and genetic findings, a final diagnosis of **splenic marginal zone lymphoma** (SMZL) was rendered.

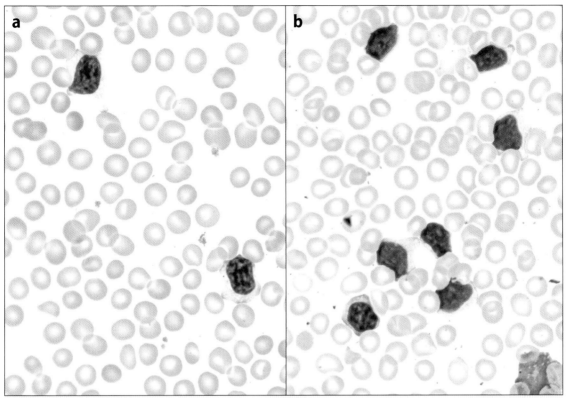

f36.1 **a** Peripheral blood & **b** bone marrow aspirate demonstrating increased small to intermediate-sized lymphocytes with condensed chromatin, inconspicuous nucleoli, and a moderate amount of cytoplasm

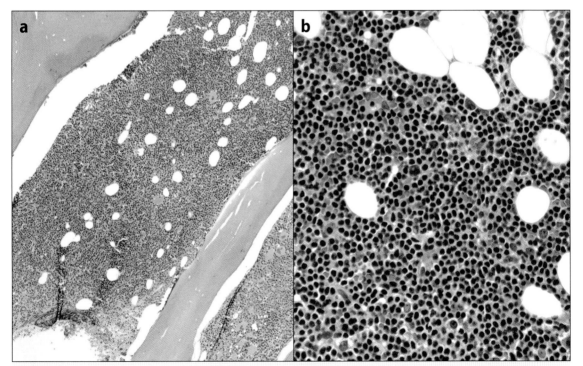

f36.2 Bone marrow core biopsy demonstrating **a** diffuse replacement of the marrow by **b** an infiltrate of small monotonous lymphocytes with dense chromatin

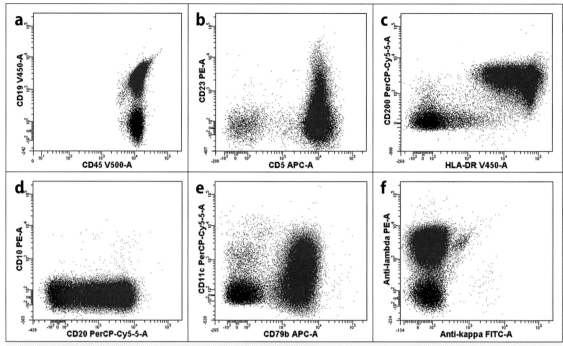

f36.3 Flow cytometry demonstrating **a** CD19 positive B-cells (highlighted in red) that are **b-e** CD5+, CD23 mostly negative, **c** CD200+, HLA-DR+, **d** CD20+, CD10–, **e** CD11c+ (partial), & CD79b+ with **f** λ-light chain restriction

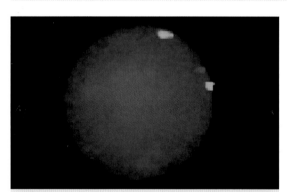

f36.4 FISH using *D7S522* (7q31, orange) & *CEP7* (centromere 7, green) showing loss of 1 orange signal with preservation of 2 green signals, consistent with deletion of 7q

Discussion SMZL is an uncommon B-cell lymphoma of older adults, with average age at diagnosis around 65 years. The disease presents with an enlarged spleen without lymphadenopathy and is typically found after workup for cytopenias or symptomatic splenomegaly. Prognosis is overall favorable, with median survival of 10-15 years, though in 10%-20% of patients, the disease may progress to diffuse large B-cell lymphoma. SMZL is felt to originate from a unique compartment of B cells in the spleen localized at the interface between the lymphoid follicle and the red pulp; these B cells are normally activated in a T-independent manner via direct binding of B-cell receptor (BCR) and toll-like receptors with microbial antigens containing repetitive units (such as polysaccharides or nucleotides). Hepatitis C virus is known to be epidemiologically linked to SMZL and some patients respond to antiviral therapy. The diagnosis is usually established based on a combination of morphology, clinical finding of splenomegaly, and genetic abnormalities, particularly del(7q), as seen in this case. SMZL is frequently a diagnosis of exclusion, rendered in a patient with splenomegaly having a small B-cell lymphoproliferative disorder detected in blood and/or marrow. In such cases, the clonal B cells do not express CD5 and CD10 and do not have the diagnostic phenotype of hairy cell leukemia (HCL; see **Case 31**) or the *MYD88* L265P mutation found in lymphoplasmacytic lymphoma (LPL; see **Case 35**).

Approximately 25% of SZML cases may express some CD5, as in this example, and the differential diagnosis will then include chronic lymphocytic leukemia/small lymphocytic lymphoma (CLL/SLL) and mantle cell lymphoma (MCL). In this case, the phenotype was inconsistent with CLL/SLL because the cells lacked CD23 and CD43 and demonstrated moderate expression of CD20, CD79b, and immunoglobulin light chain. MCL was excluded because of the absence of cyclin D1 and SOX11 shown by immunohistochemistry, as well as lack of t(11;14) *CCND1-IGH*. Rare MCL cases do not express cyclin D1 or have *CCND1* translocation; these cases should express SOX11.

t36.1 Genetic abnormalities (chromosomal aberrations & individual gene mutations) found in low-grade B-cell neoplasms that have marginal zone immunophenotype

Abnormality	SMZL	NMZL	EMZL	LPL
del(7q)	30%	not seen	5%	8%
trisomy 3	10%-20%	25%-35%	25%-30%	20%
t(11;18) *BIRC3-MALT1*	not seen	not seen	15%-50% (gastric, lung)	not seen
t(14;18) *IGH-MALT1*	not seen	not seen	15%-20% (orbit, lung)	not seen
t(1;14) *IGH-BCL10*	not seen	not seen	1%-2%	not seen
del(6q)	20%	20%	20%	20%
NOTCH2	20-25%	40%	~10%	rare
KLF2	25%-40%	10%-20%	5%-10%	rare
MYD88	5%-10%	5%-10%	5%-10%	90%
CARD11	5%-10%	5%-10%	~8%	rare
PTPRD	rare	20%	rare	rare
CCND3	7%	not seen	not seen	not seen
BIRC3 (C-IAP2)	10%	5%	rare	rare
TNFAIP3	10%	10%-20%	15%-30% (orbit) 5%-10% other	rare
MAP3K14	5%	rare	~3%	rare
IKBKB	5%	rare	rare	rare
KMT2D (MLL2)	5%-10%	35%	15%	25%
CXCR4	rare	5%	rare	25%
IGHV use	IGHV1-2*04 ~30%	IGHV4-34 ~30%	IGHV1-69: salivary IGHV3-30, 3-23: gastric IGHV4-34: orbit IGHV3,4: lung IGHV1-69,4-59: skin	IGHV3-23 (46%) IGHV3-7 (29%) mutated

EMZL, extranodal marginal zone lymphoma; LPL, lymphoplasmacytic lymphoma; NMZL, nodal marginal zone lymphoma; SMZL, splenic marginal zone lymphoma

LPL in particular is notoriously difficult to discern from SMZL because both have a similar immunophenotype and both may demonstrate plasmacytic differentiation. Morphologically, LPL is more likely to show a spectrum of differentiation from mature lymphocytes to plasmacytoid lymphocytes to plasma cells. However, this spectrum is not always present. Dutcher bodies (pseudointranuclear round to oval inclusions of immunoglobulin) are characteristic of LPL but rarely encountered in SMZL and may be helpful if present. Expression of CD5 (usually partial dim) is more often detected in LPL (~40% of cases); however, as mentioned, CD5 expression also occurs in SMZL, and currently, no immunohistochemical pattern can reliably distinguish LPL from MZL. Subtle flow cytometric findings may be helpful; in our experience, in addition to a clonal B-cell population, careful flow cytometric analysis often detects a small clonal CD19-positive plasmacytic population in cases of LPL but not typically in cases of SMZL. This plasmacytic population recovered with flow cytometry is often at a very low level and may be missed without appropriate clinical suspicion. Clinically, patients with SMZL should show evidence of splenomegaly, although enlarged spleens do occur in ~20% of patients with LPL. Therefore, differentiating the 2 disorders often requires genetic studies.

The *MYD88* L265P mutation is present in 90%-95% of LPL cases and can be helpful to separate this disorder from MZL. Nonetheless a small subset of SMZL may also contain this mutation (~5%-10%) **t36.1**. Therefore, the presence or absence of *MYD88* L265P by itself should not be used as definitive evidence of either disorder. Deletion of the long arm of chromosome 7, del(7q), is the most common chromosomal abnormality in SMZL (present in ~30% of cases) and is rarely encountered in other low-grade B-cell lymphoproliferative disorders. Therefore, the presence of del(7q) as well as absence of *MYD88* mutation helped solidify the diagnosis of SMZL in the example case. Notably, the disease-associated gene(s) on 7q is currently unknown and del(7q) does not appear to affect prognosis. Other chromosomal abnormalities observed in SMZL include deletion 6q (~20%) and trisomy of chromosomes 3 (20%), 12 (10%), and 18 (15%), as well as deletion of *TP53* on chromosome 17p (25%).

Genomic studies of SMZL demonstrate a diverse range of recurrent somatic mutations, which are best understood when examined in the context of cell signaling pathways **f36.5**. Most of the mutations enhance signaling through the NF-κB canonical or noncanonical pathways or the Notch2 pathway. Mutations of NF-κB and Notch pathway genes are not unique to SMZL, though *KLF2, NOTCH2,*

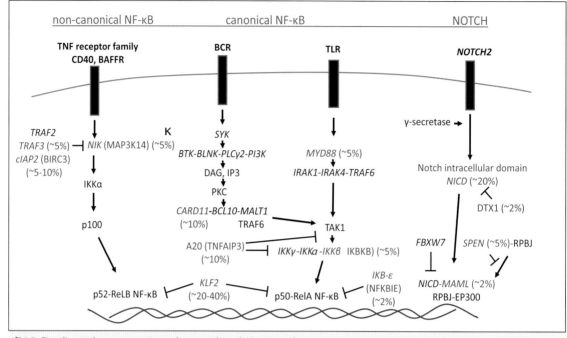

f36.5 Signaling pathway genes commonly mutated in splenic marginal zone lymphoma. Mutations occur primarily in 3 main pathways, Notch & the canonical & noncanonical NF-κB pathways, which mediate signaling for B-cell surface receptors (note that some TLRs are intracellular and use the same signaling pathways). Genes are highlighted in red and approximate frequency of the mutations are indicated in parentheses, with mutations in *NOTCH2* & *KLF2* being the most common in this disease
BCR, B-cell receptor; TLR, toll-like receptor. Arrows indicate activation of downstream pathway proteins, while T-bars indicate an inhibitory function

IKBKB, and *CARD11* alterations are more common in SMZL than in other low-grade B-cell neoplasms. As illustrated in **f36.5**, mutations affecting inhibitors are deleterious and alterations affecting constituents of a pathway are activating. In SMZL, mutations in *KLF2* (25%-40% of cases) and *NOTCH2* (20%-25%) are the most frequently observed genomic abnormalities. *KLF2* mutations may be difficult to identify because of the high GC content of this gene. In SMZLs, they are associated with 7q deletion and preferential *IGHV1-2* gene use and may co-occur with mutations in *NOTCH2* and *TNFAIP3*. Mutations in *KLF2* are uncommon in other low-grade B-cell lymphoproliferative disorders except for HCL; however, the type of *KLF2* mutation in HCL usually differs from that in SMZL. *KLF2* alterations in HCL are characterized by amino acid substitutions whereas in SMZL the *KLF2* mutations affect splicing or lead to frameshifts. *IGHV* gene use is skewed in cases of SMZL, with IGHV1-2*04 used most commonly (30% of cases). Few studies have examined the prognostic significance of genomic alterations in SMZL, although *TP53* mutation (5%-15% of cases) or deletion has been associated with decreased overall survival. *NOTCH2* mutations and unmutated *IGHV* gene status have been correlated with shorter time to first treatment.

SMZL shares some genetic abnormalities with both nodal MZL and extranodal MZL (**Case 37**). A comparison of the shared abnormalities, together with some found in LPL, is shown in **t36.1**, and demonstrates how cytogenetic and molecular analysis can aid in distinguishing these similar neoplasms. In addition to del(7q), genetic findings in the example patient included mutations in *CARD11* and *CXCR4*. The protein encoded by *CARD11* is a component of the CBM (CARD11/ BCL-10/MALT1) complex, critical for signaling in the canonical NF-κB pathway **f35.5**, and mutations in this gene occur more frequently in SMZL than LPL **t35.1**. In contrast, *CXCR4* mutations are usually seen as a secondary alteration in LPL; however, *CXCR4* mutations rarely may occur in SMZL (<1% of cases).

The patient in this case received a trial of rituximab therapy but was allergic and intolerant to the drug; therefore, a splenectomy was performed, which resolved the thrombocytopenia. The patient is currently being observed without evidence of progression of disease.

Diagnostic pearls/pitfalls
– Approximately 25% of SMZLs may express CD5. Distinguishing CD5-positive SMZL from other CD5-positive low-grade B-cell neoplasms

is a diagnostic challenge necessitating detailed immunophenotypic and molecular characterization, including evaluation for cyclin D1 and SOX11 expression to exclude MCL.

– Genetic findings help to distinguish SMZL from other low-grade B-cell neoplasms, especially LPL. The most common cytogenetic finding in SMZL is del(7q) and the most common somatic mutations involve *KLF2* and *NOTCH2*; none of these abnormalities are typically found in LPL.

– Many somatic mutations are found in SMZL and involve genes within the canonical and noncanonical NF-κB pathways as well as Notch signaling pathways.

– *MYD88* L265P is found in >90% of LPL cases but is also present in 5%-10% of SMZL, limiting the usefulness of this mutation in distinguishing SMZL from LPL when evaluated by itself.

Readings

Arcaini L, Rossi D, Paulli M. Splenic marginal zone lymphoma: from genetics to management. Blood. 2016;127(17):2072-81. **DOI: 10.1182/blood-2015-11-624312**

Baseggio L, Traverse-Glehen A, Petinataud F, et al. CD5 expression identifies a subset of splenic marginal zone lymphomas with higher lymphocytosis: a clinico-pathological, cytogenetic and molecular study of 24 cases. Haematologica. 2010;95(4):604-61. **DOI: 10.3324/haematol.2009.011049**

Bertoni F, Rossi D, Zucca E. Recent advances in understanding the biology of marginal zone lymphoma. F1000Res. 2018;7:406. **DOI: 10.12688/f1000research.13826.1**

Campos-Martín Y, Martínez N, Martínez-López A, et al. Clinical and diagnostic relevance of *NOTCH2*- and *KLF2*-mutations in splenic marginal zone lymphoma. Haematologica. 2017;102(8):e310-2. **DOI: 10.3324/haematol.2016.161711**

Cascione L, Rinaldi A, Bruscaggin A, et al. Novel insights into the genetics and epigenetics of MALT lymphoma unveiled by next generation sequencing analyses. Haematologica. 2019;104(12):e558-61. **DOI: 10.3324/haematol.2018.214957**

Clipson A, Wang M, de Leval L, et al. *KLF2* mutation is the most frequent somatic change in splenic marginal zone lymphoma and identifies a subset with distinct genotype. Leukemia. 2015;29(5):1177-85. **DOI: 10.1038/leu.2014.330**

Curiel-Olmo S, Mondéjar R, Almaraz C, et al. Splenic diffuse red pulp small B-cell lymphoma displays increased expression of cyclin D3 and recurrent CCND3 mutations. Blood. 2017;129(8):1042-5. **DOI: 10.1182/blood-2016-11-751024**

Gachard N, Parrens M, Soubeyran I, et al. IGHV gene features and *MYD88* L265P mutation separate the three marginal zone lymphoma entities and Waldenström macroglobulinemia/lymphoplasmacytic lymphomas. Leukemia. 2013;27(1):183-9. **DOI: 10.1038/leu.2012.257**

Hyeon J, Lee B, Shin SH, et al. Targeted deep sequencing of gastric marginal zone lymphoma identified alterations of *TRAF3* and *TNFAIP3* that were mutually exclusive for MALT1 rearrangement. Mod Pathol. 2018;31(9):1418-28. **DOI: 10.1038/s41379-018-0064-0**

Jaramillo Oquendo C, Parker H, et al. Systematic review of somatic mutations in splenic marginal zone lymphoma. Sci Rep. 2019;9(1):10444. **DOI: 10.1038/s41598-019-46906-1**

Jung H, Yoo HY, Lee SH, et al. The mutational landscape of ocular marginal zone lymphoma identifies frequent alterations in TNFAIP3 followed by mutations in *TBL1XR1* and *CREBBP*. Oncotarget. 2017;8(10):17038-49. **DOI: 10.18632/oncotarget.14928**

Kiel MJ, Velusamy T, Betz BL, et al. Whole-genome sequencing identifies recurrent somatic *NOTCH2* mutations in splenic marginal zone lymphoma. J Exp Med. 2012;209(9):1553-65. **DOI: 10.1084/jem.20120910**

Morice WG, Chen D, Kurtin PJ, et al. Novel immunophenotypic features of marrow lymphoplasmacytic lymphoma and correlation with Waldenström's macroglobulinemia. Mod Pathol. 2009;22(6):807-16. **DOI: 10.1038/modpathol.2009.34**

Parry M, Rose-Zerilli MJ, Gibson J, et al. Whole exome sequencing identifies novel recurrently mutated genes in patients with splenic marginal zone lymphoma. PLoS One. 2013;8(12):e83244. **DOI: 10.1371/journal.pone.0083244**

Parry M, Rose-Zerilli MJ, Ljungström V, et al. Genetics and prognostication in splenic marginal zone lymphoma: revelations from deep sequencing. Clin Cancer Res. 2015;21(18):4174-83. **DOI: 10.1158/1078-0432.CCR-14-2759**

Piris MA, Onaindía A, Mollejo M. Splenic marginal zone lymphoma. Best Pract Res Clin Haematol. 2017;30(1-2):56-64. **DOI: 10.1016/j.beha.2016.09.005**

Rossi D, Ciardullo C, Gaidano G. Genetic aberrations of signaling pathways in lymphomagenesis: revelations from next generation sequencing studies. Semin Cancer Biol. 2013;23(6):422-30. **DOI: 10.1016/j.semcancer.2013.04.002**

Rossi D, Deaglio S, Dominguez-Sola D, et al. Alteration of *BIRC3* and multiple other NF-κB pathway genes in splenic marginal zone lymphoma. Blood. 2011;118(18):4930-4. **DOI: 10.1182/blood-2011-06-359166**

Rossi D, Trifonov V, Fangazio M, et al. The coding genome of splenic marginal zone lymphoma: activation of NOTCH2 and other pathways regulating marginal zone development. J Exp Med. 2012;209(9):1537-51. **DOI: 10.1084/jem.20120904**

Salido M, Baró C, Oscier D, et al. Cytogenetic aberrations and their prognostic value in a series of 330 splenic marginal zone B-cell lymphomas: a multicenter study of the Splenic B-Cell Lymphoma Group. Blood. 2010;116(9):1479-88. **DOI: 10.1182/blood-2010-02-267476**

Spina V, Khiabanian H, Messina M, et al. The genetics of nodal marginal zone lymphoma. Blood. 2016;128(10):1362-73. **DOI: 10.1182/blood-2016-02-696757**

Thieblemont C. Improved biological insight and influence on management in indolent lymphoma. Talk 3: update on nodal and splenic marginal zone lymphoma. Hematology Am Soc Hematol Educ Program. 2017;2017(1):371-8. **DOI: 10.1182/asheducation-2017.1.371**

Treon SP, Xu L, Liu X, et al. Genomic landscape of Waldenström macroglobulinemia. Hematol Oncol Clin North Am. 2018;32(5):745-52. **DOI: 10.1016/j.hoc.2018.05.003**

Varettoni M, Zibellini S, Defrancesco I, et al. Pattern of somatic mutations in patients with Waldenström macroglobulinemia or IgM monoclonal gammopathy of undetermined significance. Haematologica. 2017;102(12):2077-85. **DOI: 10.3324/haematol.2017.172718**

Watkins AJ, Huang Y, Ye H, et al. Splenic marginal zone lymphoma: characterization of 7q deletion and its value in diagnosis. J Pathol. 2010;220(4):461-74. **DOI: 10.1002/path.2665**

Zhu S, Jin J, Gokhale S, et al. Genetic alterations of TRAF proteins in human cancers. Front Immunol. 2018;9:2111. **DOI: 10.3389/fimmu.2018.02111**

Jingwei Li & Annette S Kim

37

Extranodal marginal zone lymphoma with t(11;18)(q21;q21) *BIRC3-MALT1*

History A 58-year-old female presented with a 2-month history of progressively worsening epigastric pain and was found upon imaging to have circumferential thickening of the stomach wall and abdominal adenopathy. Esophagogastroduodenoscopy showed a large and nonobstructing ulcer in the greater curvature of the stomach. CBC results are shown at right.

Other pertinent laboratory results include an elevated IgM of 1,155 mg/dL (11.55 g/L) with borderline low IgG and IgA levels at 655 mg/dL (6.55 g/L) sand 79 mg/dL (0.79 g/L), respectively. β2-microglobulin level was mildly elevated at 2.96 mg/L. A gastric biopsy and subsequent partial gastrectomy were performed.

WBC	7.67×10^9/L
Differential	
Neutrophils	81.2%
Lymphocytes	9.0%
Monocytes	8.7%
Eosinophils	0.8%
Basophils	0.3%
HGB	13.5 g/dL
HCT	39.1%
MCV	88.4 fL
Platelets	239×10^9/L

Morphology & flow cytometry The stomach lesion was adherent to the anterior abdominal wall and an area of chronic perforation was also noted intraoperatively. Histologic sections of the stomach, duodenum, and omental tissue were extensively involved by diffuse sheets of small-sized, atypical lymphocytes with round to irregular nuclei, condensed chromatin, and moderately abundant pale cytoplasm **f37.1**, **f37.2**. Within the stomach, the lymphocytic infiltrate extensively involved the mucosa, submucosa, and gastric wall, with evidence of perforation.

Immunohistochemistry showed that the neoplastic infiltrate was positive for CD20, BCL2, and CD43 (weak), but negative for CD10, BCL6, and cyclin D1. Scattered background plasma cells showed monotypic expression for κ light chain **f37.2**. No definitive follicular dendritic meshworks were identified with a CD21 stain. The Ki-67 proliferation index was 5%. Staining for *Helicobacter pylori* was negative.

Flow cytometric analysis on a subsequent repeat biopsy 1 month later (no intervening therapy) with similar histologic findings demonstrated a population of B cells (62% of gated events, 42% of total events) that was positive for CD19 and CD20, exhibited monotypic staining for surface κ, and was negative for CD5, CD10, CD23, CD11c, CD38, and other T cell markers **f37.3**.

Genetics/molecular results Cytogenetic analysis showed a karyotype of 46,XX,t(11;18)(q21;q21)[8] **f37.4**, resulting in a *BIRC3-MALT1* fusion. Based on the morphologic, flow cytometric, and cytogenetic findings, a diagnosis of **extranodal marginal zone lymphoma of mucosa-associated lymphoid tissue (MALT lymphoma)** was rendered.

37 *Extranodal marginal zone lymphoma with t(11;18)(q21;q21) BIRC3-MALT1*

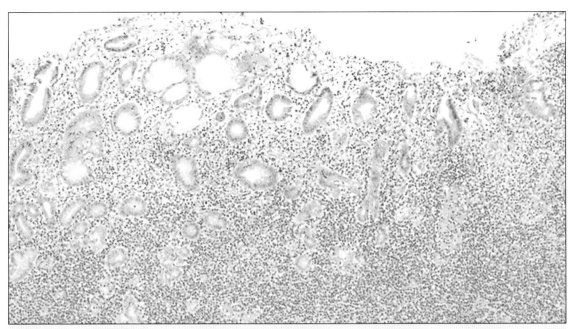

f37.1 H&E stain of the gastric biopsy shows extensive involvement by lymphoma

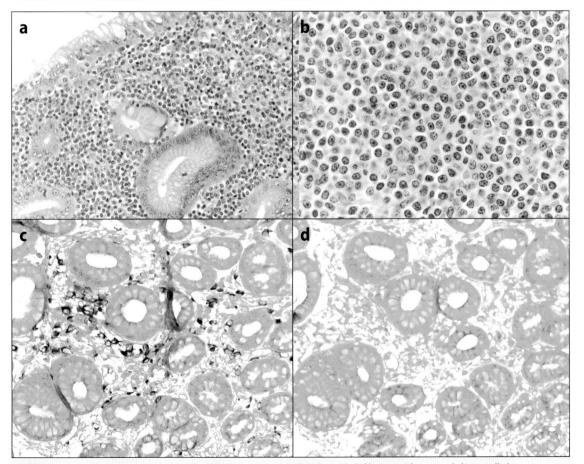

f37.2 H&E stain of the resection specimen demonstrates **a** prominent lymphoepithelial lesions with scattered plasma cells &
b monocytoid cellular morphology; ISH studies of immunoglobulin expression demonstrate **c** expression of κ light chain
& **d** absence of λ light chain expression

37 *Extranodal marginal zone lymphoma with t(11;18)(q21;q21) BIRC3-MALT1*

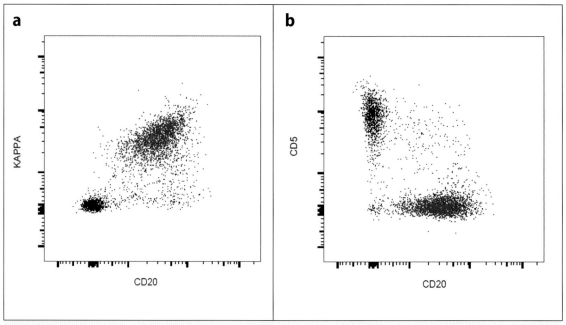

f37.3 Flow cytometric analysis of the gastric biopsy demonstrating **a** κ-restricted, CD20 positive B cells that are **b** negative for CD5 (highlighted in red)

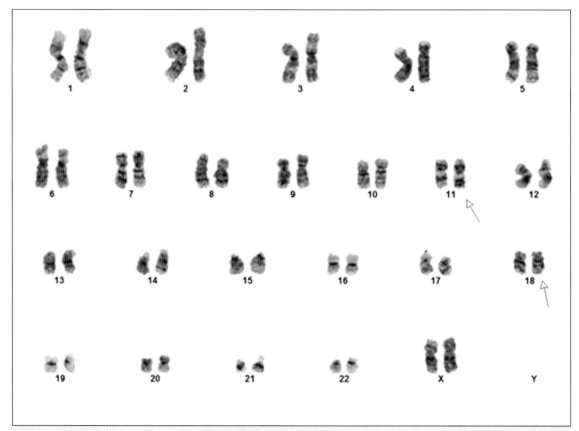

f37.4 Karyotype shows a balanced translocation between chromosomes 11 & 18 (arrows)

ISBN 978-089189-6814   ©2021 ASCP

t37.1 Recurrent translocations found in extranodal marginal zone lymphoma, with frequencies & proposed oncogenic activity based on the fusion products (adapted from Remstein et al, 2006)

Abnormality	Fusion product	Proposed oncogenic activity	Stomach	Intestine	Ocular adnexa	Salivary gland	Lung	Thyroid	Other
t(11;18)(q21;q21)	*BIRC3-MALT1*	caspase inhibition, NF-κB activation	22%	41%	7%	2%	42%	17%	1%
t(1;14)(p22;q32)	*IGH-BCL10*	deregulated *BCL10* expression, NF-κB activation	0%	7%	0%	2%	3%	0%	0%
t(14;18)(q32;q21)	*IGH-MALT1*	deregulated *MALT1* expression, NF-κB activation	2%	0%	16%	13%	9%	0%	14%
t(3;14)(p14.1;q32)	*IGH-FOXP1*	deregulated *FOXP1* expression, apoptosis inhibition	0%	0%	9%	0%	0%	33%	7%

Discussion Extranodal marginal zone lymphoma of mucosa-associated lymphoid tissue (MALT lymphoma) is defined as an extranodal lymphoma of morphologically heterogenous B cells with a post-germinal center phenotype occurring at mucosal sites. A subtype of this entity was initially described in 1965 in the Middle East as α heavy chain disease (also known as *immunoproliferative small intestinal disease*), arising in the gastrointestinal tract of young adults, with the classic findings of neoplastic B cells with plasmacytic differentiation diffusely infiltrating into mucosal epithelium and forming lymphoepithelial lesions. Since then, extranodal marginal zone lymphoma arising from other mucosal sites such as the stomach, ocular adnexa, salivary gland, lung, skin, and thyroid have been unified under the diagnostic umbrella of MALT lymphoma. There is a wide spectrum of morphology in cases of MALT lymphoma. The characteristic neoplastic marginal zone lymphocytes have small to intermediate-sized nuclei with moderately dispersed chromatin and moderate cytoplasm. Variable numbers of plasma cells may be present and some cases are composed almost exclusively of plasma cells, mimicking an extramedullary plasmacytoma. Large, immunoblast-like cells are typically seen but generally are few in number. Bystander reactive (non-neoplastic) follicles may also be present, with occasional follicular colonization by the marginal zone lymphocytes which can be identified by moth-eaten and disrupted follicular dendritic meshworks. The neoplastic lymphocytes may also invade the mucosa with formation of lymphoepithelial lesions. Immunophenotyping of the neoplastic B cells typically reveals positivity for common B-cell antigens (such as CD19 and CD20) without coexpression of CD5 or CD10; however, rarer cases may have CD5 positivity, usually dim and/or partial. In such cases, distinction from mantle cell or small lymphocytic lymphoma is important. CD43 may be aberrantly co-expressed on the B cells in ~50% of cases and, when present, can be helpful in distinguishing MALT lymphoma from reactive conditions. In cases with significant plasma cell differentiation, cytoplasmic light chain restriction is also helpful.

Although the etiology of MALT lymphoma is not well understood, inflammatory conditions characterized by chronic antigenic stimulation of various etiologies (either microbial antigens or autoimmune disease) are strongly associated with site-specific variants of MALT lymphoma and can lead to diagnostic challenges in the discrimination between chronic inflammation and lymphoma. For instance, there is a well-established etiologic link between *Helicobacter pylori* infection and MALT lymphoma arising in the stomach, as well as *Borrelia burgdoferi* and cutaneous MALT lymphoma. Eradication of the microorganism by antibiotics leads to a marked decline of antigen-driven growth of the neoplastic process and even regression in some cases. Furthermore, *Chlamydia psittaci* has been associated with ocular adnexal and lung MALT lymphomas in European and Japanese studies. MALT lymphoma has also been associated with Sjögren disease and Hashimoto thyroiditis. Immunoglobulin heavy chain (*IGH*) gene rearrangement studies can help distinguish between chronic inflammation and lymphoma, although it should be noted that even using primers against all 3 *IGH* framework regions, *IGH* clonality studies may be falsely negative in 12%-14% of cases because of somatic hypermutation. NGS studies, which are more heavily multiplexed, may allow for improved recognition of the clonal population in those cases.

Interestingly, although the MALT lymphomas that arise at various sites may share morphologic and immunophenotypic similarities, there are also site-specific molecular cytogenetic abnormalities. There are 4 known recurrent balanced translocations in MALT lymphomas **t37.1**. Each of these balanced translocations has a predilection for different anatomic sites. For instance, the t(11;18)(q21;q21) variant of MALT lymphoma is most commonly found in the lung (42%), intestine (41%), and stomach (22%). In contrast, the t(14;18)(q32;q21) variant is most commonly associated with the salivary gland (13%), ocular adnexa (16%), and skin (9%). Of note, this fusion is between *IGH* and *MALT1* and is distinct from the t(14;18)(q32;q21) *IGH-BCL2* found in follicular lymphoma; the 2 fusions can be distinguished using FISH probes but not metaphase cytogenetics. The t(3;14)(p14.1;q32) variant of MALT lymphoma is primarily found in the thyroid (33%) and ocular adnexa (9%). The t(1;14)(p22;q32) variant is perhaps the most uncommon and is seen in <10% of MALT lymphomas arising in the intestine, lung, and salivary gland. In addition to translocations, recurrent aneuploidies are also found in MALT lymphomas, with trisomy 3 and 18 most commonly seen in intestinal cases. Genetic abnormalities at 6q23 including deletion or mutation in *TNFAIP3*, a negative regulator of NF-κB, occur in up to 30% of MALT lymphomas but are also found in other B-cell lymphomas, including other types of marginal zone lymphoma (see **Case 36**). In addition to the aforementioned recurrent translocations, several case reports have described MALT lymphomas having t(3;14)(q27;q32) and t(6;14)(p21.1q32), involving *IGH* translocation partners *BCL6* and *CCND3*, respectively.

The most commonly identified chromosomal translocation in gastric MALT lymphoma is t(11;18)(q21;q21) *BIRC3-MALT1*, seen in up to 22% of cases and exemplified in this patient. The translocation generates a functional cIAP2-MALT1 fusion protein with an N-terminal region BIR (*B*aculovirus *I*nhibitor of apoptosis protein *R*epeat) domain and a C-terminal region caspase-like domain. The fusion product is thought to exert its oncogenic activity via multiple pathways. For instance, cIAP2 inhibits the biological activity of caspases and is believed to be an apoptosis inhibitor. The cIAP2-MALT1 fusion product is also capable of inappropriately activating NF-κB through B-cell receptor-independent dimerization of MALT1. Indeed, activation of NF-κB is the final common pathway of 3 of 4 recurrent MALT-associated translocations as well as of recurrent somatic mutations, especially in *TNFAIP3*. Activation of this pathway stimulates the expression of genes involved in cell survival and proliferation in MALT lymphomas. The *BIRC3-MALT1* fusion is specific for MALT lymphomas and is more frequently associated with stage IIE at diagnosis. Its acquisition marks a transition from *H pylori*-dependent growth, when antibiotics may be useful, to independent growth requiring chemotherapy for successful treatment.

Diagnostic pearls/pitfalls

- MALT lymphomas can be morphologically heterogeneous and may include small to medium-sized lymphocytes, monocytoid-appearing cells, few to numerous plasma cells, as well as occasional immunoblast-like cells.
- Site-specific antigenic stimulation and inflammation set the stage for the development of MALT lymphomas, making it sometimes difficult to distinguish lymphoma from chronic inflammation based on histologic findings. Evidence of B-cell clonality by immunophenotyping or molecular studies is helpful in these cases.

ISBN 978-089189-6814

– The 4 most common translocations associated with MALT lymphomas are: t(11;18)(q21;q21), t(1;14)(p22;q32), t(14;18)(q32;q21), and t(3;14) (p14.1;q32), and each translocation is associated with specific anatomic sites **t37.1**.

– Gastric MALT lymphomas with t(11;18) *BIRC3-MALT1* will not respond to antibiotic treatment directed against *H pylori*.

Readings

Aigelsreiter A, Gerlza T, Deutsch AJ, et al. *Chlamydia psittaci* infection in nongastrointestinal extranodal MALT lymphomas and their precursor lesions. Am J Clin Pathol. 2011;135(1):70-5. **DOI: 10.1309/AJCPXMDRT1SY6KIV**

Akyüz N, Albert-Konetzny N, Pott C et al. MALT1 sequencing analyses in marginal zone B-cell lymphomas reveal mutations in the translocated *MALT1* allele in an *IGH-MALT1*-positive MALT lymphoma. Leuk Lymphoma. 2017;58(10):2480-4. **DOI: 10.1080/10428194.2017.1296144**

Cook JR, Isaacson PG, Chott A, et al. (2017) Extranodal marginal zone lymphoma of mucosa-associated lymphoid tissue (MALT lymphoma). In: Swerdlow SH, Campo E, Harris NL, et al. World Health Organization Classification of Tumours of Haematopoietic and Lymphoid Tissues. 4th ed. Lyon, France: IARC Press; 2017:259-62. **ISBN: 9789283244943**

Cuneo A, Bigoni R, Roberti MG, et al. Molecular cytogenetic characterization of marginal zone B-cell lymphoma: correlation with clinicopathologic findings in 14 cases. Haematologica. 2001;86(1):64-70. **DOI: https://doi.org/10.3324/%25x**

Du MQ. MALT lymphoma : recent advances in aetiology and molecular genetics. J Clin Exp Hematop. 2007;47(2):31-42. **DOI: 10.3960/jslrt.47.31**

Elton L, Carpentier I, Staal J, et al. MALT1 cleaves the E3 ubiquitin ligase HOIL-1 in activated T cells, generating a dominant negative inhibitor of LUBAC-induced NF-κB signaling. FEBS J. 2016;283(3):403-12. **DOI: 10.1111/febs.13597**

Gehring T, Seeholzer T, Krappmann D. BCL10: Bridging CARDs to immune activation. Front Immunol. 2018;9:1539. **DOI: 10.3389/fimmu.2018.01539**

Isaacson P, Wright DH. Malignant lymphoma of mucosa-associated lymphoid tissue: a distinctive type of B-cell lymphoma. Cancer. 1983;52(8):1410-6. **DOI: 10.1002/1097-0142(19831015)52:8<1410::aid-cncr2820520813>3.0.co;2-3**

Kim AS, Wu CJ, Lovitch SB. Molecular genetic aspects of non-Hodgkin lymphomas. In: Greer JP, Arber DA, Appelbalm FR, et al, eds. Wintrobe's Clinical Hematology. 14th ed. Philadelphia, PA: Wolters Kluwer Health; 2018;Chap 88:1843-79. **ISBN: 978-1496347428**

Patzelt T, Keppler SJ, Gorka O, et al. Foxp1 controls mature B cell survival and the development of follicular and B-1 B cells. Proc Natl Acad Sci USA. 2018;115(12):3120-5. **DOI:10.1073/pnas.1711335115**

Ramot B, Shahin N, Bubis JJ. Malabsorption syndrome in lymphoma of small intestine: a study of 13 cases. Isr J Med Sci. 1965;1:221-6. **PMID: 14279068**

Remstein ED, Dogan A, Einerson RR, et al. The incidence and anatomic site specificity of chromosomal translocations in primary extranodal marginal zone B-cell lymphoma of mucosa-associated lymphoid tissue (MALT lymphoma) in North America. Am J Surg Pathol. 2006;30(12):1546-53. **DOI: 10.1097/01.pas.0000213275.60962.2a**

Roggero E, Zucca E, Mainetti C, et al. Eradication of *Borrelia burgdorferi* infection in primary marginal zone B-cell lymphoma of the skin. Hum Pathol. 2000;31(2):263-8. **DOI: 10.1016/s0046-8177(00)80233-6**

Shanmugam V, Kim AS. Lymphomas. In: Tafe JL, Arcila ME, eds. Genomic Medicine: A Practical Guide. New York, NY: Springer; 2020;chap 16:253-315. **ISBN: 978-3030229214**

Streubel B, Simonitsch-Klupp I, and Müllauer L, et al. Variable frequencies of MALT lymphoma-associated genetic aberrations in MALT lymphomas of different sites. Leukemia. 2004;18(10):1722-6. **DOI: 10.1038/sj.leu.2403501**

Wotherspoon AC, Ortiz-Hidalgo C, Falzon MR, et al. *Helicobacter pylori*-associated gastritis and primary B-cell gastric lymphoma. Lancet. 1991;338(8776):1175-6. **DOI: 10.1016/0140-6736(91)92035-z**

Erika M Moore

38

High grade B-cell lymphoma with *MYC* & *BCL2* & *BCL6* rearrangements

History A 62-year-old female presented with night sweats and abdominal pain. Imaging revealed abdominal lymphadenopathy **f38.1**, and a CT-guided core biopsy specimen of the enlarged lymph nodes was obtained.

Morphology & flow cytometry The lymph node biopsy demonstrated cores of tissue containing a diffuse lymphoid infiltrate of predominantly large cells with irregular nuclear contours, vesicular chromatin, and single to multiple nucleoli. Mitotic figures and single cell apoptosis were prominent **f38.2**.

Immunostains demonstrated that the large atypical cells were positive for CD20, CD10, BCL6, and BCL2. MYC was positive in ~50% of the B-cell infiltrate and Ki-67 appeared to be positive in >60% of the B-cell portion of the infiltrate **f38.3**.

Flow cytometry demonstrated a CD10 positive, CD19 dim, κ-restricted B-cell population comprising 19% of total events **f38.4**.

Genetics/molecular results Paraffin FISH studies performed on the lymph node core were positive for rearrangements of *MYC*, *BCL2*, and *BCL6*: nuc ish(BCL6x2)(5' BCL6 sep 3' BCL6x1) [76/300], (MYCx2)(5' MYC sep 3'MYCx1) [72/300], (BCL2x2) (5' BCL2 sep 3' BCL2x1) [57/200] **f38.5**.

Based on the morphologic, flow cytometric, and genetic findings, a diagnosis of **high-grade B-cell lymphoma with *MYC* and *BCL2* and *BCL6* rearrangements** was rendered.

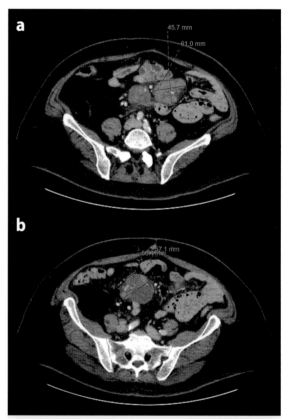

f38.1 Abdominal CT with contrast reveals intra-abdominal lymphadenopathy, including **a** 45 × 61mm & **b** 57.1 × 58.4 mm lymph nodes

ISBN 978-089189-6814

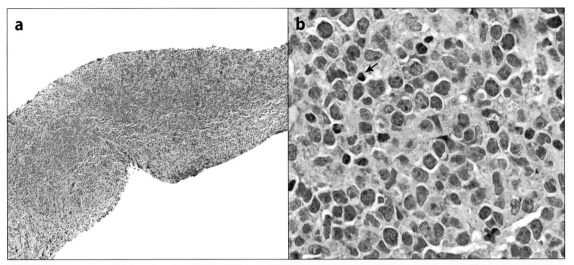

f38.2 Lymph node core biopsy with **a** a diffuse atypical lymphoid infiltrate at low power; **b** higher-power view reveals large atypical cells with irregular nuclear contours, vesicular chromatin & prominent nucleoli; arrow indicates single cell apoptosis

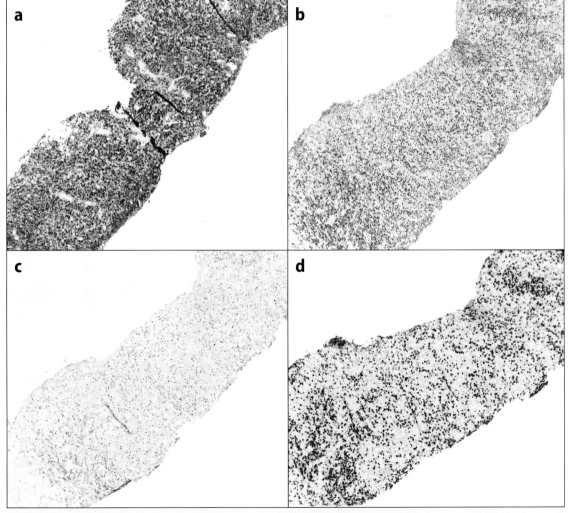

f38.3 Immunohistochemistry reveals the lymphoma cells are positive for **a** BCL2, **b** BCL6, **c** MYC & **d** Ki-67

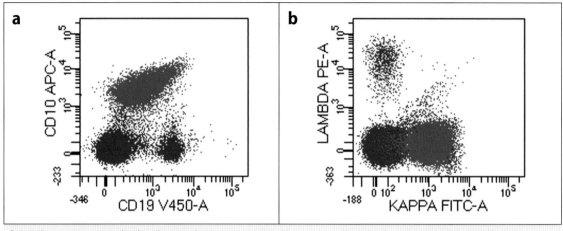

f38.4 Flow cytometry, gated on lymphocytes, demonstrating 19% **a** CD10-positive, CD19-dim, **b** κ-restricted B cells (highlighted in purple)

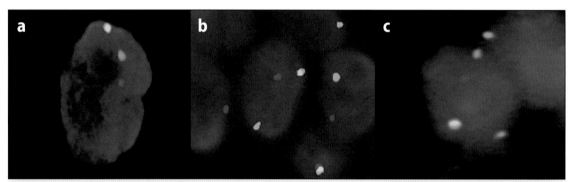

f38.5 FISH studies show the presence of *BCL2* (18q21), *BCL6* (3q27) & *MYC* (8q24) gene rearrangements as evidenced by separate red & green signals present after hybridization with break-apart (yellow) probes

Discussion A thorough evaluation of large B-cell lymphomas generally involves clinical context, histology, immunophenotype, and genetic studies. Large B-cell lymphoma may arise de novo, result from progression of a lower grade process such as chronic lymphocytic leukemia/small lymphocytic lymphoma or follicular lymphoma (transformation), or more rarely, be associated with an immunocompromised state and/or viral infection. Morphologically, a number of distinct entities may present with diffuse sheets of atypical B lymphocytes that are intermediate to large in size; some of these entities are compared in **t38.1**. A properly fixed specimen is essential for evaluating cell size and chromatin features, and adequate immunophenotyping is necessary for determining cell of origin (COO), which has prognostic impact in de novo DLBCL, not otherwise specified (NOS). Sub-classification of DLBCL according to COO was originally performed using gene expression studies which demonstrated that lymphomas having a non-germinal center (non-GC) profile, or "activated B-cell" profile, appear to have a poorer prognosis than lymphomas with a GC profile. Several algorithms using immunohistochemistry (IHC) have since been developed as simpler, surrogate methods for determining COO. The most common of these is the Hans algorithm, in which CD10+BCL6+/−MUM+/− or CD10−BCL6+MUM1− defines GC origin and CD10−BCL6+MUM1+, CD10−BCL6−MUM1+, or CD10−BCL6−MUM1− defines non-GC origin. In recent years, COO has also been

t38.1 Comparison of morphologic, IHC & genetic features of large B-cell lymphomas

	DLBCL, NOS	Burkitt lymphoma	Lymphoblastic lymphoma	HGBCL, DH, or TH	HGBCL, NOS
Morphology of lymphocytes	large, pleomorphic, variable nuclear features	intermediate size, monomorphic, often with multiple small nucleoli	intermediate size, monomorphic, blastic appearance with stippled chromatin	DLBCL, Burkitt-like, or blastoid	blastoid or Burkitt-like
IHC	TdT–, CD10 variable*, MYC & BCL2 variable†	TdT–, CD10+, BCL6+, BCL2–, Ki67 95%-100%	TdT+, often CD10+, high Ki-67	TdT–, usually GC origin*, MYC & BCL2 variable	TdT–, often BCL6+, MYC & BCL2 variable
Gene rearrangement	may have gene rearrangements but not *MYC* with *BCL2* and/or *BCL6*	*MYC*	may have gene rearrangements but usually not *MYC* with *BCL2* and/or *BCL6*‡	*MYC* with *BCL2* and/or *BCL6*	may have gene rearrangements but not *MYC* with *BCL2* and/or *BCL6*

DH, double hit; DLBCL, diffuse large B-cell lymphoma; GC, germinal center; HGBCL, high-grade B-cell lymphoma; IHC, immunohistochemical; NOS, not otherwise specified; TH, triple hit
*See text for details on the evaluation of GC or non-GC origin
†The term "double-expressor DLBCL" refers to cases expressing both MYC & BCL2 by IHC
‡Rare cases of lymphoblastic lymphoma may have DH gene rearrangements

determined by low density gene expression array in some academic centers.

"High-grade B-cell lymphoma" (HGBCL) is a new entity in the 2017 World Health Organization (WHO) classification of hematopoietic neoplasms and has 2 subcategories: HGBCL, NOS, and HGBCL with *MYC* and *BCL2* and/or *BCL6* rearrangements. This entity replaces the former "B-cell lymphoma, unclassifiable, with features intermediate between diffuse large B-cell lymphoma (DLBCL) and Burkitt lymphoma" and provides an official diagnostic category for so-called "double" or "triple" hit lymphomas, which have a rearrangement of the *MYC* gene co-occurring with rearrangement of the *BCL2* and/or *BCL6* genes.

Morphologically, HGBCL may have larger cells resembling DLBCL, NOS, or intermediate-sized cells resembling Burkitt lymphoma. The specific diagnosis of HGBCL with *MYC* and *BCL2* and/or *BCL6* rearrangements rests upon the results of cytogenetic studies, most often FISH using break-apart probes for these genes. Although the diagnosis is uncommon (<10% of all large B-cell lymphomas in some studies), it carries significant prognostic and therapeutic implications and thus accurate diagnosis is critical. Patients tend to do poorly with standard chemotherapy regimens typically used for patients with DLBCL, NOS (eg, rituximab, cyclophosphamide, doxorubicin hydrochloride, vincristine [previously called oncovin], prednisolone [R-CHOP]) and will usually require more aggressive therapy at diagnosis. Several studies indicate that IHC for CD10, BCL2, BCL6, MUM1, MYC, and/or

Ki-67 cannot reliably predict which cases will have gene rearrangements and therefore, IHC is not sufficient as a screening method for double or triple hit lymphoma.

Multiple studies have demonstrated that most, but not all, double or triple hit lymphomas tend to be of GC origin (based on gene expression analysis or the Hans algorithm). Larger institutions tend to perform FISH for *MYC*, *BCL2*, and *BCL6* rearrangements on all cases of large B-cell lymphoma; however, if resources are limited, testing only GC-type lymphomas could be an acceptable strategy with the acknowledgment that rare cases may be missed. Another conservative approach is to screen all large B-cell lymphomas for *MYC* rearrangement, then proceed to test for *BCL2* and *BCL6* rearrangements if the *MYC* result is positive. It is important to note that FISH probes for *MYC* vary in sensitivity and optimal strategies for detection of *MYC* rearrangement include using multiple probe sets, such as using both a *MYC* break-apart probe and dual-color, dual-fusion probes for *IGH-MYC*. Each of these individual probe sets may fail to detect a small number of *MYC*-rearranged cases and using both types ensures detection of all *MYC* rearrangements.

The term "double-expressor" has been used to describe cases of large B-cell lymphoma that co-express MYC and BCL2 protein. This term is often confused with the moniker "double hit"; the latter is defined cytogenetically by the presence of gene rearrangements, while "double-expressor" refers to protein expression detected by IHC. Many, but not all, double or triple hit lymphomas are also double-expressors, but most double-expressors are not double or triple hit lymphomas. Double-expressor lymphomas tend to have a relatively poor prognosis independent of *MYC, BCL2*, and *BCL6* gene rearrangement status and independent of COO. Although there are no official numerical cut-offs of percent positive cells to determine whether a case is considered positive for MYC or BCL2 expression by IHC, a 40% threshold (of positive lymphoma cells) for MYC and 50% for BCL2 are generally used, based on the initial studies defining the double-expressor phenotype. Evaluation of MYC and BCL2 by IHC to determine double-expressor status should be a standard part of the work-up of all large B-cell lymphomas.

HGBCL, NOS, is a diagnosis that is reserved for rare cases of B-cell lymphoma that have morphologic and/or immunophenotypic features intermediate between DLBCL and Burkitt lymphoma or have a blastoid morphology, but do not have *MYC* and *BCL2* and/or *BCL6* rearrangements. The HGBCL, NOS, designation is not intended to be used for cases that have a typical DLBCL morphology with high MYC or Ki-67 expression alone, or for DLBCL-appearing cases with an isolated *MYC* gene rearrangement. According to 2017 WHO criteria, these cases should be classified as DLBCL, NOS. The HGBCL, NOS, designation also does not include blastoid-appearing cases of mantle cell lymphoma and cases of B-lymphoblastic leukemia/lymphoma. Morphologically, most cases of HGBCL, NOS, typically resemble Burkitt lymphoma but tend to be more pleomorphic and/or have an immunophenotype that is not typical for Burkitt lymphoma.

Diagnostic pearls/pitfalls

– Distinguishing HGBCL from DLBCL, NOS, is critical because of the therapeutic and prognostic implications.
– The presence of *MYC* and *BCL2* and/or *BCL6* rearrangements cannot be reliably predicted with immunohistochemical stains. Cases with lower MYC and/or Ki67 expression by IHC can have gene rearrangements detected by FISH, and vice versa.
– Screening all cases of large B-cell lymphoma with FISH for *MYC, BCL2*, and *BCL6* rearrangements is recommended, because the presence of double or triple hit lymphoma usually requires more aggressive chemotherapy.
– *MYC* rearrangements may be missed if only using the *MYC* break-apart probe or dual-color, dual-fusion *IGH/MYC* probe. Testing with both probes minimizes the chance of a false-negative result.
– Double/triple hit lymphomas and double-expressor lymphomas are separate concepts and not synonymous. A lymphoma may meet the criteria for either a double/triple hit or double-expressor, both, or neither.

Readings

Alizadeh AA, Eisen MB, Davis RE, et al. Distinct types of diffuse large B-cell lymphoma identified by gene expression profiling. Nature. 2000;403(6769):503-11. **DOI: 10.1038/35000501**

Hans CP, Weisenburger DD, Greiner TC, et al. Confirmation of the molecular classification of diffuse large B-cell lymphoma by immunohistochemistry using a tissue microarray. Blood. 2004;103(1):275-82. **DOI: 10.1182/blood-2003-05-1545**

Johnson NA, Slack GW, Savage KJ, et al. Concurrent expression of *MYC* and *BCL2* in diffuse large B-cell lymphoma treated with rituximab plus cyclophosphamide, doxorubicin, vincristine, and prednisone. J Clin Oncol. 2012;30:3452-9. **DOI: 10.1200/JCO.2011.41.0985**

Landsburg DJ, Nasta SD, Svoboda J, Morrissette JJD, Schuster SJ. "Double-hit" cytogenetic status may not be predicted by baseline clinicopathological characteristics and is highly associated with overall survival in B cell lymphoma patients. Br J Haematol. 2014;166:369-74. **DOI: 10.1111/bjh.12901**

Landsburg DJ, Schuster SJ. Who should be tested for double-hit lymphoma? J Oncol Pract. 2016;12:243-4. **DOI: 10.1200/JOP.2015.010595**

Petrich AM, Gandhi M, Jovanovic B, et al. Impact of induction regimen and stem cell transplantation on outcomes in double-hit lymphoma: a multicenter retrospective analysis. Blood. 2014;124:2354–2361. Histopathology. 2012;61(6):1214-8. **DOI: 10.1182/blood-2014-05-578963**

Scott DW, King RL, Staiger AM, et al. High-grade B-cell lymphoma with *MYC* and *BCL2* and/or *BCL6* rearrangements with diffuse large B-cell lymphoma morphology. Blood. 2018;131(18):2060-4. **DOI: 10.1182/blood-2017-12-820605**

Swerdlow SH. Diagnosis of "double hit" diffuse large B-cell lymphoma and B-cell lymphoma, unclassifiable, with features intermediate between DLBCL and Burkitt lymphoma: when and how, FISH versus IHC. Hematology Am Soc Hematol Educ Program. 2014;2014:90-9. **DOI: 10.1182/asheducation-2014.1.90**

Swerdlow SH, Campo E, Harris NL, et al. World Health Organization Classification of Tumours of Haematopoietic and Lymphoid Tissues. 4th ed. Lyon, France: IARC Press, 2017. **ISBN: 9789283244943**

Yoon N, Ahn S, Yong Yoo H, et al. Cell-of-origin of diffuse large B-cell lymphomas determined by the Lymph2Cx assay: better prognostic indicator than Hans algorithm. Oncotarget. 2017;8(13):22014-22. **DOI: 10.18632/oncotarget.15782**

Bryan Rea

39

Primary mediastinal large B-cell lymphoma with 9p24.1 amplification

History A 29-year-old male with no significant past medical history presented with unexplained bruising on his upper arm and was found to have a 14 cm anterior mediastinal mass **f39.1**, along with upper extremity deep venous thrombosis. Additional imaging revealed no other sites of disease or significant lymphadenopathy. Fine needle aspiration demonstrated an abnormal lymphoid infiltrate but was ultimately nondiagnostic, and an open biopsy was performed for more definitive assessment.

Morphology & flow cytometry The mediastinal mass biopsy showed a dense lymphoid infiltrate composed of intermediate to large lymphoid cells with fewer interspersed smaller lymphoid cells, plasmacytoid cells, and granulocytes. The large cells had large nuclei with irregular nuclear contours, prominent nucleoli, and a moderate amount of cytoplasm. Faint sclerotic bands were prominent throughout the infiltrate **f39.2**.

IHC/ISH stains showed that the large cells were positive for CD20, CD79a, and PAX5, but negative for CD3, CD5, AE1/AE3, and EBER. A subset of the large cells was positive for CD30, CD23, and PD-L1 **f39.3**. Flow cytometric studies demonstrated an atypical population of B cells that was surface immunoglobulin negative, CD19 positive, CD20 bright positive, CD5 negative, and CD10 negative, in a background of some polytypic B cells **f39.4**. Overall, the findings were consistent with a diagnosis of large B-cell lymphoma and were very suspicious for **primary mediastinal large B-cell lymphoma (PMBL)**.

Genetics/molecular results To further support a diagnosis of PMBL, FISH studies for amplification of the 9p24.1 region (using a JAK2 probe) were performed and were positive **f39.5**. Therefore, the combined morphologic,

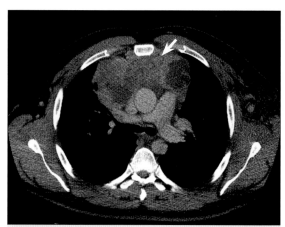

f39.1 Radiograph of the chest reveals a 14 cm anterior mediastinal mass (arrow)

immunophenotypic, and genetic features were consistent with a diagnosis of **primary mediastinal large B-cell lymphoma**.

Discussion Primary (thymic) mediastinal large B-cell lymphoma (PMBL) is a distinct subset of large B-cell lymphoma with unique clinical, morphologic, immunophenotypic, and genetic features. PMBL is relatively uncommon and accounts for ~2%-3% of all non-Hodgkin lymphomas. It occurs most commonly in young adults (median age, ~35 years) and has been shown to have a female predominance.

The classic presentation of PMBL includes a bulky anterior mediastinal mass that is rapidly progressive and often gives rise to associated compressive symptoms leading to superior vena cava syndrome. There may be local invasion into adjacent structures, such as the lung, chest wall, and pleura; however, widely disseminated disease at presentation is uncommon. Bone marrow

ISBN 978-089189-6814

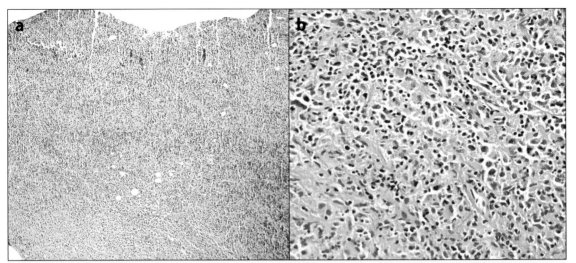

f39.2 a Sections of the mediastinal mass show a diffuse, dense lymphoid infiltrate on low power; **b** higher power demonstrates the lymphoid infiltrate is composed of moderately numerous intermediate to large cells in a background of fewer smaller lymphocytes, histiocytes & plasma cells; faint bands of sclerosis are also easily identified

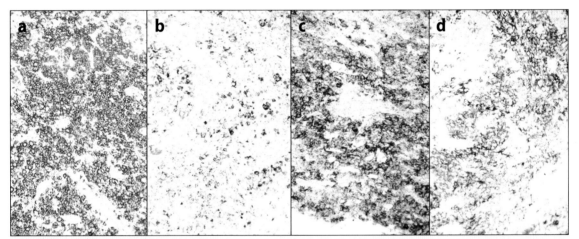

f39.3 Immunohistochemical staining demonstrates that the large cells are positive for **a** CD20, with partial positivity for **b** CD30, **c** CD23 & **d** PDL1

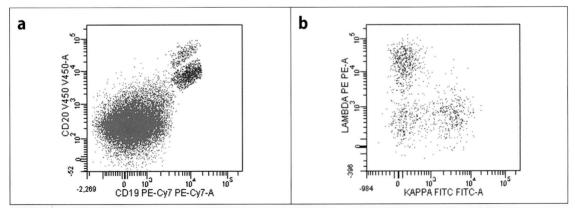

f39.4 Flow cytometric studies identify an abnormal **a** CD19 positive, CD20 positive, **b** surface light chain negative B-cell population (red); background polytypic B cells (blue) & presumptive T cells (orange) are shown for reference

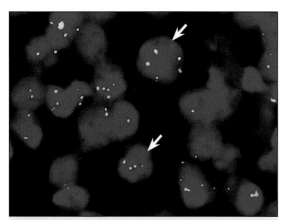

f39.5 FISH using a break-apart JAK2 probe (yellow or juxtaposed green & orange) identified amplification of the region 9p24.1; a large proportion of cells contained 3, 4, 5, or 6 copies of the probe; cells with 5 copies are specifically highlighted (arrows); image courtesy of Mary Ann West

and/or cerebrospinal fluid involvement is not typically identified at diagnosis. The lack of widespread involvement is sometimes helpful in the differential diagnosis of an otherwise systemic diffuse large B-cell lymphoma (DLBCL) with mediastinal involvement.

There is a somewhat wide spectrum of morphologic features, but many cases, similar to the current case, demonstrate a diffuse proliferation of intermediate to large cells associated with sclerosis/compartmentalization **f39.2**. With this morphology, the primary differential diagnosis is typically DLBCL. Occasionally, the large cells may have features that mimic Reed-Sternberg cells, making the distinction between PMBL and classic Hodgkin lymphoma (cHL) difficult on morphologic grounds alone. It should also be noted that true "gray zone" lymphomas with features intermediate between large B-cell lymphoma and cHL do exist, and these rare cases should be classified separately as B-cell lymphoma, unclassifiable, with features intermediate between DLBCL and Hodgkin lymphoma.

Importantly, there are some immunophenotypic features that, while not entirely specific, aid in establishing a diagnosis of PMBL as compared to its morphologic mimics. PMBL, unlike cHL, tends to express all of the B-cell antigens/transcription factors including CD19, CD20, CD22, CD79a, PAX5, BOB1, and OCT2. PMBL also frequently shows significant or subset expression of CD30, CD23, MAL, and PD-L1, antigens which are expressed only in a minority of DLBCL cases. Finally, flow cytometric studies often identify a surface immunoglobulin-negative population, as seen in this case, though surface immunoglobulin expression is detected in some cases.

The genetic features of PMBL have been well-studied and show significant overlap with cHL. As exemplified in the current case, amplifications at 9p24.1 are a common occurrence and seen in ~50%-70% of all cases **f39.5**. This locus includes *JAK2*, *CD274* (PDL1), and *PDCD1LG2* (PDL2). JAK/STAT pathway dysregulation and overexpression of PD-L1 and PD-L2 are thought to play a major role in allowing PMBL cell survival and immune escape. Other common abnormalities include rearrangements with *CIITA*, an activator of MHC class II genes, gains at the 2p16 region involving REL (a member of the NF-κB pathway), as well as other somatic mutations involving the JAK/STAT and NF-κB pathways. Specific genes that have been identified as recurrently mutated in a significant proportion of PMBL include *TNFAIP3*, *STAT6*, *SOCS1*, *XPO1*, and *PTPN1*. In addition, gene rearrangements of BCL2, BCL6, and *MYC*, relatively common in DLBCL, are rare in PMBL. Because of the aforementioned molecular overlap with cHL, these genetic features are most useful from a diagnostic perspective when the primary differential diagnosis is a DLBCL with mediastinal involvement, and in general, gene expression profiling (GEP) studies have indicated that it is possible to distinguish these entities by molecular characteristics. Although GEP technologies may not be readily performed on routine clinical specimens, intriguingly, recent studies have indicated that a molecular classification assay performed on formalinfixed paraffin-embedded specimens can be useful in differentiating PMBL from DLBCL.

It is important to accurately distinguish PMBL from DLBCL and cHL because all 3 entities are treated quite differently and have different survival characteristics. PMBL is treated more aggressively than standard DLBCL, such as with a DA-EPOCH-R type regimen. Overall survival is generally favorable. In the immunotherapy era, given the molecular pathogenesis of PMBL, there is also possibly a role for JAK2 inhibitors, anti-CD30 therapy, and/or PD-1/PD-L1 targeting, and investigations into these therapies are ongoing. A summary of the key features described herein are found in **t39.1**.

Diagnostic pearls/pitfalls

– PMBL is a distinct clinicopathologic entity but demonstrates morphologic overlap with DLBCL and occasionally cHL. In addition to thorough immunophenotyping, the clinical history and radiographic findings can aid in differentiating from these entities.

ISBN 978-089189-6814 ©2021 ASCP

t39.1 Key features of primary mediastinal large B-cell lymphoma, diffuse large B-cell lymphoma, NOS & classic Hodgkin lymphoma

	Primary mediastinal large B-cell lymphoma	Diffuse large B-cell lymphoma, NOS	Classic Hodgkin lymphoma
Presentation	young adults, isolated bulky mediastinal mass	variable, but usually older patients, disseminated disease	variable, mediastinal involvement most common in NS subtype
Morphology	large cells, faint sclerosis, rarely Reed-Sternberg-like cells	variable but typically sheets of large mononuclear cells, rarely Reed-Sternberg-like cells	Reed-Sternberg cells, mixed inflammatory background, thick sclerotic bands in NS subtype
Key phenotypic features	pan B-cell antigens +; variable CD23, CD30, MAL, PD-L1/2; negative for EBV	pan B-cell antigens +; usually CD23, CD30, MAL, PD-L1/2 negative	CD45–, CD20–, PAX5+ (often dim), CD15+, CD30+, MUM1+, may be EBV+
Genetics	9p24 & 2p16 amplification, PDL1/2 and CIITA rearrangement, JAK/STAT, NF-κB pathway gene mutations	*BCL2*, *BCL6*, or *MYC* rearrangements, variety of other chromosomal changes/somatic mutations, with little gene expression overlap with PMBL	9p24 & 2p16 amplification, JAK/STAT, NF-κB pathway gene mutations, similar to PMBL
Frontline therapy	DA-EPOCH-R	R-CHOP	ABVD

+, positive; –, negative; NOS, not otherwise specified; NS, nodular sclerosis

- PMBL morphologically resembling cHL is not synonymous with so-called "gray zone lymphoma," which is a distinct separate entity in the WHO 2017 classification of hematologic neoplasms.
- Genetic features, such as amplification of 9p24.1 identified by FISH, in combination with a typical phenotype and clinical presentation, can aid in accurate diagnosis of PMBL.
- Accurate classification of PMBL is essential, because treatment and prognosis differ in comparison to DLBCL and cHL.

Readings

Dubois S, Viailly PJ, Mareschal S, et al. Next-generation sequencing in diffuse large B-cell lymphoma highlights molecular divergence and therapeutic opportunities: a LYSA study. Clin Cancer Res. 2016;22(12):2919-28. **DOI: 10.1158/1078-0432.CCR-15- 2305**

Dunleavy K, Pittaluga S, Maeda LS, et al. Dose-adjusted EPOCH-rituximab therapy in primary mediastinal B-cell lymphoma. N Engl J Med. 2013;368(15):1408-16. **DOI: 10.1056/ NEJMoa1214561**

Green MR, Monti S, Rodig SJ, et al. Integrative analysis reveals selective 9p24.1 amplification, increased PD-1 ligand expression, and further induction via *JAK2* in nodular sclerosing Hodgkin lymphoma and primary mediastinal large B-cell lymphoma. Blood. 2010;116(17):3268-77. **DOI: 10.1182/ blood-2010-05-282780**

Martelli M, Ferreri A, Di Rocco A, et al. Primary mediastinal large B-cell lymphoma. Crit Rev Oncol Hematol. 2017;113:318-27. **DOI: 10.1016/j.critrevonc.2017.01.009**

Mottok A, Woolcock B, Chan FC, et al. Genomic alterations in CIITA are frequent in primary mediastinal large B cell lymphoma and are associated with diminished MHC class II expression. Cell Rep. 2015;13(7):1418-31. **DOI: 10.1016/j.celrep.2015.10.008**

Mottok A, Wright G, Rosenwald A, et al. Molecular classification of primary mediastinal large B-cell lymphoma using routinely available tissue specimens. Blood. 2018;132(22):2401-5. **DOI: 10.1182/blood-2018-05-851154**

Rosenwald A, Wright G, Leroy K, et al. Molecular diagnosis of primary mediastinal B cell lymphoma identifies a clinically favorable subgroup of diffuse large B cell lymphoma related to Hodgkin lymphoma. J Exp Med. 2003;198(6):851-62. **DOI: 10.1084/jem.20031074**

Savage KJ, Monti S, Kutok JL, et al. The molecular signature of mediastinal large B-cell lymphoma differs from that of other diffuse large B-cell lymphomas and shares features with classical Hodgkin lymphoma. Blood. 2003;102(12):3871-9. **DOI: 10.1182/blood-2003-06-1841**

Swerdlow SH, Campo E, Harris NL, et al, eds. World Health Organization Classification of Tumours of Haematopoietic and Lymphoid Tissues. 4th ed. Lyon, France: IARC Press; 2017. **ISBN: 9789283244943**

Twa DD, Chan FC, Ben-Neriah S, et al. Genomic rearrangements involving programmed death ligands are recurrent in primary mediastinal large B-cell lymphoma. Blood. 2014;123(13):2062-5. **DOI: 10.1182/blood-2013-10-535443**

Ramya Gadde & Erika M Moore

40

Large B-cell lymphoma with *IRF4* rearrangement

History An 8-year-old girl presented with sore throat, cough, difficulty swallowing, upper abdominal pain, joint pains, and fatigue. Her peripheral blood CBC was within normal limits and EBV serology titers were negative. PET/CT imaging revealed hypermetabolic activity involving the bilateral palatine tonsils (SUV of 11.4 on the right side and 7.4 on the left side) **f40.1**, but no adenopathy or organomegaly was noted. A biopsy of the right tonsil was obtained.

Morphology & flow cytometry Histologic sections of the right tonsil showed a diffuse atypical lymphoid proliferation consisting of pleomorphic large lymphoid cells with a scant to moderate amount of cytoplasm, vesicular nuclei, and occasional prominent nucleoli. Large areas of necrosis and frequent apoptotic bodies were also present **f40.2**.

Immunohistochemistry demonstrated that the large, atypical cells were positive for CD20, PAX5, CD5, BCL6, and BCL2 and negative for CD10. MUM1 was strongly and diffusely expressed in the B cells and the Ki67 proliferation index was high (>90%) **f40.3**. A MYC immunostain was negative in the neoplastic B cells.

Flow cytometric studies performed at an outside institution reportedly demonstrated a CD5 positive, CD10 negative, CD19 dim, CD20 positive, surface κ light chain restricted B-cell population comprising approximately 19% of total events.

Genetics/molecular results Paraffin FISH studies performed on the tonsil biopsy were negative for rearrangements of *MYC*, *BCL2*, and *BCL6* but positive for a *DUSP22/IRF4* rearrangement **f40.4**.

Based on the morphologic, flow cytometric, and genetic findings, a diagnosis of **large B-cell lymphoma with *IRF4/MUM1* rearrangement** was rendered.

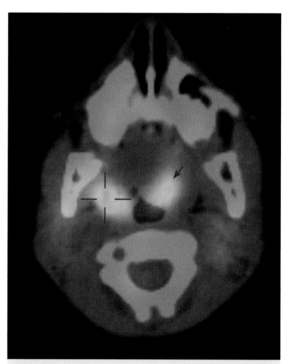

f40.1 Dual PET/CT image demonstrating hypermetabolic activity in both the right & left tonsils (red cross & red arrow)

Discussion Large B-cell lymphoma with *IRF4* (LBCL-*IRF4*) rearrangement is a novel entity recently included in the 2017 WHO classification of lymphoid tumors. This lymphoma typically presents in the pediatric and young adult population, usually in the head or neck region, and particularly within the Waldeyer ring. These cases characteristically harbor a rearrangement in the *IRF4* gene that results in strong expression of IRF4 (*i*nterferon *r*egulatory *f*actor *4*, also known as *mu*ltiple *m*yeloma 1, or MUM1), which can be detected using immunohistochemistry. LBCL-*IRF4* is typically localized in presentation, but involvement

ISBN 978-089189-6814

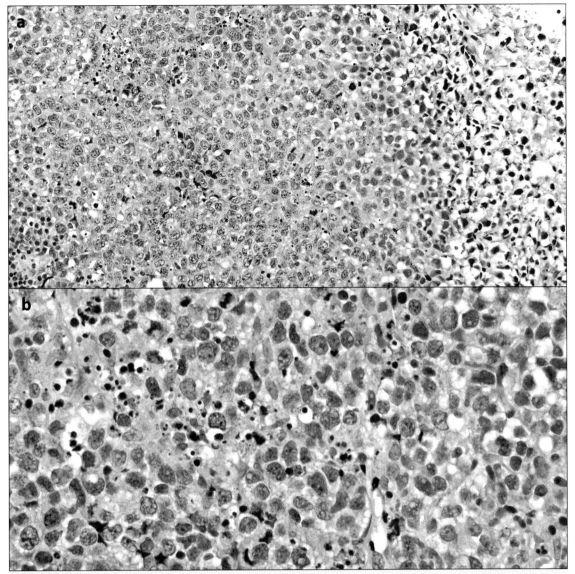

f40.2 Tonsil biopsy demonstrating a diffuse atypical lymphoid infiltrate **a** at 20× & **b** at higher power view, 40×; the atypical cells are large with irregular nuclear contours, vesicular chromatin & prominent nucleoli; apoptotic bodies are also present

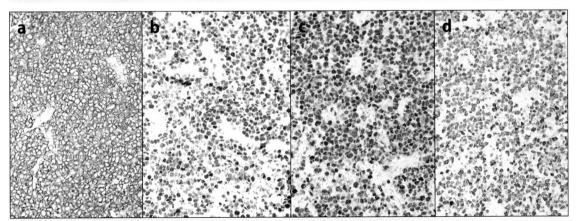

f40.3 The lymphoma cells are positive for **a** CD20, **b** BCL6, & **c** MUM1; **d** Ki67 shows a high proliferation index (>90%)

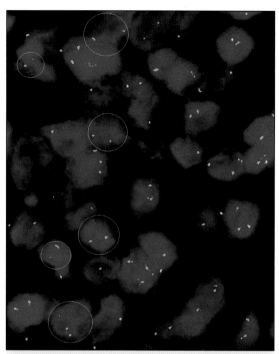

f40.4 FISH analysis for rearrangement at the *DUSP22/IRF4* locus on chromosome 6 using a break-apart probe set; presence of separate red & green signals (circled examples) indicates rearrangement of *DUSP22/IRF4*, which are adjacent genes located at 6p25.3

of abdominal lymph nodes and bowel has been rarely reported. *IRF4/MUM1*, a 19.7 kb gene located at the 6p25.3 locus, encodes the IRF4/MUM1 protein, which is a transcription factor that plays an important role in the proliferation and differentiation of B cells. Among B-lineage cells, IRF4/MUM1 is strongly expressed in post-germinal center B cells and plasma cells.

Histologically, most cases of LBCL-*IRF4* appear as diffuse large B-cell lymphoma (DLBCL), although some may resemble grade 3B follicular lymphoma or a combination of both. In addition to strong positivity for IRF4/MUM1, cases typically express pan B-cell antigens (CD20, CD79a, and PAX-5) as well as BCL6. The Ki-67 proliferation index is often high. CD10 and BCL2 are also positive in ~2/3 of cases, which may suggest a germinal center phenotype for these lymphomas, despite the strong expression of IRF4/MUM1. For this reason, it is useful to evaluate large B-cell lymphomas or grade 3B follicular lymphomas which co-express CD10, BCL6, and IRF4/MUM1 for *IRF4* rearrangements. Although many cases demonstrate germinal center B-cell origin by gene expression profiling (or by immunohistochemical algorithms; see also **Case 38**), the gene expression signature of these cases is somewhat unique and distinct

from both germinal center B cells (GCB) and activated B cells (ABC).

The *IRF4* rearrangement is usually cryptic by karyotype analysis but can be detected with FISH studies using a break-apart probe for *DUSP22/IRF4*. In the majority of cases, the fusion partner is the immunoglobulin (Ig) heavy chain gene, *IGH* (85% of cases), although rare cases of translocations with the Ig light chain genes (*IGK* and *IGL*) have been reported. In addition to an *IRF4* rearrangement, some cases have additional rearrangements of *BCL6* but not *BCL2* or *MYC* (although extremely rare cases with concurrent *MYC* rearrangement have been identified and are being investigated). Very rare cases have also been noted, that have features otherwise consistent with LBCL-*IRF4* but do not have a detectable *IRF4* translocation. Molecular analysis of LBCL-*IRF4* cases has shown frequent mutations in *IRF4* as well as genes that are typically mutated in ABC-type DLBCL and involving the NF-κB pathway (*CARD11*, *CD79B*, and *MYD88*).

When encountering an abnormal follicular lymphoid proliferation in a pediatric patient, pediatric-type follicular lymphoma (PTFL; see **Case 34**) should be considered in the differential diagnosis along with LBCL-*IRF4*, as they have overlapping clinical features. Both lymphomas tend to occur in younger patients and are usually localized, most often occurring in the head and neck region or tonsils. PTFL has an entirely follicular pattern with large, expansile or serpiginous follicles containing sheets of centroblasts (histology similar to grade 3B adult follicular lymphoma), often with many tingible-body macrophages. In contrast, although LBCL-*IRF4* can also be entirely follicular in appearance, the follicles tend not to be serpiginous and lack tingible-body macrophages. Areas of DLBCL preclude a diagnosis of PTFL but not LBCL-*IRF4*. Distinction between the 2 entities is important as patients with localized PTFL tend to do well with excision alone without the need for additional therapy while LBCL-*IRF4* is typically treated with chemotherapy, with or without radiation.

In practice, the combination of rapidly enlarging tonsils in children/young adults, along with histology demonstrating a follicular or diffuse growth pattern of large atypical B cells, should prompt evaluation with MUM1 immunostain, and if positive, further testing using FISH for the detection of an *IRF4* rearrangement should be performed. Accurate diagnosis is essential, as LBCL-*IRF4* cases tend to have more indolent behavior,

ISBN 978-089189-6814

t40.1 Comparison of morphologic, IHC & genetic features of follicular & diffuse large lymphoid infiltrates in children/young adults

	Reactive follicular hyperplasia	Pediatric-type follicular lymphoma	Large B-cell lymphoma with *IRF4* rearrangement	DLBCL, NOS
Histology	follicles predominantly distributed in the nodal cortex with polarization & distinct mantle zones	expansile or serpiginous follicles with intermediate-sized blastoid cells; grade 3B morphology, with tingible body macrophages imparting a starry sky appearance	follicular or diffuse growth pattern composed of medium to large neoplastic cells with centroblast-like morphology; generally devoid of tingible body macrophages	diffuse growth pattern composed of medium to large pleomorphic cells
IHC	absence of BCL2 & MUM1 in follicles	absence of BCL2 & MUM1 in follicles	strong diffuse MUM1; may be positive for BCL6, CD5 (~30%), BCL2 (~60%) & CD10 (~60%)	pan B-cell markers with variable CD10, BCL6, MUM1, MYC, and BCL2 expression; do not typically see co-expression of CD10, BCL6 & MUM1
Genetic studies	none	negative for *BCL2*, *BCL6* & *IRF4* rearrangements, may have deletion of 1p36 and/or mutations in *MAP2K1*, *TNFRS14*, or *IRF8*	*IRF4* rearrangement with or without *BCL6* rearrangements. Frequent mutations in *IRF4* & NF-κB pathway genes (*CARD11*, *CD79B*, *MYD88*)	often rearrangements in *BCL2* or *BCL6* genes; negative for *IRF4* rearrangements

with increased response to therapy and better prognosis, as compared to DLBCL, not otherwise specified (DLBCL, NOS). Younger age and tonsillar location in particular are associated with a more favorable outcome.

The patient in this case decided not to receive chemotherapy and is currently under close clinical follow-up.

Diagnostic pearls/pitfalls

- Cases of LBCL-*IRF4* may demonstrate an entirely follicular growth pattern (which resembles grade 3B follicular lymphoma), an entirely diffuse growth pattern, or have both follicular and diffuse components.
- FISH to detect an *IRF4* rearrangement should be considered in large B-cell lymphomas with co-expression of CD10, BCL6, and IRF4/MUM1, particularly when occurring in younger patients in the head and neck.
- *IRF4* rearrangements are best detected by break-apart FISH probes for *DUSP22/IRF4*, as they are typically cryptic by karyotype and can have different fusion partners, although *IGH* is the most common.
- Distinction of LBCL-*IRF4* from DLBCL, NOS, is critical given the more indolent behavior of LBCL-*IRF4*.
- Cases of pediatric-type follicular lymphoma tend to have serpiginous-appearing follicles and many tingible body macrophages, features that can help distinguish this entity from LBCL-*IRF4* with follicular histology.

Readings

Liu Q, Salaverria I, Pittaluga S, et al. Follicular lymphomas in children and young adults: a comparison of the pediatric variant with usual follicular lymphoma. Am J Surg Pathol 2013 Mar;37(3):333-43. **DOI: 10.1097/PAS.0b013e31826b9b57**

Pittaluga S, Harris NL, Siebert R, et al. Large B-cell lymphoma with *IRF4* rearrangement. In: Swerdlow SH, Campo E, Harris NL, et al. World Health Organization Classification of Tumours of Haematopoietic and Lymphoid Tissues. 4th ed. Lyon, France: IARC Press; 2017. **ISBN: 9789283244943**

Quintanilla-Martinez L, Sander B, Chan JK, et al. Indolent lymphomas in the pediatric population: follicular lymphoma, *IRF4*/MUM1+ lymphoma, nodal marginal zone lymphoma and chronic lymphocytic leukemia. Virchows Arch 2016;468(2):141-57. **DOI: 10.1007/s00428-015-1855-z**

Ramis-Zaldivar JE, Gonzalez-Farré B, Balagué O, et al. Distinct molecular profile of *IRF4*-rearranged large B-cell lymphoma. Blood. 2020 Jan 23;135(4):274-286. **DOI: 10.1182/blood.2019002699**

Salaverria I, Philipp C, Oschlies I, et al. Translocations activating *IRF4* identify a subtype of germinal center-derived B-cell lymphoma affecting predominantly children and young adults. Blood 2011;118(1):139-147. **DOI: 10.1182/blood-2011-01-330795**

Verma A, Epari S, Gujral S, et al. An unusual presentation of large B-cell lymphoma with interferon regulatory factor 4 gene rearrangement. Indian J Pathol Microbiol 2018;61: 271-4. **DOI: 10.4103/IJPM.IJPM_194_17**

Vincent G, Richebourg S, Cloutier S, et al. Large B-cell lymphoma with *IRF4* rearrangement: from theory to practice, Am J Surg Pathol: Reviews & Reports 2019 Oct; 24(5):240-3. **DOI: 10.1097/PCR.0000000000000329**

Wada DA, Law ME, Hsi ED, et al. Specificity of *IRF4* translocations for primary cutaneous anaplastic large cell lymphoma: a multicenter study of 204 skin biopsies. Mod Pathol 2011;24(4):596-605. **DOI: 10.1038/modpathol.2010.225**

Erika M Moore

41

Plasma cell myeloma with rearrangement of *CCND1*

History A 73-year-old male with a past medical history of renal cell carcinoma and colon cancer presented with 2 months of lower sternal chest pain. CT showed a T6 lytic lesion concerning for metastatic disease. He underwent biopsy of the T6 lesion and a subsequent bone marrow biopsy. CBC results are shown at right.

Serum protein electrophoresis identified a 0.1 g/dL monoclonal IgA λ paraprotein and a 0.2 g/dL monoclonal free λ paraprotein. Serum free light chain studies demonstrated 566 mg/dL free λ light chain and 0.71 mg/dL free κ light chain.

Morphology & flow cytometry The T6 biopsy showed sheets of plasma cells with λ light chain restriction by IHC. The bone marrow aspirate smear demonstrated markedly increased plasma cells including occasional binucleate forms **f41.1**. The bone marrow core biopsy was 50% cellular with sheets of λ-restricted plasma cells which comprised 80% of the total marrow cellularity **f41.2**. The plasma cells expressed cyclin D1 by IHC **f41.3**.

Flow cytometry showed 0.7% abnormal plasma cells which were CD38 bright, CD138 positive, CD19 negative, CD56 subset positive, partial dim CD20, and cytoplasmic λ light chain restricted **f41.4**.

Based on the overall findings, a diagnosis of **plasma cell myeloma** was rendered.

WBC	4.5×10^9/L
RBC	3.65×10^{12}/L
HGB	12.8 g/dL
HCT	38.1%
MCV	104 fL
RDW	13.4%
Platelets	235×10^9/L

Genetics/molecular results Cytogenetics showed a normal male karyotype but FISH studies were positive for *IGH-CCND1* translocation in 17% of nuclei **f41.5**. FISH studies were negative for numerical abnormalities of 1p/1q, 3, 7 and 11, as well as negative for del(17p).

Discussion In the 2017 World Health Organization classification of hematologic neoplasms, plasma cell myeloma is defined by either ≥60% clonal plasma cells in the bone marrow, or ≥10% clonal plasma cells in the bone marrow or plasmacytoma with >1 of the following myeloma-defining events: hypercalcemia, renal insufficiency, anemia, bone lesion on imaging, or serum free light chain ratio ≥100. This definition is based on the 2014 International Myeloma Working Group diagnostic criteria. So-called "smoldering" (or asymptomatic) myeloma is defined by a serum monoclonal protein ≥30 g/L or a urinary monoclonal protein ≥500 mg/24 hours or clonal bone marrow plasma cells of 10%-59% and the absence of myeloma-defining events. Patients with smoldering myeloma

ISBN 978-089189-6814   ©2021 ASCP

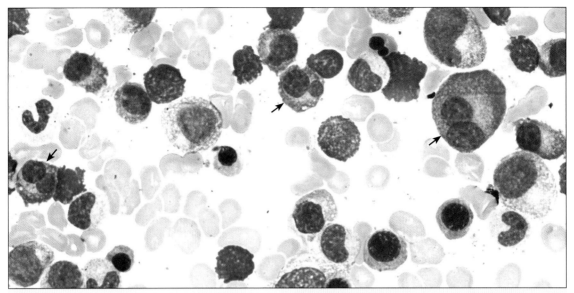

f41.1 Bone marrow aspirate showing increased, atypical plasma cells, including binucleate forms (arrows)

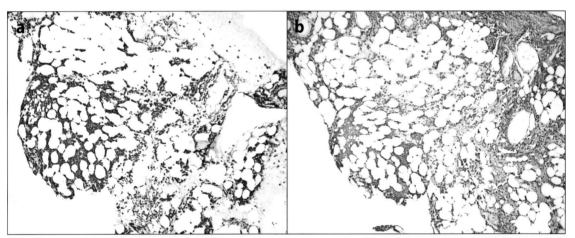

f41.2 Bone marrow core biopsy: **a** CD138 immunostain demonstrating sheets of plasma cells comprising ~80% of the total marrow cellularity; **b** λ light chain stain showing λ restriction in the plasma cells

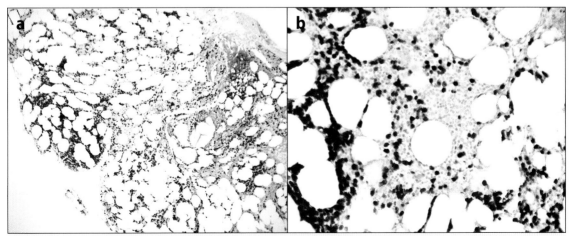

f41.3 Bone marrow core biopsy cyclin D1 stain demonstrating positivity in the plasma cells, **a** 100× & **b** 400×

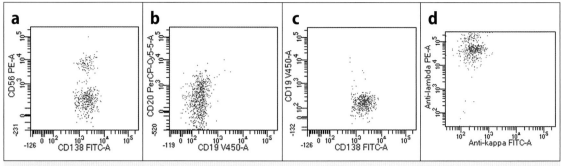

f41.4 Flow cytometry (gated on 0.7% CD38 bright, CD138+ plasma cells) demonstrates that the plasma cells have **a** partial CD56 expression, **b** partial CD20 expression, **c** lack of CD19 & **d** cytoplasmic λ restriction

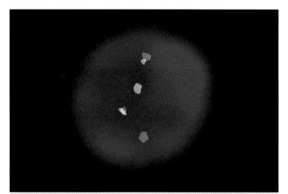

f41.5 Non-selected FISH studies demonstrate an *IGH-CCND1* translocation in 32/250 cells (17%); dual-color, dual-fusion probes with *IGH* (14q32) in green & *CCND1* (11q13) in orange show 2 dual-fusion (yellow) signals consistent with *IGH-CCND1*

usually do not need treatment until the criteria for plasma cell myeloma are met. Finally, monoclonal gammopathy of undetermined significance (MGUS) is a pre-myeloma condition defined by serum or urinary monoclonal proteins at levels below those seen in smoldering myeloma, or clonal bone marrow plasma cells <10% and absence of end-organ damage. Because these diagnostic criteria rely heavily on clinical and radiologic features, it can be difficult to definitively categorize cases having clonal bone marrow plasma cells between 10% and 60% if other information is not readily available. In these situations, a pathologist diagnosis of "plasma cell neoplasm" may be sufficient, with a suggestion to correlate with the clinical and radiologic features for further classification.

In addition to light chain restriction, abnormal surface antigen expression is found in >95% of plasma cell neoplasms and can be readily assessed using flow cytometry. Malignant plasma cells often lack or only dimly express CD45, CD19, CD27, and CD81, and/or have aberrant expression of CD56, CD200, CD117, or CD20, among other antigens. CD20

expression, in particular, is associated with myeloma cases having t(11;14) *CCND1-IGH*, as seen in this case. Although flow cytometry is a useful tool for qualitative characterization of malignant plasma cells, this technique does not accurately quantify plasma cells in liquid specimens due to loss of these cells during standard staining and analysis procedures. While usually not necessary to assess for a malignant plasma cell population, IHC for CD56 or CD117 may help identify myeloma cells in tissue sections. Normally absent in benign plasma cells, cyclin D1 expression can also be detected by IHC in some myeloma cases, especially those which harbor a t(11;14) *CCND1-IGH* translocation or multiple copies of *CCND1*, and cyclin D1 may serve as a useful marker for malignant plasma cells, especially in follow-up biopsies.

Cytogenetic abnormalities are detected in >90% of myeloma cases when evaluated by FISH and are important for risk stratification. It is important to note that cytogenetic abnormalities in myeloma cells are often not detected by standard karyotype analysis, given the low proliferative rate of these cells. In addition, unless a large number of plasma cells is present in the aspirate, FISH studies may also be falsely negative; therefore, plasma cell enrichment is recommended before performing FISH on bone marrow aspirates. Hyperdiploidy is the most frequent genetic aberration in myeloma, occurring in ~45% of cases, and most commonly manifests as trisomies of the odd numbered chromosomes 3, 5, 7, 9, 11, 15, 19, and 21. Translocations involving *IGH* are the second most common abnormality, usually with one of seven gene partners: *CCND1* (16%), *CCND2*, *CCND3*, *MAF*, *MAFA*, *MAFB*, and *FGFR3/NSD2* (15%). Hyperdiploidy and *IGH* translocations are considered primary cytogenetic abnormalities, occurring earlier in the disease, while additional secondary genetic/molecular aberrations

t41.1 Mayo stratification of myeloma & risk-adapted therapy (mSMART) genetic risk stratification of plasma cell myeloma (2013)

Standard risk (60%)	Intermediate risk (20%)	High risk (20%)
hyperdiploidy t(11;14) *CCND1-IGH* t(6;14) *CCND3-IGH* all others	t(4;14) *FGFR3-IGH* del(13) (by karyotype) hypodiploidy	t(14;16) *IGH-MAF* t(14;20) *IGH-MAFB* del(17p) high risk GEP signature

*A subsequent study from the Mayo Clinic demonstrated that gain of 1q is also independently associated with advanced disease stage, a high tumor burden, and decreased overall survival

include del(17p), del(13), gain(1q), del(1p), *MYC* rearrangements, and mutations in *KRAS, NRAS,* and *BRAF*. Genetic characterization by FISH at diagnosis is especially important for risk stratification and therapy. Hyperdiploidy, *IGH-CCND1*, and *IGH-CCND3* all confer a standard risk prognosis, while hypodiploidy and *FGFR3* translocation are intermediate risk, and del(17p) and rearrangements including *MAF* and *MAFB* are high risk **t41.1**. Gene expression profiles (GEP) have also been used to stratify patients into a high-risk group; however, to date, these are not routinely used outside clinical trial settings.

Although myeloma is generally considered to be incurable, newer therapy options continue to improve overall survival. More recent developments include use of immune-modulating agents and monoclonal antibody-targeted therapy to plasma cell antigens such as CD38 (eg, daratumumab). Awareness of these treatment modalities is especially important when evaluating follow-up bone marrow specimens for minimal residual disease. Plasma cells in patients who have received these monoclonal antibody therapies may have these antigens masked, resulting in difficulty identifying plasma cells through immunophenotyping.

Diagnostic pearls/pitfalls
– Myeloma cells are often characterized by aberrant antigen expression that may be detected with flow cytometry.
– FISH analysis of myeloma cells is important for prognostication purposes. A typical myeloma FISH panel includes probes to evaluate for hyperdiploidy (usually probes for chromosomes 3, 7, and 11), *IGH* translocation(s), 1p/1q abnormalities, and 17p deletion. Using a single *IGH* break-apart FISH probe initially is an economical and efficient way to screen cases for *IGH* fusion. Positive cases can then be reflexed to assays using partner-specific dual-color/dual-fusion probes.
– Karyotype analysis is often not sensitive in detecting chromosomal abnormalities of myeloma cells, because of their low proliferation rate in culture.

– CD20-positive, small (lymphoid-like) plasma cells are often seen in myeloma cases with t(11;14) *IGH-CCND1*, and these plasma cells will express cyclin D1 on IHC.
– Cyclin D1 positivity is not unique to plasma cell myeloma and is also present in most cases of mantle cell lymphoma and some cases of hairy cell leukemia. Normal endothelial cells and histiocytes also express cyclin D1 so when evaluating the immunostain in the bone marrow, it is important to make sure the positive cells identified have plasma cell morphology.

Readings
Chesi M, Bergsagel PL. Molecular pathogenesis of multiple myeloma: basic and clinical updates. Int J Hematol. 2013;97(3):313-23. **DOI: 10.1007/s12185-013-1291-2**

Hoyer JD, Hanson CA, Fonseca R, et al. The (11;14)(q13;q32) translocation in multiple myeloma. A morphologic and immunohistochemical study. Am J Clin Pathol. 2000;113(6):831-7. **DOI: 10.1309/4W8E-8F4K-BHUP-UBE7**

Mikhael JR, Dingli D, Roy V, et al. Management of newly diagnosed symptomatic multiple myeloma: updated Mayo Stratification of Myeloma and Risk-Adapted Therapy (mSMART) consensus guidelines 2013. Mayo Clin Proc. 2013;88(4):360-76. **DOI:10.1016/j.mayocp.2013.01.019**

Rajkumar SV. Multiple myeloma: 2016 update on diagnosis, risk-stratification, and management. Am J Hematol. 2016;91(7):719-34. **DOI: 10.1002/ajh.24402**

Rajkumar SV, Dimopoulos MA, Palumbo A, et al. International Myeloma Working Group updated criteria for the diagnosis of multiple myeloma. Lancet Oncol. 2014;15(12):e538-48. **DOI: 10.1016/S1470-2045(14)70442-5**

Robillard N, Avet-Loiseau H, Garand R, et al. CD20 is associated with a small mature plasma cell morphology and t(11;14) in multiple myeloma. Blood. 2003;102(3):1070-1. **DOI: 10.1182/blood-2002-11-3333**

Swerdlow SH, Campo E, Harris NL, et al. World Health Organization Classification of Tumours of Haematopoietic and Lymphoid Tissues. 4th ed. Lyon, France: IARC Press; 2017. **ISBN: 9789283244943**

Erika M Moore

42

T-cell large granular lymphocytic leukemia with *STAT3* mutation

History A 73-year-old male with a past medical history of rheumatoid arthritis and splenomegaly presented for evaluation of pancytopenia. CBC results are shown at right.

A bone marrow biopsy with peripheral smear review was performed.

Morphology & flow cytometry Review of the peripheral blood smear demonstrated leukopenia with a predominance of large granular lymphocytes **f42.1**. The bone marrow was normocellular for age with trilineage hematopoiesis but increased lymphocytes were noted by manual differential count of the aspirate smears. IHC stains showed increased interstitial CD3-positive T cells, sometimes forming linear arrays indicative of intrasinusoidal infiltration. Additional stains showed that the T cells expressed TIA1 and granzyme B **f42.2**.

Flow cytometry was significant for an abnormal CD4-negative, CD8-negative T-cell population that was positive for surface CD3, CD2, CD7, and T-cell receptor (TCR) γ/δ, negative for CD16 and CD56, and dim to negative for CD5. Additional analysis for natural killer (NK) cell antigens, including killer immunoglobulin-like receptors (KIRs), demonstrated that the T-cell population expressed moderate CD94 and CD158a/h (KIR2DL1/DS1) restriction **f42.3**.

Based on the morphologic and flow cytometric findings, a diagnosis of **γ/δ T-cell large granular lymphocytic leukemia** was rendered.

WBC	2.4×10^9/L
Differential	
Neutrophils	4%
Bands	2%
Lymphocytes	72%
Monocytes	21%
RBC	2.37×10^{12}/L
HGB	8.3 g/dL
HCT	24.6%
MCV	104 fL
RDW	16.2%
Platelets	132×10^9/L

ISBN 978-089189-6814

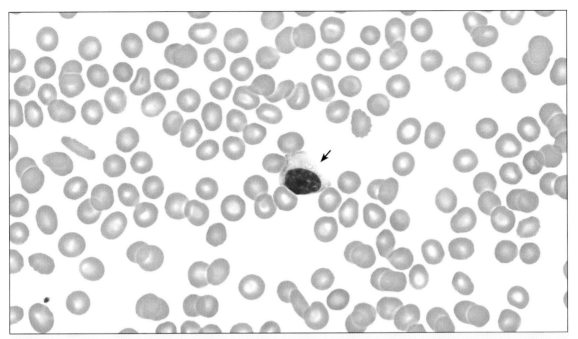

f42.1 Peripheral blood smear demonstrating a large granular lymphocyte (arrow)

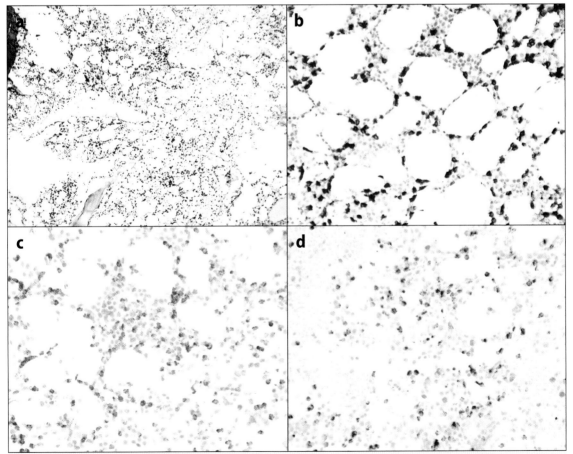

f42.2 IHC on the core biopsy; **a** at low magnification, CD3 demonstrates a T-cell infiltrate, which at higher magnification **b** can be seen forming linear arrays indicative of intrasinusoidal involvement; the infiltrate is also positive for **c** TIA1 & **d** granzyme B

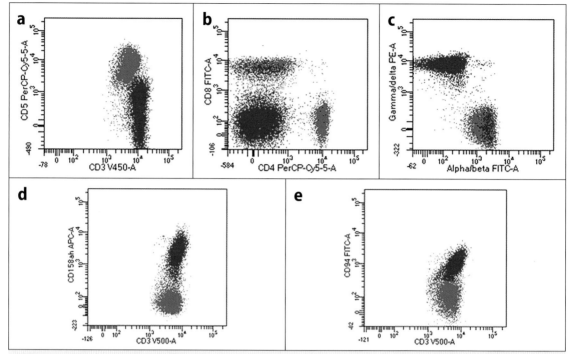

f42.3 Flow cytometry (gated on CD3+ T cells) demonstrating an abnormal T-cell population (highlighted in red) that is **a** CD5 dim to negative, **b** CD4−, CD8−, **c** TCR γ/δ+, with **d** KIR restriction for CD158a/h as well as **e** abnormal expression of CD94

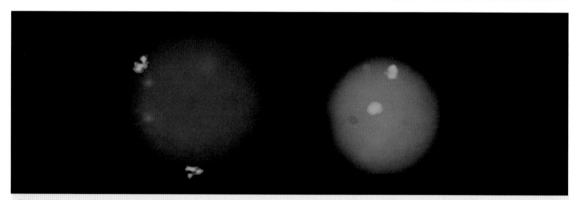

f42.4 FISH studies for chromosome 7 abnormalities using probes *D7S522* (7q31, orange) & *CEP7* (7 centromere, green) are normal & do not demonstrate isochromosome 7q

Genetics/molecular results Karyotype analysis was normal and FISH studies for chromosome 7 abnormalities were negative **f42.4**. Molecular studies demonstrated a clonal TCR gene rearrangement **f42.5** and the presence of a *STAT3* p.D661Y (c.1981G>T) mutation with a variant allele frequency of 4% **f42.6**.

Discussion T-cell large granular lymphocytic (T-LGL) leukemia is a lymphoproliferative disorder of mature T cells, defined by a clonal increase in peripheral blood cytotoxic T cells (large granular lymphocytes) which persists for at least 6 months. Although no minimum absolute cell count is required for diagnosis,

ISBN 978-089189-6814   ©2021 ASCP

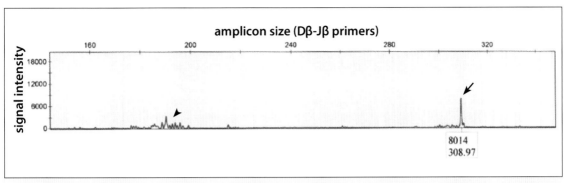

f42.5 T-cell receptor (TCR) clonality analysis with multiplex PCR showing clonal *TCRβ* rearrangement with a 309 bp product (arrow); amplified products from background polyclonal T cells are indicated by the arrowhead; note that *TCRβ* gene rearrangement occurs early in T-cell ontogeny & therefore can be detected in γ/δ T cells

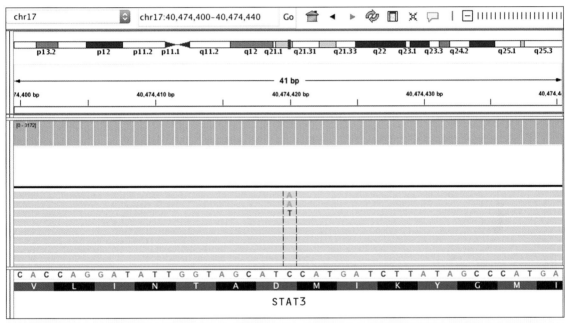

f42.6 Somatic variant analysis using a targeted lymphoid NGS panel; annotated reads mapped to the *STAT3* locus demonstrate low-level p.D661Y (c.1981G>T), highlighted in green (hg19, Integrative Genomics Viewer browser, showing the reverse strand) [see **fA.8**, p312]

the large granular lymphocytes usually constitute at least 2×10^9/L or >50% of circulating lymphocytes. T-LGL leukemia is rare (comprising <5% of mature lymphocytic leukemias) and generally occurs in older patients. The majority of cases are indolent, with most morbidity arising from associated severe neutropenia and/or anemia. Splenomegaly is common because of T-cell infiltration of the spleen. T-LGL is strongly associated with autoimmune disorders, particularly rheumatoid arthritis, as well as polyclonal hypergammaglobulinemia and autoimmune cytopenias, including pure red cell aplasia. Approximately 5%-10% of patients have a concurrent B-cell lymphoproliferative disorder or myelodysplastic syndrome. Although there are no well-defined diagnostic criteria in the 2017 World Health Organization classification, suggested criteria

t42.1 Major & minor diagnostic criteria for T-cell large granular lymphocytic leukemia

Major criteria	Flow studies reveal >50% of the total peripheral blood or bone marrow surface CD3-positive T cells have ≥2 of the following:
	   CD8+ (may be dim)
	   uniform expression of CD16 or CD57 (>75% of cells positive)
	   loss of CD5 expression (partial or complete)
	   uniform expression of ≥1 of the KIRs CD158a, CD158b, and CD158e

	intrasinusoidal bone marrow or splenic infiltration by cytotoxic lymphocytes positive for CD8 and ≥1 of the cytotoxic markers TIA-1, granzyme B, granzyme M, or perforin
	T-cell clonality by flow analysis of TCR Vβ expression or molecular genetic analysis of T-cell receptor gene rearrangements
	STAT3 gene mutation in exons 20 or 21
Minor criteria	peripheral blood granular lymphocytes (morphology) or CD8-positive T cells (flow cytometry) either >2 × 10⁹/L or >80% of total lymphocytes
	unexplained persistence of cell population for >6 months
	positive rheumatoid factor, antinuclear antibodies, or polyclonal hypergammaglobulinemia
	unexplained neutropenia (<1.8 × 10⁹/L) and/or anemia (<10 g/dL)
	peripheral blood absolute NK-cell count <0.1 × 10⁹/L or <5% of total lymphocytes
	STAT5b gene mutation in exons encoding the SH2 domain

Adapted from Morice WG [2017] T-cell and NK-cell large granular lymphocyte proliferations. In: Jaffe ES, Arber DA, Campo E, Harris NL, Quintanilla-Martinez L. Hematopathology, 2nd ed, 599-607. ISBN: 9780323296137

are listed in **t42.1**. Per these guidelines, a diagnosis of T-LGL leukemia requires at least 3 major criteria or 2 major plus 2 minor criteria.

Morphologic review of the peripheral blood typically demonstrates increased large granular lymphocytes that contain mature nuclei and abundant pale cytoplasm with small, fine to coarse azurophilic granules that are variably conspicuous. These are generally easier to identify on the peripheral smear than on the bone marrow aspirate smears. In the bone marrow core biopsy, the clonal lymphocytes typically form a subtle, interstitial and/or single file intrasinusoidal infiltrate that is best identified by IHC.

Essentially all T-LGL leukemias express surface CD3 and the NK cell-associated antigens CD16 and/or CD57, and although most are positive for CD8 and TCR α/β, rare cases of CD4-positive T-LGL leukemia or TCR γ/δ-positive T-LGL leukemia have been described, as in this example case. Most T-LGL leukemias demonstrate T-cell phenotypic abnormalities, such as decreased or absent CD5 and/or CD7 expression, and less commonly, decreased CD2 expression. CD56 expression is seen in a small subset of cases and may be associated with more aggressive disease. As seen in this example case, evaluation of NK-cell receptor expression can be helpful in assessing clonality, because ~1/3 of T-LGL leukemias will have homogeneous expression of members of the KIR family, including CD158a, b,

or e, with CD158b expression seen most commonly. Uniform expression of the NK-cell receptor CD94, sometimes in combination with NKG2A, may also be seen. It should be noted that most T cells do not normally express the aforementioned NK-cell receptor antigens, so lack of expression of these antigens is not evidence for atypia. Immunostains performed on the bone marrow for CD8 and the cytotoxic markers, TIA-1 and granzyme B, characteristically highlight linear arrays of cells due to the frequent intrasinusoidal distribution of the T cells in T-LGL leukemia.

Clonality can be detected either by analyzing for restricted expression TCR Vβ or TCRβ constant chain 1 (TRBC1) by flow cytometry or molecular evaluation of TCR gene rearrangements. Both flow cytometric and molecular findings must be interpreted in context, as clonal T-cell populations can be seen in non-neoplastic settings such as viral infection, bone marrow reconstitution, or aging, and the presence of a clonal T-cell population should not be used in isolation as evidence of a T-cell lymphoproliferative disorder. Furthermore, small cytotoxic T-cell populations with phenotypic atypia can be seen by flow cytometry in normal patients and do not necessarily signify a diagnosis of T-LGL leukemia.

There are no recurrent cytogenetic abnormalities present in T-LGL leukemia but molecular testing has demonstrated that up to half of all cases harbor an activating *STAT3* mutation, usually present in exon 20 or 21. These mutations result in constitutive activation of the JAK/STAT signaling pathway, which is necessary for TCR signaling, leading to increased cytokine production, cytotoxic activity, and resistance to apoptosis. A small number of *STAT3* mutation–negative cases have a *STAT5b* mutation. In some studies, *STAT3* mutation-positive T-LGL leukemias are more likely to need treatment and have a higher association with pure red cell aplasia. *STAT5b* mutations are reportedly associated with CD4-positive cases and more aggressive disease.

In the rarer TCR γ/δ T-LGL leukemia cases, such as this case, a diagnosis of hepatosplenic T-cell lymphoma (HSTCL; see **Case 44**) must be excluded. HSTCL is typically of TCR γ/δ origin and is also associated with splenomegaly and an intrasinusoidal infiltration pattern in the bone marrow; however, unlike the more subtle linear formation of T cells in T-LGL leukemia, T cells in HSTCL often cause distention of the sinusoids. In contrast to the indolent nature of T-LGL leukemia, HSTCL is a much more aggressive disease, with a median survival of less than 2 years. Cases of HSTCL do not typically express CD57 and granzyme B and may simultaneously express multiple KIR isoforms. *STAT3* and *STAT5b* mutations have also been described in a significant number of HSTCL cases, but unlike T-LGL leukemias which lack a characteristic cytogenetic abnormality, isochromosome 7q is present in most cases of HSTCL and can be excluded by FISH, as seen in this case.

Diagnostic pearls/pitfalls
- Most cases of T-LGL leukemia are CD8-positive and TCR α/β-positive but rarely, they may be CD4-positive or TCR γ/δ-positive.
- T-LGL leukemias typically form a very subtle intrasinusoidal infiltrate in the bone marrow that may not be recognizable on hematoxylin-eosin stain. IHC on the core biopsy specimen is recommended in any case being evaluated for T-LGL leukemia.
- Evaluation of natural killer cell receptor expression by flow cytometry can be helpful in identifying abnormal T-cell large granular lymphocyte populations.
- Older individuals may have persistent, reactive or clonally expanded, small atypical CD8-positive T-cell populations in blood. These populations often have decreased CD5 or CD7 expression by flow cytometry but usually comprise <5% of cells and should not be confused with the presence of T-LGL leukemia.

– TCR γ/δ-positive T-LGL leukemia, which is typically indolent, must be differentiated from aggressive hepatosplenic T-cell lymphoma. Both can have similar immunophenotypes, an intrasinusoidal pattern in the marrow, and *STAT3* or *STAT5b* mutations, but the detection of isochromosome 7q suggests a diagnosis of HSTCL.

Readings

Andersson EI, Tanahashi T, Sekiguchi N, et al. High incidence of activating *STAT5B* mutations in CD4-positive T-cell large granular lymphocyte leukemia. Blood. 2016;128(20):2465-8. **DOI: 10.1182/blood-2016-06-724856**

Belhadj K, Reyes F, Farcet JP, et al. Hepatosplenic gamma delta T-cell lymphoma is a rare clinicopathologic entity with poor outcome: report on a series of 21 patients. Blood. 2003;102:4261-9. **DOI: 10.1182/blood-2003-05-1675**

Ishida F, Matsuda K, Sekiguchi N, et al. STAT3 gene mutations and their association with pure red cell aplasia in large granular lymphocyte leukemia. Cancer Sci. 2014;105(3):342-6. **DOI: 10.1111/cas.12341**

Jaffe ES, Arber DA, Campo E, Harris NL, Quintanilla-Martinez L. Hematopathology. 2nd ed. Philadelphia, PA: Elsevier Inc; 2017. **ISBN: 9780323296137**

Koskela HL, Eldfors S, Ellonen P, et al. Somatic *STAT3* mutations in large granular lymphocytic leukemia. N Engl J Med. 2012;366:1905-13. **DOI: 10.1056/NEJMoa1114885**

Lamy T, Moignet A, Loughran TP. LGL leukemia: from pathogenesis to treatment. Blood. 2017;129(9):1082-94. **DOI: 10.1182/blood-2016-08-692590**

Morice WG. The immunophenotypic attributes of NK cells and NK-cell lineage lymphoproliferative disorders. Am J Clin Pathol. 2007;127:881-6. **DOI: 10.1309/Q49CRJ030L22MHLF**

Morice WG, Kurtin PJ, Leibson PJ, et al. Demonstration of aberrant T-cell and natural killer–cell antigen expression in all cases of granular lymphocytic leukaemia. Br J Haematol. 2003;120:1026-36. **DOI: 10.1046/j.1365-2141.2003.04201.x**

Morice WG, Kurtin PJ, Tefferi A, et al. Distinct bone marrow findings in T-cell granular lymphocytic leukemia revealed by paraffin section immunoperoxidase stains for CD8, TIA-1, and granzyme B. Blood. 2002;99:268-27. **DOI: 10.1182/blood.v99.1.268**

Rajala HL, Eldfors S, Kuusanmaki H, et al. Discovery of somatic *STAT5b* mutations in large granular lymphocytic leukemia. Blood. 2013;121:4541-50. **DOI: 10.1182/blood-2012-12-474577**

Rajala HL, Olson T, Clemente MJ, et al. The analysis of clonal diversity and therapy responses using *STAT3* mutations as a molecular marker in large granular lymphocytic leukemia. Haematologica. 2015;100(1):91-9. **DOI: 10.3324/haematol.2014.113142**

Swerdlow SH, Campo E, Harris NL, et al. World Health Organization Classification of Tumours of Haematopoietic and Lymphoid Tissues. 4th ed. Lyon, France: IARC Press; 2017. **ISBN: 9789283244943**

43

Erika M Moore & Rose C Beck

T-cell prolymphocytic leukemia with inv(14)

History An 88-year-old male was referred to an oncologist for leukocytosis detected during an evaluation for constipation and diarrhea. CBC results are shown at right.

A peripheral blood smear review with flow cytometry was performed.

Morphology & flow cytometry The blood smear showed lymphocytosis composed of mature lymphocytes with distinct nucleoli and occasional irregular nuclear contours **f43.1**. By flow cytometry, the atypical lymphocytes were T cells that had normal levels of CD2, CD3, CD4, CD5, and CD7, dim expression of CD25, and were negative for CD8 and CD56 **f43.2**. Flow cytometry also revealed that the atypical T cells expressed T-cell receptor (TCR) α/β, with uniform absence of TCR β constant 1 (TRBC1) and restricted use of TCR Vβ12 by Vβ chain analysis, consistent with a clonal T-cell population. The morphologic and flow cytometric findings indicated a diagnosis of T-cell lymphoproliferative disorder.

Serologies for antibodies against human T-cell lymphotropic virus (HTLV) types 1/2 were performed and were negative. A bone marrow biopsy with genetic studies was then performed for further characterization. The bone marrow aspirate demonstrated normal trilineage hematopoiesis with 59% small lymphocytes similar to those seen in blood; the lymphocytes were visible in the core section as loose aggregates, highlighted by immunostains for CD3, TCL-1, and S100 **f43.3**. Based on the overall morphologic, immunophenotypic, and clinical findings, a diagnosis of **T-cell prolymphocytic leukemia** (T-PLL) was rendered.

WBC	23.3×10^9/L
Differential	
Neutrophils	24%
Lymphocytes	70%
Monocytes	3%
Eosinophils	3%
HGB	13.8 g/dL
MCV	96 fL
Platelets	239×10^9/L

Because of his age, the patient refused treatment with cytotoxic agents and was given supportive and palliative care as needed. The WBC rose to 88.9×10^9/L within 4 months of diagnosis, with the development of a skin rash; a biopsy was consistent with cutaneous involvement by T-PLL. The patient died shortly thereafter.

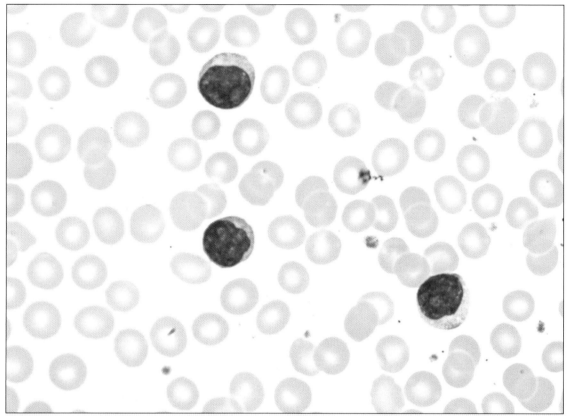

f43.1 Atypical mature lymphocytes in peripheral blood with nucleoli & occasional irregular nuclei

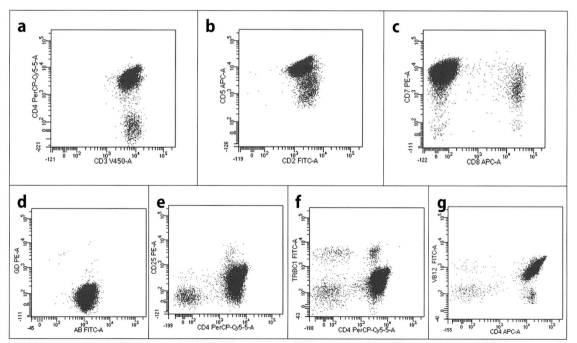

f43.2 a-e Flow cytometry performed on blood & gated on CD3+ cells, demonstrating a predominant CD4+ T-cell population that expresses normal levels of CD2, CD5, CD7, and T-cell receptor (TCR) α/β & dim expression of CD25; clonality is demonstrated by **f** uniform lack of TRBC1 expression & **g** restricted use of TCR Vβ12

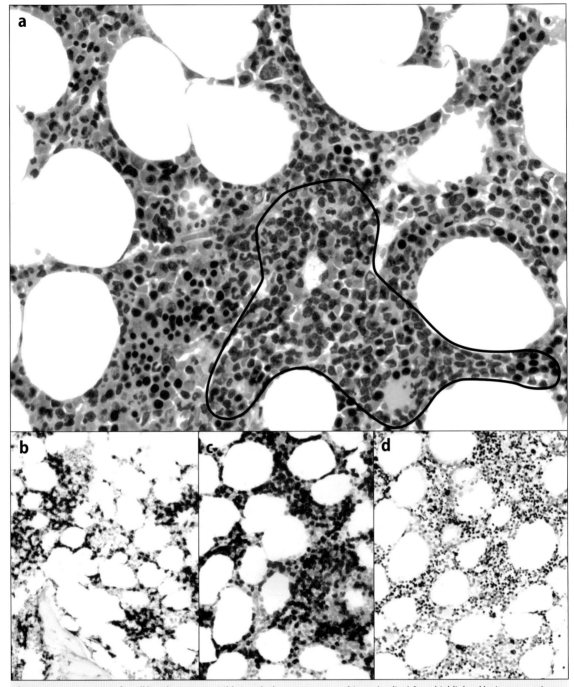

f43.3 Loose aggregates of small lymphocytes are visible in **a** the bone marrow core biopsy (outline) & are highlighted by immunostains for **b** CD3, **c** TCL1 & **d** S100

Genetics/molecular results The karyotype of the bone marrow was complex, with multiple subclones including abnormal metaphases having 43-45 chromosomes. FISH for inv(14) was positive **f43.4**.

ISBN 978-089189-6814   ©2021 ASCP

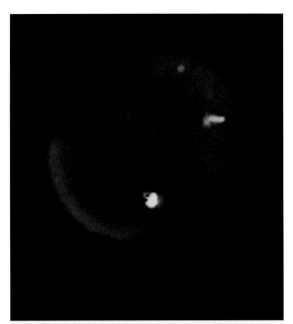

f43.4 FISH using break apart probes for 14q11.2 (*TRA/D*) demonstrating 1 normal yellow fusion signal & 1 set of separate orange & green signals, indicative of a rearrangement at 14q11.2 & consistent with inversion 14

Discussion T-cell prolymphocytic leukemia (T-PLL) is a rare, mature T-cell leukemia involving the peripheral blood, bone marrow, lymph nodes, liver, spleen, and sometimes skin (25% of patients). T-PLL is characterized by a proliferation of small to intermediate sized prolymphocytes and generally occurs in older adults with a median age of 65; most patients present with lymphadenopathy and hepatosplenomegaly. It has an aggressive clinical course with a median survival of 1-2 years. The WBC is typically very high at presentation, with an absolute lymphocyte count usually >100 × 10⁹/L, whereas the red cell and platelet counts are often low due to bone marrow infiltration. The neoplastic cells are small to intermediate in size with a high nuclear to cytoplasmic ratio, condensed chromatin, no granules, occasional cytoplasmic blebbing, and

variable nuclear morphology. The nuclear contours range from round to very irregular or even cerebriform, and although nucleoli are typically prominent, they may be inconspicuous. The bone marrow may have a nodular, interstitial, or diffuse pattern of involvement. Organ and lymph node involvement is typically diffuse, although the infiltrate may spare follicles in the lymph node. Because T-PLL is a mature T-cell neoplasm, it is negative for T-lymphoblast markers such as CD1a, TdT, and CD10, and usually positive for CD2, CD3, CD5, and CD7, although CD3 may be dimly expressed. Most cases are CD4-positive/CD8-negative, and somewhat unique to T-PLL, a subset of cases coexpress CD4 and CD8; few cases are CD8-positive. By immunohistochemistry, TCL1 will highlight the cells, as can S100, as seen in this case. Cytotoxic markers such as granzyme B, TIA1, and perforin are typically negative. CD52 tends to be strongly expressed and if present, is an important target of alemtuzumab, a therapeutic anti-CD52 monoclonal antibody.

The vast majority of T-PLL cases have a rearrangement of chromosome 14, involving the TCR α (*TRA*) gene and *TCL1A* and *TCL1B* genes: inv(14)(q11q32) or t(14;14)(q11;q32). Another, less frequent translocation seen is t(X;14)(q28;q11) involving *TRA* and *MTCP1*, which is homologous to *TCL1A/B*. Chromosome 8 abnormalities are also common. Cases of T-PLL often harbor mutations in the JAK/STAT signaling pathway, including mutations in *JAK1*, *JAK2*, and *STAT5B*, all of which result in constitutive activation of this pathway which is necessary for TCR signaling. JAK/STAT pathway mutations tend to be mutually exclusive. *ATM* mutations are also quite prevalent in T-PLL, in addition to 11q23 deletions (which includes the *ATM* locus) and patients with ataxia-telangiectasia with germline *ATM* mutations are predisposed to develop T-PLL. Although data are limited and the prognosis of T-PLL is poor overall, 1 study found that *JAK3* mutations in particular were associated with inferior survival.

t43.1 Comparison of typical immunophenotypes found in circulating mature T-cell neoplasms

Disorder	CD3	CD4	CD8	CD5	CD7	CD25	TCR α/β	TCR γ/δ
T-prolymphocytic leukemia	+	+*	occasional + (~15%)	+	+ (often strong)	– or dim	+	-
Sézary syndrome	+	+	–	+	– or dim	–/+	+	rare +
adult T-cell leukemia/lymphoma	+	+	rare +	+	– or dim	+ (often strong)	+	–
T-large granular lymphocyte leukemia	+	rare +	+	+ (often dim)	+ (often dim)	–	+	rare +

+, positive; –, negative
*About 25% of T-PLL cases are double positive for CD4 & CD8

Several T-cell lymphoproliferative disorders can be confused with T-PLL **t43.1**. A more commonly encountered T-cell leukemia is T-cell large granular lymphocytic (T-LGL) leukemia; however, T-LGL leukemia typically presents with a much lower WBC count than T-PLL, and the neoplastic cells have abundant cytoplasm and visible cytoplasmic granules, with positivity for CD8 (usually) and expression of cytotoxic markers. T-PLL should also be differentiated from Sézary syndrome, given the possible cerebriform nuclear morphology and propensity to involve the skin. Patients with Sézary syndrome typically have a prior history of mycosis fungoides (cutaneous T-cell lymphoma), and CD7 expression by Sézary cells is usually dim or absent, as opposed to the dim to moderate levels seen in T-PLL **t43.1**. Finally, it is also important to document negative serologic studies for HTLV-1, the causative agent of adult T-cell leukemia/lymphoma, which can have unusual presentations and may mimic other T-cell disorders, including T-PLL.

Historically, molecular studies for TCR gene rearrangement have been the most frequently used method for detection of T-cell clonality; however, several flow cytometric assays can provide similar information much more rapidly, although with some limitations. TCR Vβ analysis by flow cytometry uses antibodies directed against the most common gene families of the TCR Vβ region to identify T-cell clones via restricted Vβ gene usage. Because of lack of coverage by available antibodies, this method will not detect every single clonal population, but does capture ~70% of Vβ gene usage and can be especially useful in cases not having atypical T-cell antigen loss. Another more recently described flow cytometric tool

for identifying T-cell lymphoproliferative disorders is evaluation of TCR β-chain constant region (TRBC) usage. α/β T cells exclusively express either TRBC1 or TRBC2, similar to the way B cells express κ or λ light chain. By evaluating the percentage of T cells expressing TRBC1, a presumptive clonal T-cell population can be identified which restrictively expresses or lacks TRBC1 (a clinical TRBC2 antibody is not presently available, so the 2 cannot be analyzed directly). Although only a few studies have been published thus far, these initial data suggest that a clonal population is likely present if greater than ~90% or less than ~10% of the T cells express TRBC1. Of note, neither TCR Vβ nor TRBC1 analysis can be used for T-cell disorders of γ/δ origin, or those lacking expression of the TCR β chain (as seen in many T-lymphoblastic leukemia/lymphomas). This example case demonstrated both uniform lack of TRBC1 expression and restricted Vβ12 gene usage, consistent with a clonal T-cell population.

Diagnostic pearls/pitfalls

- T-PLL can have variable nuclear morphology and may mimic other T-cell lymphoproliferative disorders, such as Sézary syndrome.
- Among mature T-cell neoplasms, coexpression of CD4 and CD8 is a somewhat unique, albeit infrequent, feature of T-PLL and can be helpful in diagnosis. Most T-PLL cases solely express CD4, while fewer express CD8.
- T-PLL is characterized by chromosomal abnormalities of the *TRA* and *TCL1A/B* loci on chromosome 14 as well as frequent mutations in *ATM* and genes in the JAK/STAT signaling pathway.
- Both TCR Vβ analysis and TRBC1 evaluation by flow cytometry are helpful tools to rapidly identify clonal T-cell populations.

Readings

Beck RC, Stahl S, O'Keefe CL, et al. Detection of mature T-cell leukemias by flow cytometry using anti-T-cell receptor Vβ antibodies. Am J Clin Pathol. 2003;120(5):785-94. **DOI: 10.1309/835B-04QX-GNNF-NRJU**

Kiel M, Velusamy T, Rolland D, et al. Integrated genomic sequencing reveals mutational landscape of T-cell prolymphocytic leukemia. Blood. 2014;124(9):1460-72. **DOI: 10.1182/blood-2014-03-559542**

López C, Bergmann AK, Paul U, et al. Genes encoding members of the *JAK-STAT* pathway or epigenetic regulators are recurrently mutated in T-cell prolymphocytic leukaemia. Br J Haematol. 2016;173(2):265-73. **DOI: 10.1111/bjh.13952**

Novikov ND, Griffin GK, Dudley G, et al. Utility of a simple and robust flow cytometry assay for rapid clonality testing in mature peripheral T-cell lymphomas. Am J Clin Pathol. 2019;151(5):494-503. **DOI: 10.1093/ajcp/aqy173**

Schrader A, Crispatzu G, Oberbeck S, et al. Actionable perturbations of damage responses by *TCL1/ATM* and epigenetic lesions form the basis of T-PLL. Nat Commun. 2018;9(1):697. **DOI: 10.1038/s41467-017-02688-6**

Shi M, Jevremovic D, Otteson GE, et al. Single antibody detection of T-cell receptor αβ clonality by flow cytometry rapidly identifies mature T-cell neoplasms and monotypic small CD8-positive subsets of uncertain significance. Cytometry B Clin Cytom. 2020;98(1):99-107. **DOI: 10.1002/cyto.b.21782**

Stengel A, Kern W, Zenger M, et al. Genetic characterization of T-PLL reveals 2 major biologic subgroups and *JAK3* mutations as prognostic marker. Genes Chromosomes Cancer. 2016;55(1):82-94. **DOI: 10.1002/gcc.22313**

Swerdlow SH, Campo E, Harris NL, et al. World Health Organization Classification of Tumours of Haematopoietic and Lymphoid Tissues. 4th ed. Lyon, France: IARC Press; 2017. **ISBN: 9789283244943**

Howard Meyerson

44

Hepatosplenic T-cell lymphoma with iso(7q)

History A 21-year-old male with a 7-year history of ulcerative colitis previously treated with azathioprine presented with left flank pain and early satiety. The patient recently had an acute Epstein-Barr virus (EBV) infection but symptoms persisted for several months. CBC results are shown at right.

Because of marked splenic enlargement, a splenectomy was performed, and a bone marrow aspirate and biopsy were performed several days later.

Morphology & flow cytometry Sections of the spleen showed diffuse sinusoidal infiltration of the red pulp by intermediate-sized lymphoid cells with pale cytoplasm, oval to irregular nuclei, and occasional small nucleoli **f44.1**. A peripheral blood smear revealed 10% atypical, moderately enlarged lymphocytes with slightly pale, oval nuclei, and deeply basophilic cytoplasm. The bone marrow aspirate was aspicular and hemodilute but contained similar atypical lymphocytes as those seen on the peripheral smear **f44.2a**. The trephine biopsy was 90% cellular with extensive sinusoidal and interstitial infiltration by cells similar to those seen in the spleen; these cells were positive for CD3 **f44.2b**. Flow cytometric analysis of the spleen and bone marrow both revealed an atypical population of lymphoid cells that was positive for CD2, CD3, CD7, CD8, CD56, CD16 (partial), and TCR γ/δ, and negative for CD4, CD5, CD25, CD30, CD57, and HLA-DR **f44.3**. Killer immunoglobulin-like receptor (KIR) expression was negative. EBV was negative by in situ hybridization performed on the splenic tissue. Based on the morphologic and flow cytometric findings, a diagnosis of **hepatosplenic T-cell lymphoma** (**HSTCL**) was rendered.

WBC	7.9×10^9/L
Differential	
Polymorphonuclear leukocytes	42%
Lymphocytes	41%
Monocytes	16%
Eosinophils	1%
HGB	11.9 g/dL
HCT	35.4
MCV	87 fL
RDW	14.8%
Platelets	42×10^9/L

ISBN 978-089189-6814 ©2021 ASCP

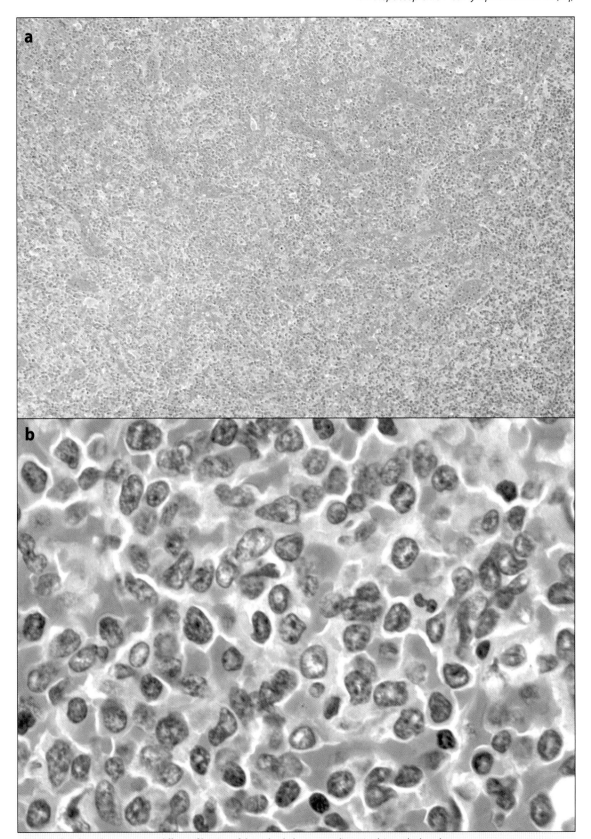

f44.1 a, b Spleen demonstrating diffuse infiltration of the red pulp by intermediate-sized, irregular lymphocytes

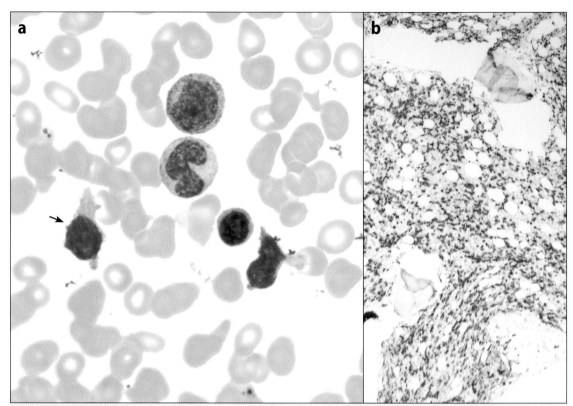

f44.2 a Bone marrow aspirate smear is hemodilute but contains occasional irregular lymphocytes (arrow); **b** CD3 stain performed on the bone marrow core biopsy highlights diffuse interstitial & intrasinusoidal infiltration by T cells

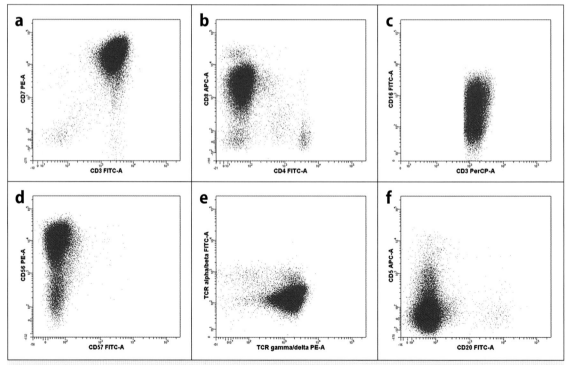

f44.3 Flow cytometry performed on the spleen demonstrates an abnormal population of T cells that is **a** CD3+, CD7+, **b** CD4–, CD8+, **c** CD16+(partial), **d** CD56+, CD57–, **e** TCR γ/δ+, TCR α/β–, and **f** mostly negative for CD5

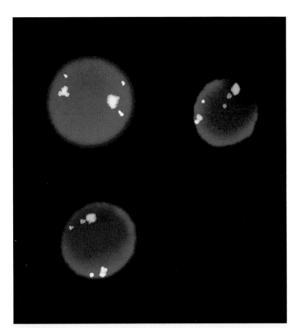

f44.4 Single-color FISH probes *D7S522* (7q31, orange) & *CEP7* (7 centromere, green) demonstrating 3 orange signals, consistent with an extra copy of 7q31; this signal pattern can be seen with iso(7q), which was observed by karyotype

Genetics/molecular results Cytogenetic analysis of the bone marrow cells revealed an isochromosome of the long arm of chromosome 7 in 5 of 20 metaphase cells. FISH using *CEP7* (chromosome 7 centromere probe) and *D7S522* (7q31) revealed that 18% of cells had 2 *CEP7* signals and 3 *D7S522* signals **f44.4**, consistent with the iso(7q) observed by karyotype.

Discussion The differential diagnosis in this case includes causes of splenomegaly associated with T-cell processes versus those related to EBV infection and/or immunosuppression. This includes T-cell lymphoproliferative disorders such as T-cell large granular lymphocytic (T-LGL) leukemia and peripheral T-cell lymphoma, not otherwise specified, reactive florid γ/δ T-cell proliferation of the spleen and EBV-related disorders such as systemic chronic active EBV infection (CAEBV) of T and NK cells, systemic EBV-positive T-cell lymphoma of childhood and EBV-associated hemophagocytic lymphohistiocytosis. Clinical, morphologic, and genetic features of these process are listed in **t44.1**. Although the lack of EBV in the tumor cells excluded the EBV-associated diagnoses in this case, it is important to recognize these rare entities, in particular EBV-associated hemophagocytosis, which is often related to an underlying immunodeficiency. Molecular analysis for an immunodeficiency is therefore needed in the evaluation of such cases.

HSTCL is a clinically aggressive, often fatal, T-cell neoplasm of TCR γ/δ or cytotoxic T cells. The disease is notable for producing marked splenomegaly, often associated with hepatomegaly, with histologic analysis showing a striking sinusoidal pattern of infiltration in affected organs. Bone marrow is universally involved and lymph nodes only rarely. Circulating lymphoma cells are present more frequently than generally believed, with cells detectable in ~50% of patients. The disease occurs more often in younger individuals, particularly men, and has a known increased occurrence in individuals with inflammatory bowel disease treated with azathioprine for several years prior to disease presentation. Phenotypically, HSTCL cells express TCR γ/δ receptor more often than TCR α/β, so much so that the initial terminology for the neoplasm was "hepatosplenic γ/δ T cell lymphoma," before rare cases expressing TCR α/β were described. The lymphoma cells are typically negative for CD5 and always negative for CD4. CD8 may or may not be expressed.

T-LGL leukemia may also involve the spleen and bone marrow and may be difficult to distinguish from HSTCL due to immunophenotypic overlap (see **Case 42**). Most T-LGL leukemia cases are positive for CD8 and TCR α/β, although rare cases express TCR γ/δ. Cytotoxic protein expression and CD57 are useful to distinguish between the 2 entities, as HSTCL is typically positive for TIA1 but lacks perforin and granzyme B, and is negative for CD57, whereas T-LGL leukemia typically expresses all cytotoxic markers and often is at least partially positive for CD57. The cells of HSTCL have been reported to have unusual expression of multiple KIRs, whereas T-LGL leukemia cells may express a single KIR in up to 50% of cases. Compared to HSTCL, T-LGL leukemia occurs more frequently in older individuals with a history of autoimmune disease and has a more indolent behavior. Histologically, the cells of T-LGL leukemia are generally smaller and less pleomorphic than those of HSTCL. EBV is not associated with either neoplasm, while the presence of iso(7q) is unique to HSTCL.

Marked reactive γ/δ T-cell populations may occur in the spleen and may be confused with HSTCL. Clonality testing by TCR gene rearrangement studies may be helpful to identify a clonal population, although the presence of a T-cell clone is not equivalent to malignancy. In this example case, extensive bone marrow involvement and the presence of a clonal cytogenetic abnormality excluded a reactive process.

t44.1 Comparison of EBV-associated T-cell proliferations with T-LGL leukemia & HSTCL

Disorder	EBV	Clinical	Morphology	Flow cytometry	TCR	Cytogenetic/ molecular
EBV– associated HLH	+	HLH-2004 criteria (5/8 of fever, splenomegaly, cytopenias, ↑ triglycerides or ↓ fibrinogen,↑ sCD25, ↑ ferritin, hemophagocytosis, ↓ NK activity, EBV+, no LPD, child > adult	hemophagocytosis in BM, spleen or LN, few EBV+ T cells	↑ % of activated CD8+ T cells (CD38 bright, HLA-DR+, CD7 dim), no aberrancy	usually polyclonal, occasionally clonal	germline mutations: FHL-associated (*PRF1, UNC13D, STX11, STXBP2*); IMD-associated (*GS2, LYST, HPS, XLP1, XLP2, XIAP, MAGT1, ITK, CD27, SLC7A7*)
Systemic CAEBV of T & NK cells	+	no IMD, mono-like illness >3 mo, hepatosplenomegaly, cytopenias, EBV-DNA load >10²·⁵/µg, most common in Asia, may progress to T or NK lymphoma	EBV+ T or NK cells in blood, nonspecific, nonlymphomatous infiltrates in tissues	infected cells CD4+ > CD8+ or NK, phenotypic findings otherwise not well defined	~50% clonal	somatic mutations in ~60%; *DDX3X* 16%, *KMT2D* 5%; *BCOR/BCORL1* 4%; *KDM6A* 4%
Systemic EBV- associated T-cell lymphoma of childhood	+	very aggressive lymphoma occurring shortly after EBV infection on spectrum with systemic CAEBV of T & NK cells, no IMD, most common in Asia	liver, spleen sinusoidal EBV+ T cell infiltrates of small lymphs, depleted B-cell zones in spleen & LN, hemophagocytosis	CD8+, CD56–, TIA1+, T cells	clonal	somatic mutations in *STAT3, KMT2D, DDX3X, NOTCH1* & *TET2* reported
T-LGL leukemia	–	indolent lymphoproliferative disorder, splenomegaly, immune cytopenias, hypergammaglobulinemia, arthralgias, rheumatoid factor+, elderly	lymphocytosis of slightly enlarged granular lymphocytes, splenic red pulp sinusoidal involvement, interstitial BM involvement	TCR α/β >>TCR γ/δ, CD8+, CD5 dim/–, CD57part, CD16+/–, CD56–/+, cytotoxic protein+, KIR restricted (50%)	clonal	somatic mutations: *STAT3* ~40%; *TNFAIP3* ~8%, *STAT5b* 15–50% of CD4+ cases; others (rare): *PRPT, BCL11b, SLIT2, NRP1, IGFN1, MUC4, ARL13B, KMT2D, FAT4, PCLO, TTN, TYRP1, IGSF3, USH2A, CCT6P1*
HSTCL	–	marked hepatosplenomegaly, young males, very poor prognosis, associated with immunosuppression in IBD with azathioprine	liver, spleen, BM sinusoidal infiltrate by medium-sized slightly irregular lymphoid cells, circulating cells in ~40%-50% of cases	TCR γ/δ > TCR α/β, CD3 dim/+, CD4–, CD5–, CD8–/+, CD16+, CD56+/–, CD57–, TIA1+, granzyme B–/+, perforin–	clonal	cytogenetic: iso(7q) or +7q (~50%), trisomy 8 (25%) Molecular: *STAT3* 10%, *STAT5B* 30%, *PIK3CD* 10%, *SETD2* 25%, *INO80* 20%, *ARID1B* 20%, *TET3* 15%, *SMARCA2* 10%, *TP53* 10%, *UBR5* 10%

+, positive; –, negative; ↑, increased; ↓, decreased; BM, bone marrow; CAEBV, chronic active EBV; EBV, Epstein-Barr virus; FHL, familial hemophagocytic lymphohistiocytosis; HLH, hemophagocytic lymphohistiocytosis; HSTCL, hepatosplenic T-cell lymphoma; IBD, inflammatory bowel disease; IMD, immunodeficiency; KIR, Killer immunoglobulin-like receptor; LN, lymph node; BM, bone marrow; LPD, lymphoproliferative disorder; mono, mononucleosis; NK, natural killer; TCR, T-cell receptor; T-LGL, T-cell large granular lymphocytic

In over half of all HSTCL cases, the lymphoma cells carry an iso(7q) or have extra copies of 7q. The detection of this abnormality is essentially pathognomonic for HSTCL. An isochromosome is a structural abnormality in which the arms of the chromosome are near mirror images of each other due to duplication of one arm, commonly the q arm. The chromosomal abnormality comes about during cell division because of either an abnormal transverse, rather than longitudinal, separation of the sister chromatids, or U-type joining of sister chromatid arms due to an abnormal break in and deletion of the other chromatid arms. In addition to iso(7q), trisomy 8 is seen as a secondary aberration in ~25% of cases of HSTCL. Losses in chromosome 10q and gains in chromosome 1q may also occur. In one study, whole exome sequencing of 68 HSTCL cases revealed recurrent mutations, most commonly in chromatin-modifying genes (62%) including *SETD2, INO80, ARID1B,* and *TET3*. Additional recurrent mutations were seen in JAK/STAT signaling pathway genes, most frequently *STAT5B* (30%), and less often, *STAT3* (10%) and *PIK3CD* (10%). *TP53* (10%) and *UBR5* (10%) are also recurrently mutated. Mutations in *STAT5B* and *STAT3* overlap with those seen in T-LGL leukemia, limiting the usefulness of molecular analysis for distinguishing between these 2 disorders. The clinical impact of somatic mutations in HSTCL is currently unclear.

In summary, this is a case of HSTCL in a young man with inflammatory bowel disease previously treated with azathioprine. A recent EBV infection confounded the clinical presentation; however, the diagnosis was established by morphologic examination and immunophenotyping, as well as detection of iso(7q).

Diagnostic pearls/pitfalls

- HSTCL has a striking sinusoidal growth pattern in the liver, spleen, and bone marrow.
- HSTCL is uniquely associated with iso(7q) as a recurring genetic abnormality. On FISH, iso(7q) manifests as an extra copy of the 7q probe.
- HSTLC shares immunophenotypic features with γ/δ T-LGL leukemia and can be distinguished from T-LGL leukemia by lack of CD57 expression and cytotoxic (other than TIA1), as well as clinical history and presentation.
- The incidence of this aggressive disease is increased in young men and individuals with inflammatory bowel disease treated with azathioprine.

Readings

Aguilera NS, Auerbach A. T-cell lymphoproliferative processes in the spleen. Semin Diagn Pathol. 2020 Jan;37(1):47-56. **DOI: 10.1053/j.semdp.2019.12.003**

Arai A. Advances in the study of chronic active Epstein-Barr virus infection: clinical features under the 2016 WHO classification and mechanisms of development. Front Pediatr. 2019;7:14. **DOI: 10.3389/fped.2019.00014**

Coppe A, Andersson EI, Binatti A, et al. Genomic landscape characterization of large granular lymphocyte leukemia with a systems genetics approach. Leukemia. 2017;31(5):1243-6. **DOI: 10.1038/leu.2017.49**

Dong J, Chong YY, Meyerson HJ. Hepatosplenic alpha/beta T-cell lymphoma: a report of an S100-positive case. Arch Pathol Lab Med. 2003;127(3):e119-22. **DOI: 10.1043/0003-9985(2003)127<e119:HTLARO >2.0.CO;2**

Horwitz SM, Ansell S, Ai WZ, et al. NCCN Guidelines Insights: T-Cell Lymphomas, Version 1.2021. J Natl Compr Canc Netw. 2020 Nov 2;18(11):1460-1467.0 **DOI: 10.6004/jnccn.2020.0053**

Kim WY, Montes-Mojarro IA, Fend F, Quintanilla-Martinez L. Epstein-Barr virus-associated T and NK-cell lymphoproliferative diseases. Front Pediatr. 2019;7:71. **DOI: 10.3389/fped.2019.00071**

Kimura H, Fujiwara S. Overview of EBV-associated T/NK-Cell lymphoproliferative diseases. Front Pediatr. 2019 Jan 4;6:417. **DOI: 10.3389/fped.2018.00417**

Macon WR, Levy NB, Kurtin PJ, et al. Hepatosplenic alpha/beta T-cell lymphomas: a report of 14 cases and comparison with hepatosplenic gamma/delta T-cell lymphomas. Am J Surg Pathol. 2001;25(3):285-96. **DOI: 10.1097/00000478-200103000-00002**

McKinney M, Moffitt AB, Gaulard P et. al. The genetic basis for hepatosplenic T cell lymphoma. Cancer Discov. 2017;7(4):369-79. **DOI: 10.1158/2159-8290.CD-16-0330**

Montes-Mojarro IA, Kim WY, Fend F, et al. Epstein-Barr virus positive T and NK-cell lymphoproliferations: morphological features and differential diagnosis. Semin Diagn Pathol. 2020 Jan;37(1):32-46. **DOI: 10.1053/j.semdp.2019.12.004**

Nicolae A, Xi L, Pittaluga S, Abdullaev Z, et al. Frequent *STAT5B* mutations in γδ hepatosplenic T-cell lymphomas. Leukemia. 2014;28(11):2244-8. **DOI: 10.1038/leu.2014.200**

Pro B, Allen P, Behdad A. Hepatosplenic T-cell lymphoma: a rare but challenging entity. Blood. 2020 Oct 29;136(18):2018-2026. **DOI: 10.1182/blood.2019004118**

Teramo A, Barilà G, Calabretto G, et al. *STAT3* mutation impacts biological and clinical features of T-LGL leukemia. Oncotarget. 2017;8(37):61876-89. **DOI: 10.18632/oncotarget.18711**

Yabe M, Medeiros LJ, Wang SA, et al. Distinguishing between hepatosplenic T-cell lymphoma and γδ T-cell large granular lymphocytic leukemia: a clinicopathologic, immunophenotypic, and molecular analysis. Am J Surg Pathol. 2017;41(1):82-93. **DOI: 10.1097/PAS.0000000000000743**

Yabe M, Miranda RN, Medeiros LJ. Hepatosplenic T cell lymphoma: a review of clinicopathologic features, pathogenesis, and prognostic factors. Hum Pathol. 2018;74:5-16. **DOI: 10.1016/j.humpath.2018.01.005**

Zhang S, Bayerl MG. Florid splenic γ/δ T-cell proliferation in patients with splenomegaly and cytopenias: a "high stakes" diagnostic challenge. Hum Pathol. 2017;66:216-21. **DOI: 10.1016/j.humpath.2017.01.015**

Christopher Ryder

45

Anaplastic large cell lymphoma, ALK-negative, with rearrangement of *DUSP22*

History An 86-year-old male with a past medical history of Parkinson disease and atrial fibrillation presented for evaluation of a left parotid mass that had been enlarging over the past year. Imaging studies showed a 4 cm round mass in the tail of the left parotid gland **f45.1**, as well as findings suggestive of local soft tissue and lymph node extension/involvement. Following a concerning but nondiagnostic fine-needle aspiration, an excisional biopsy was performed for definitive diagnosis.

Morphology & flow cytometry The parotid biopsy showed an atypical infiltrate composed predominantly of pleomorphic, medium-sized to large cells including cells with eccentric, kidney-shaped nuclei, 1 or more prominent nucleoli, and abundant eosinophilic cytoplasm, as well as scattered large, multinucleated cells **f45.2**. Mitotic figures, numerous interspersed single-cell apoptotic bodies, and few small areas of necrosis were also present. Immunohistochemical stains showed the lymphoma cells to be positive for CD2, CD3, CD4, CD5, CD45 (LCA), and CD30 (strong and diffuse) and negative for CD7, CD8, CD20, epithelial membrane antigen (EMA), anaplastic lymphoma kinase (ALK), and pan-keratins **f45.3**. Flow cytometric studies performed on a portion of the specimen identified an atypical population of CD45-positive (bright), CD30-positive, surface CD3-negative, CD2-positive, CD4-positive, CD5-positive, CD7-negative cells that were large based on forward scatter characteristics and showed increased side scatter **f45.4**. The overall morphologic and immunophenotypic findings were consistent with a diagnosis of **anaplastic large cell lymphoma, ALK-negative** (ALK– ALCL).

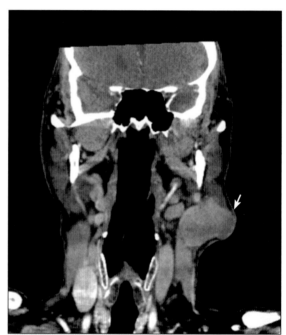

f45.1 Coronal CT image of the head & neck demonstrates a large parotid mass (arrow)

ISBN 978-089189-6814 ©2021 ASCP

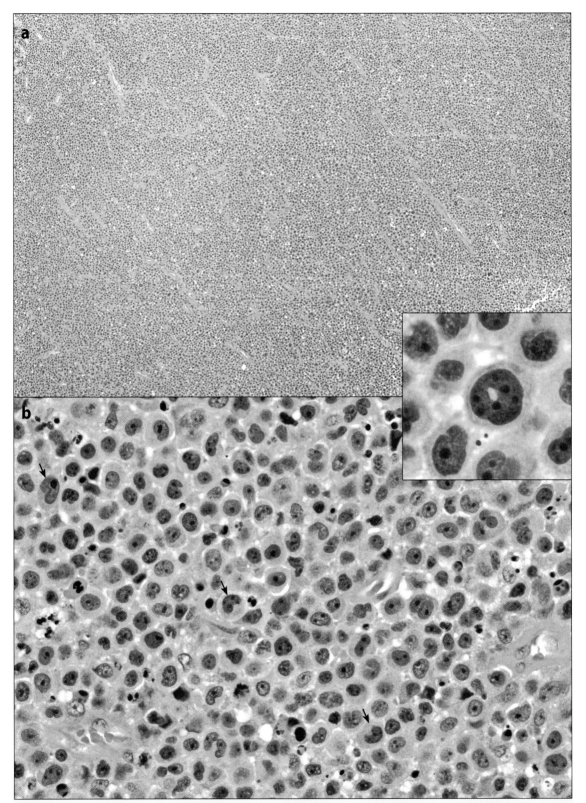

f45.2 **a** Low-power view of the parotid biopsy specimen demonstrating architectural effacement by a monotonous proliferation; **b** higher-power view of the biopsy showing sheets of large cells, including hallmark cells (arrows), with frequent apoptotic bodies & a single "doughnut" cell (inset)

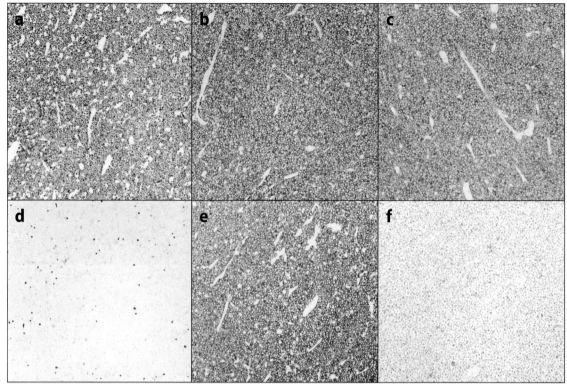

f45.3 Immunostains for **a** CD3, **b** CD5 & **c** CD4 confirm T-cell lineage with additional stains demonstrating **d** loss of CD7, **e** strong, diffuse CD30 expression & **f** lack of ALK protein expression

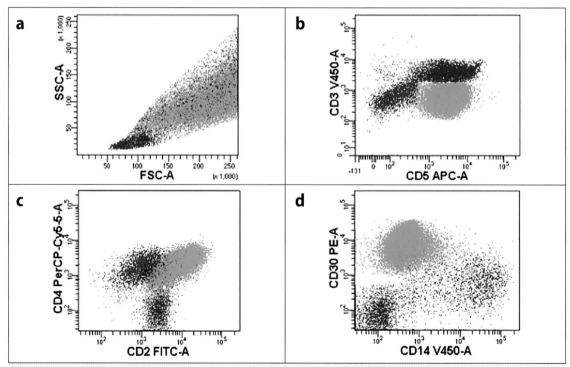

f45.4 Flow cytometric histograms demonstrating a population of abnormal cells (green) with **a** high forward scatter & increased side scatter characteristics, which **b** lack surface CD3, and are positive for CD5, **c** CD2, CD4, and **d** CD30; background small T-cells (red) & monocyte/macrophages (blue) are shown for comparison

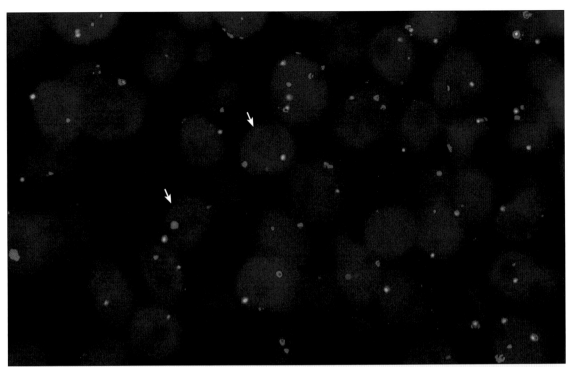

f45.5 Paraffin FISH image showing break-apart probe for the *DUSP22-IRF4* locus at chromosome 6p25.3, with cells denoted by the arrows demonstrating 1 normal yellow signal as well as separate orange & green signals, indicative of a gene rearrangement in the 6p25 region

t45.1 Types of ALCL recognized in the 2017 WHO classification of hematopoietic neoplasms

Disease	Typical sites of involvement	Clinical behavior	Recurrent translocations
Primary cutaneous ALCL	skin, regional lymph nodes	favorable	*DUSP22* (~25%) lack of *ALK* translocation
Systemic ALCL, ALK+	lymph nodes, bone, skin, soft tissue	favorable	involving *ALK*, most often t(2;5) *NPM1-ALK*
Systemic ALCL, ALK–	lymph nodes, bone, skin, soft tissue	more aggressive except in cases with *DUSP22* translocation	*DUSP22* (~30%) *TP63* (~10%) lack of *ALK* translocation
Breast implant-associated ALCL (provisional entity)	seroma associated with breast implant, regional lymph nodes	favorable	lack of *ALK* translocation

ALCL, anaplastic large cell lymphoma; ALK, anaplastic lymphoma kinase; WHO, World Health Organization

Genetics/molecular results Due to the reported prognostic significance and relative frequency of rearrangement involving the *DUSP22-IRF4* locus in ALK-negative ALCL, FISH studies were performed and were positive **f45.5**. Genetic testing for translocations involving *ALK* or *TP63* was not performed.

Discussion Anaplastic large cell lymphoma (ALCL) encompasses a group of systemic and primary cutaneous T-cell lymphoproliferative disorders having shared morphologic and phenotypic features but with distinct clinical and genetic characteristics **t45.1**. Systemic

ALCL accounts for ~3% of non-Hodgkin lymphomas in adults and ~10% of childhood lymphomas. Despite the higher incidence of ALCL in children, >80% of ALCLs occur in the adult population, with a male predominance across all age groups.

Most systemic ALCLs express ALK protein due to one of several recurrent translocations, most commonly t(2;5)(p23;q35) *NPM1-ALK*, which is present in ~80% of ALK-positive ALCL cases. Cases of ALCL without *ALK* translocation or expression of ALK (ALK-negative ALCL) are morphologically indistinguishable from their

ALK-positive counterparts. However, ALK-negative ALCL is classified as a distinct entity because it exhibits different clinical features than ALK-positive ALCL. More specifically, ALK-positive ALCL tends to occur in younger patients (median age at diagnosis of ~30 years versus ~55 years for ALK-negative ALCL) and carries a more favorable prognosis, with an overall 5-year survival of ~80% vs ~50% for ALK-negative ALCL.

Systemic ALCL occurs most frequently in lymph nodes, where it often demonstrates a sinusoidal distribution but can completely efface the nodal architecture in more advanced lesions. Extranodal sites include skin, bone, and soft tissue; bone marrow involvement occurs in at least 15%-20% of systemic ALCL, with rates as high as 40% based on immunohistochemical analysis. Extranodal involvement is less common in ALK-negative ALCL vs ALK-positive disease.

All forms of ALCL by definition exhibit CD30 expression and may demonstrate a spectrum of morphology, but all cases should have a population of large atypical cells having moderate-to-abundant eosinophilic cytoplasm, a prominent Golgi zone, and horseshoe-shaped nuclei with open chromatin and prominent nucleoli (so-called "hallmark" cells, named for their presence in all morphologic variants). A related cytological variant is the "doughnut" cell which appears to have a nuclear inclusion caused by sectioning through a deeply invaginated nucleus **f45.2 (inset)**.

Due to variations in morphology (especially in ALK-positive ALCL), the differential diagnosis may include peripheral T-cell lymphoma, not otherwise specified (PTCL, NOS), Hodgkin lymphoma, diffuse large B-cell lymphoma with anaplastic morphology, and even nonhematopoietic neoplasms including melanoma and carcinoma. Because of this potentially broad differential, confirmation of T-cell lineage is critical for the diagnosis of ALCL. Comprehensive immunophenotyping is often necessary, as loss of T-cell-associated antigens (especially CD3 and CD7) is frequent. Up to 20% of ALCLs show a "null" phenotype, lacking all common T-cell antigens, but a clonal T-cell receptor gene rearrangement is nearly universal. Expression of CD3 may be discrepant between flow cytometry and immunohistochemistry (as in this case), due to cytoplasmic but not surface expression. The vast majority of ALCLs are CD4-positive; the rare CD8-positive cases are associated with atypical morphology and worse outcome. Despite being typically CD4-positive, ALCLs often express one or more cytotoxic markers (granzyme B, TIA1, and/or perforin). Other markers include HLA-DR, EMA, MUM1/IRF4, fascin, and clusterin. ALK-negative ALCL tends to have higher rates of CD3 and CD2 expression but less frequent expression of EMA and myeloid antigens (eg, CD13 and CD33) than ALK-positive disease.

It is important to distinguish cutaneous dissemination of systemic ALK-negative ALCL from primary cutaneous ALCL, which also lacks ALK expression, due to differing clinical behavior. This distinction typically requires correlation with radiologic and physical exam findings. In addition, primary cutaneous ALCL may involve draining regional lymph nodes; this finding does not define systemic disease. Differentiating between ALK-negative ALCL and PTCL, NOS, may also be challenging. Strong, diffuse CD30 staining is requisite for ALK-negative ALCL but may be present in a subset of PTCL, NOS. Although gene expression studies report reproducible discrimination between ALK-negative ALCL and PTCL, NOS, this testing is not currently clinically available. Therefore, the cytologic and immunophenotypic features must be sufficient to render a diagnosis of ALK-negative ALCL.

While ALK-positive ALCL is defined by recurrent translocations involving *ALK*, ALK-negative ALCL is genetically heterogeneous. Two recurrent translocations of prognostic importance involve the *DUSP22-IRF4* locus on chromosome 6p25.3 and *TP63* on chromosome 3q28. Rearrangements of *DUSP22* occur in ~30% of ALK-negative ALCL and show favorable outcomes similar to those for ALK-positive ALCL. Of note, *DUSP22* rearrangements also occur in a subset of primary cutaneous ALCL and lymphomatoid papulosis. Translocations of *TP63* are less common, occurring in <10% of ALK-negative ALCL and portend an aggressive disease course, with a 5-year survival rate of <20%. Although p63 protein expression is demonstrable in *TP63*-translocated disease, this finding is not specific to *TP63*-translocated cases. Rearrangements of *DUSP22* and *TP63* are thought to be mutually exclusive in ALK-negative ALCL (though rare reports describe co-existence in cases of PTCL, NOS, and primary cutaneous ALCL); they are not observed in ALK-positive ALCL. So-called "triple negative" cases of ALK–negative ALCL (without rearrangements of *ALK*, *DUSP22*, or *TP63*) show intermediate outcomes.

As demonstrated in this case **f45.2**, *DUSP22*-rearranged ALK-negative ALCL typically displays "common" variant morphology (i.e., sheet-like growth of large anaplastic cells), with frequent doughnut cells and lower occurrence of large, pleomorphic cells. *DUSP22*-rearranged cases also tend to express CD3 more often, with lower incidence of expression of EMA and cytotoxic markers, relative to other ALK-negative and ALK-positive ALCLs.

Gene expression profiling studies show JAK/STAT activation in both ALK-positive and many ALK-negative ALCLs. Whereas constitutively active ALK drives JAK/STAT activation in ALK-positive ALCL, mutations in *JAK1*, *STAT3*, and/or components of the NF-κB pathway drive this phenotype in a subset of ALK-negative cases. Interestingly, *DUSP22*-rearranged ALK-negative ALCLs have been found to lack JAK/STAT pathway activation. A recent report highlighted recurrent mutations involving the musculin gene in ALK-negative ALCL, which are strongly associated with *DUSP22* rearrangement.

CD30 has become a therapeutic target in ALCL, and this patient was initially treated with single-agent brentuximab vedotin (anti-CD30 monoclonal antibody drug conjugate), with a plan for consolidative radiotherapy. Other approaches for eligible patients with systemic ALCL include aggressive chemotherapy regimens such as cyclophosphamide-doxorubicin-vincristine-prednisone (CHOP) and CHOP + etoposide (CHEOP).

Diagnostic pearls/pitfalls

– Because of histologic and clinical variation, cases of ALCL may elicit a broad differential diagnosis and may require extensive immunophenotyping and genetic studies as well as clinical correlation for correct diagnosis.
– ALK-negative ALCL in particular must be distinguished from CD30-positive PTCL, NOS, and primary cutaneous CD30-positive lymphoproliferative disorders, the latter of which can involve local lymph nodes. Distinction between cutaneous involvement by systemic ALK-negative ALCL and primary cutaneous ALCL is typically not possible by histology alone.
– Differentiating ALK-negative ALCL from CD30-positive PTCL, NOS, is particularly problematic. Diagnosis of ALK-negative ALCL requires strong, diffuse expression of CD30 and appropriate morphologic features (eg, hallmark cells, sinusoidal pattern).

– Identification of *DUSP22* rearrangement in ALK-negative ALCL indicates a favorable clinical course that is similar to that of ALK-positive ALCL, whereas *TP63* gene rearrangement in ALK-negative ALCL portends a poor outcome.
– Flow cytometric analysis can be challenging because ALCL cells are often large with increased side scatter as well as loss of surface CD3 and other T-cell antigens. Therefore, examination of cells falling outside typical T-cell or lymphocyte gating parameters is usually necessary.

Readings

Abramov D, Oschlies I, Zimmermann M, et al. Expression of CD8 is associated with non-common type morphology and outcome in pediatric anaplastic lymphoma kinase-positive anaplastic large cell lymphoma. Haematologica. 2013;98:1547-53. **DOI: 10.3324/haematol.2013.085837**

Agnelli L, Mereu E, Pellegrino E, et al. Identification of a 3-gene model as a powerful diagnostic tool for the recognition of ALK-negative anaplastic large-cell lymphoma. Blood. 2012;120:1274-81. **DOI: 10.1182/blood-2012-01-405555**

Bovio IM, Allan RW. The expression of myeloid antigens CD13 and/or CD33 is a marker of ALK+ anaplastic large cell lymphomas. Am J Clin Pathol. 2008;130:628-34. **DOI: 10.1309/PLN1NA4QB2PC1CMQ**

Crescenzo R, Abate F, Lasorsa E, et al; European T-Cell Lymphoma Study Group; T-Cell Project: Prospective Collection of Data in Patients with Peripheral T-Cell Lymphoma and the AIRC 5xMille Consortium "Genetics-Driven Targeted Management of Lymphoid Malignancies." Convergent mutations and kinase fusions lead to oncogenic *STAT3* activation in anaplastic large cell lymphoma. Cancer Cell. 2015;27:516-32. **DOI: 10.1016/j.ccell.2015.03.006**

Feldman AL, Dogan A, Smith DI, et al. Discovery of recurrent t(6;7) (p25.3;q32.3) translocations in ALK-negative anaplastic large cell lymphomas by massively parallel genomic sequencing. Blood. 2011;117:915-9. **DOI: 10.1182/blood-2010-08-303305**

Hapgood G, Savage KJ. The biology and management of systemic anaplastic large cell lymphoma. Blood. 2015;126:17-25. **DOI: 10.1182/blood-2014-10-567461**

Karai LJ, Kadin ME, Hsi ED, et al. Chromosomal rearrangements of 6p25.3 define a new subtype of lymphomatoid papulosis. Am J Surg Pathol. 2013;37:1173-81. **DOI: 10.1097/PAS.0b013e318282d01e**

Kesler MV, Paranjape GS, Asplund SL, Mckenna RW, Jamal S, Kroft SH. Anaplastic large cell lymphoma: a flow cytometric analysis of 29 cases. Am J Clin Pathol. 2007;128:314-22. **DOI: 10.1309/GUHKGAJEJ72CEAL7**

David Zemmour & Annette S Kim

46

Angioimmunoblastic T-cell lymphoma with *RHOA* mutation

History A 68-year-old male presented with fatigue, weight loss, splenomegaly, and generalized lymphadenopathy. CBC results showed anemia and lymphopenia, with the results shown at right.

The anemia was presumed to be secondary to a warm autoimmune hemolytic anemia, because the lactate dehydrogenase concentration was moderately elevated at 300 U/L, direct Coombs test was positive for IgG/complement, and a warm autoantibody was identified by elution. CT and PET detected splenomegaly and scattered lymphadenopathy in both the thorax and upper abdomen, with mild to moderate fluorodeoxyglucose uptake. An excisional biopsy of an axillary lymph node was subsequently performed.

Morphology & flow cytometry The lymph node was enlarged (1.8 cm in greatest dimension) with focal capsular breach. The normal architecture was effaced by a vaguely nodular infiltrate of lymphocytes and a diffuse vascular hyperplasia with arborization **f46.1**. The lymphocytes were variable in size with numerous small cells as well as admixed medium to large cells having oval to slightly irregular nuclei, vesicular to open chromatin, and occasional multiple small nucleoli.

WBC	9.1×10^9/L
Differential	
Neutrophils	85%
Lymphocytes	10.8%
Monocytes	4%
Basophils	0.2%
HGB	9.8 g/dL
MCV	93.2 fL
Platelets	230×10^9/L

IHC revealed that the neoplastic infiltrate was predominantly composed of T cells positive for CD3, CD4, CD5, and PD1, with partial loss of CD7 and subset positivity for CXCL13 **f46.2a** & **f46.2b**. CD10 was negative on the T cells. Clusters of B cells were marked with CD20 and PAX5, including fewer large cells that were often aggregated. CD35 highlighted floridly expanded and disrupted follicular dendritic cell meshworks **f46.2c**. Epstein-Barr encoding region (EBER) in situ hybridization marked rare cells **f46.2d**. The Ki-67 proliferation index was 50%. A staging bone marrow biopsy was negative for lymphoma.

Flow cytometric analysis of the lymph node specimen and of peripheral blood did not identify an abnormal B- or T-cell population.

ISBN 978-089189-6814

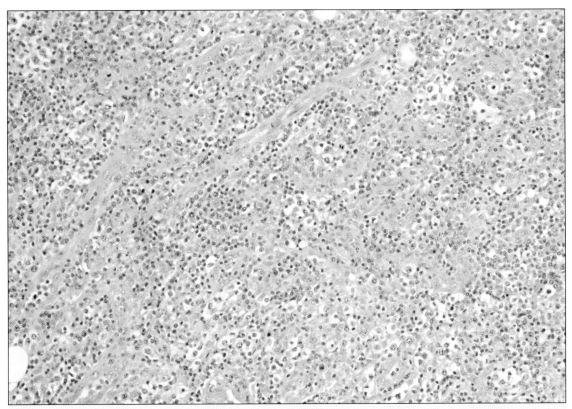

f46.1 H&E stain of the axillary lymph node showing effacement of normal architecture & diffuse vascular hyperplasia with arborization

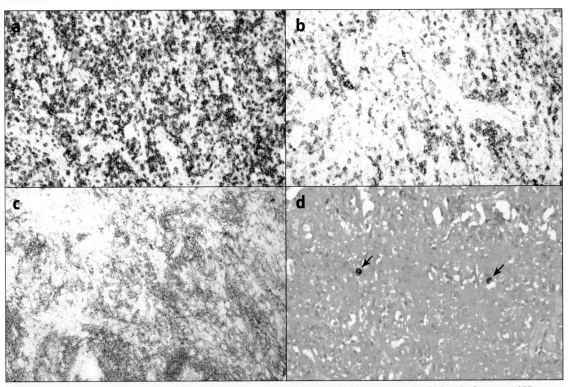

f46.2 Stains performed on the axillary lymph node showing **a** numerous variably sized CD3-positive T cells that also **b** expressed PD1; **c** floridly expanded & disrupted follicular dendritic cell meshwork by CD35 staining; **d** rare cells are EBER-positive (arrows)

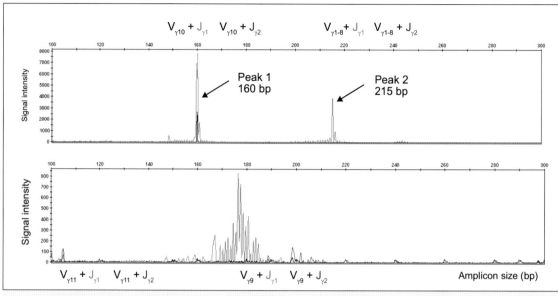

f46.3 T-cell receptor γ (TCRγ) clonality analysis with multiplex PCR showing clonal TCRγ rearrangements with $V\gamma_{1-8}$-$J\gamma_1$ primers (215 bp) and $V\gamma_{10}$-$J\gamma_1$ primers (160 bp)

Genetics/molecular results T-cell receptor (TCR) clonality analysis was performed with multiplex polymerase chain reaction (PCR) targeting the $V\gamma_{1-8}$, $V\gamma_9$, $V\gamma_{10}$, and $V\gamma_{11}$ regions. A clonal TCRγ rearrangement was detected using the $V\gamma_{1-8}$-$J\gamma_1$ (215 bp) and $V\gamma_{10}$-$J\gamma_1$ (160 bp) primer sets **f46.3**. A clonal immunoglobulin heavy chain gene rearrangement was not detected.

Cytogenetic analysis of the unstimulated lymph node cells showed hyperploidy with extra copies of chromosomes X, 5, 7, 19 and 20: 48-51,XY,+X,+5,+7, add(14)(p11.2)[2], +19[3], +20[6][cp8]/46,XY[2].

NGS of targeted exons in 447 cancer genes and 191 regions across 60 genes for rearrangement detection identified several variants in the lymph node specimen **f46.4**:

RHOA c.50G>T p.G17V (6% variant allele frequency [VAF] in 308 reads)
IDH2 c.514_515delAGinsCA p.R172Q (5% VAF in 486 reads)
TET2 c.3686T>C p.L1229P (7% VAF in 632 reads)
TET2 c.3898T>A p.F1300I (5% VAF in 340 reads)

No structural variants were detected. The genetic information supported the final morphologic and immunophenotypic diagnosis of **angioimmunoblastic T-cell lymphoma**.

Discussion Angioimmunoblastic T-cell lymphoma (AITL) is the most commonly occurring distinct subtype of T-cell lymphoma (15%-20%), excluding peripheral T-cell lymphoma, not otherwise specified (PTCL, NOS), but represents only 1%-2% of all non-Hodgkin lymphomas. It affects more men than women and its incidence peaks in the seventh and eighth decades of life. Along with the typical symptoms of lymphoma (hepatosplenomegaly, lymphadenopathy), patients also show a wide array of more systemic findings reflecting dysregulation of B-cell immunity: fever, rash, polyarthritis, polyclonal hypergammaglobulinemia, autoimmune hemolytic anemia, autoimmune antibodies (eg, rheumatoid factor, anti-smooth muscle antibodies), and immunodeficiency. The cell of origin in AITL is well-established as the T cell of follicular helper type (Tfh), a critical T cell that resides in reactive follicles to potentiate the antibody response. AITL is strongly associated with the presence of Epstein Barr virus (EBV), though the virus is only detected in bystander B cells.

Morphologically, the lymph node architecture is effaced to varying degrees. At one end of the spectrum, follicles are preserved in a heterogeneous inflammatory background composed of macrophages, eosinophils, and plasma cells, making the differential diagnosis with reactive follicular hyperplasia difficult. In addition, neoplastic AITL cells are typically small to medium-sized with minimal cytologic abnormalities and are often difficult to identify in the inflammatory

ISBN 978-089189-6814   ©2021 ASCP

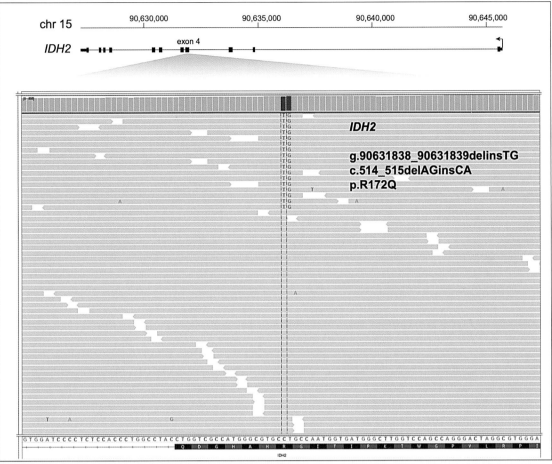

f46.4 Somatic variant analysis using NGS; mapped reads to the *IDH2* locus with 2-bp mismatch highlighting the unusual *IDH2* p.R172Q variant found in angioimmunoblastic T-cell lymphoma (hg19, Integrative Genomics Viewer browser) [see **fA.8**, p312]

background. At the other end of the spectrum, the lymph node architecture may be completely effaced, with minimal inflammation and larger neoplastic cells with pale cytoplasm, reminiscent of PTCL, NOS. In almost all cases, however, AITL shows prominent hyperplasia of high endothelial venules, often surrounded by clusters of neoplastic lymphocytes with clear cell morphology, and increased, often disorganized, follicular dendritic cell meshworks. EBV-positive B cells are also present in nearly all cases and range from immunoblasts to atypical, Reed-Sternberg-like morphology.

Immunophenotypically, the neoplastic cells are CD3-positive T cells, almost exclusively CD4-positive rather than CD8-positive, and variably retain other T-cell markers such as CD2, CD5, and CD7. This bland immunophenotype and low numbers of lymphoma cells can make this entity challenging to identify using flow cytometry alone, because many reactive conditions present with elevated CD4-CD8 ratios. The neoplastic

T-cell population may be masked by normal T cells, and careful subgating using the flow cytometer software may be necessary to identify the atypical population. AITL is classified as a subtype of PTCL of Tfh phenotype, requiring the expression of at least 2 of the following Tfh markers: PD1, CD10, BCL6, CXCL13, CXCR5, CD40LG, SAP1, or ICOS. The prominent follicular dendritic cell meshwork is best appreciated by staining with CD21, CD23, or CD35.

Molecular testing may be necessary to distinguish and consolidate the diagnosis of AITL, especially in cases morphologically similar to reactive follicular hyperplasia or to PTCL, NOS. TCR clonality is a critical piece of evidence for the diagnosis of T-cell malignancy and can be assessed using targeted PCR or NGS. A clonal TCR rearrangement is indeed identified in >95% of AITL cases, as seen in this case. In some cases, the scattered EBV-positive B cells may also be clonal by immunoglobulin gene rearrangement studies.

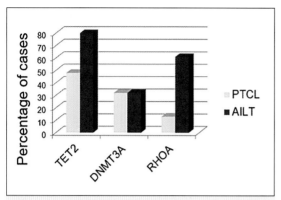

f46.5 Frequency of recurrent somatic variants (*TET2, DNMT3A, RHOA*) in angioimmunoblastic T-cell lymphoma & peripheral T-cell lymphoma, not otherwise specified

Recurrent cytogenetic abnormalities have been described in AITL. Gains of 9p23, 5q, 22q, 19, 11q11-q14, and loss of 13q are common but not specific (also seen in PTCL, NOS). Gains of 11q13 involve either *CCND1* or *GSTP1*, and gains of 13q22 might involve *MYCBP2*, a MYC regulator.

AITL is included in the larger category of PTCL with a Tfh phenotype that includes follicular T-cell lymphoma and nodal PTCL with Tfh phenotype. In these Tfh lymphomas, 2 gene rearrangements are recurrently detected and involve critical genes in the TCR signaling pathway: *ITK-SYK* and *CTLA4-CD28* in 18% (rare specifically in AITL) and 58% of cases, respectively. Although SYK overexpression is commonly seen with IHC across PTCLs, the *ITK-SYK* fusion is specific to PTCL of follicular origin. The fusion replaces the autoinhibitory SH2 and SH3 domains of ITK and its kinase domain with the SYK kinase domain. The *CTLA4-CD28* rearrangement is not specific and can also be seen in PTCL, NOS, as well as extranodal natural killer/T cell lymphoma. FISH for these rearrangements, however, is not readily available in clinical laboratories.

Somatic gene variants can be useful to diagnose AITL and monitor disease. The most frequent mutations involve *RHOA, CD28*, and epigenetic genes such as *TET2, DNMT3A*, and *IDH2*. *RHOA* is a small GTPase physiologically involved in the dynamics of the actin and stress fibers upon TCR stimulation. *RHOA* is more frequently mutated in AITL (53%-68% of cases compared to 12%-18% of cases of PTCL, NOS; **f46.5**) and is thought to be a driver mutation in this disorder. The most common *RHOA* mutation, p.G17V, is a dominant-negative mutation resulting in a protein product that lacks the ability to bind GTP but increases TCR signaling strength by binding to the VAV1 adapter. CD28 is a transmembrane protein acting as a costimulatory signal for TCR activation and is involved in the differentiation, homeostasis, and activation of T cells. *CD28* hotspot mutations (p.D124 and p.T195) are found in only 10%-11% of AITL cases but are almost never found in other lymphomas. Several genes involved in epigenetic regulation are also frequently mutated in AITL, often in conjunction with *RHOA* variants, and point to the stem cell origin of these lesions. *TET2* encodes an epigenetic eraser catalyzing the successive oxidation of methylcytosine first to 5-hydroxymethylcytosine and ultimately to removal of the methylation mark. It is mutated in up to 83% of AITL cases but also frequently mutated in other hematopoietic malignancies, including PTCL, NOS. It often co-occurs with mutations in another enzyme involved in DNA methylation, encoded by *DNMT3A*. In addition, mutations in *IDH2* at the hotspot p.R172 are observed in 45% of AITL. *IDH2* encodes a key enzyme in the citric acid cycle that catalyzes the conversion of isocitrate to α-ketoglutarate; however, variant *IDH2* is thought to increase the level of 2-hydroxyglutarate which inhibits TET2, dysregulating the epigenetic landscape. *IDH2* mutations are also commonly associated with gliomas and acute myeloid leukemia, where their prognostic role is well-established, contrary to AITL. In this case, the presence of *RHOA* and *IDH2* hotspot mutations in combination with *TET2* variants supported the diagnosis of AITL.

Diagnostic pearls/pitfalls

– AITL can be difficult to distinguish from PTCL, NOS. Expanded follicular dendritic cell meshworks and a prominent vasculature are important morphologic features of AITL.

– The Tfh origin of AITL can be established by the expression of at least 2 Tfh markers, including PD1, CD10, BCL6, CXCL13, CXCR5, CD40LG, SAP1, and ICOS.

– The tyrosine kinase SYK is often upregulated in PTCL, but *ITK-SYK* rearrangements are specific to PTCL of Tfh origin.

– *ITK-SYK* and *CTLA4-CD28* rearrangements may be present in AITL but FISH is not widely available.

– TCR repertoire analysis (using PCR or NGS) can establish the clonal nature of a T-cell lymphoma and can be used to monitor disease over time.

– Although no mutations are specific for AITL, *RHOA, IDH2, TET2*, and *CD28* variants are relatively more frequent in AITL than in PTCL, NOS. *DNMT3A* mutations are also recurrent in AITL but are also seen as or more frequently in PTCL, NOS.

ISBN 978-089189-6814 ©2021 ASCP

Readings

Attygalle AD, Feldman AL, Dogan A. *ITK/SYK* translocation in angioimmunoblastic T-cell lymphoma. Am J Surg Pathol. 2013;37:1456-7. **DOI: 10.1097/PAS.0b013e3182991415**

Cairns RA, Iqbal J, Lemonnier F, et al. *IDH2* mutations are frequent in angioimmunoblastic T-cell lymphoma. Blood. 2012;119:1901-3. **DOI: 10.1182/blood-2011-11-391748**

Couronné L, Bastard C, Bernard OA. *TET2* and *DNMT3A* mutations in human T-cell lymphoma. N Engl J Med. 2012;366:95-6. **DOI: 10.1056/NEJMc1111708**

Feldman AL, Sun DX, Law ME, et al. Overexpression of Syk tyrosine kinase in peripheral T-cell lymphomas. Leukemia. 2008;22:1139-43. **DOI: 10.1038/leu.2008.77**

Fujisawa M, Sakata-Yanagimoto M, Nishizawa S, et al. Activation of *RHOA-VAV1* signaling in angioimmunoblastic T-cell lymphoma. Leukemia. 2018;32:694-702. **DOI: 10.1038/leu.2017.273**

Kim AS, Wu CJ, Lovitch SB. Molecular genetic aspects of non-Hodgkin Lymphomas. In: Greer JP, Arber DA, Appelbalm FR, eds, et al. Wintrobe's Clinical Hematology. 14th ed. Philadelphia, PA: Wolters Kluwer Health. 2018;chap 88:1843-1879. **ISBN: 978-1496347428**

Lee SH, Kim JS, Kim J, et al. A highly recurrent novel missense mutation in CD28 among angioimmunoblastic T-cell lymphoma patients. Haematologica. 2015;100:e505-7. **DOI: 10.3324/haematol.2015.133074**

Rohr J, Guo S, Huo J, et al. Recurrent activating mutations of CD28 in peripheral T-cell lymphomas. Leukemia. 2016;30:1062-70. **DOI: 10.1038/leu.2015.357**

Sakata-Yanagimoto M, Enami T, Yoshida K, et al. Somatic *RHOA* mutation in angioimmunoblastic T cell lymphoma. Nat Genet. 2014;46:171-5. **DOI: 10.1038/ng.2872**

Sholl LM, Do K, Shivdasani P, et al. Institutional implementation of clinical tumor profiling on an unselected cancer population. JCI Insight. 2016;1(19):e87062. **DOI: 10.1172/jci.insight.87062**

Shanmugam V, Kim AS. Lymphomas. In: Tafe JL, Arcila ME, eds. Genomic Medicine: A Practical Guide. New York, NY: Springer. 2020;chap 16:253-315. **ISBN: 978-3030229214**

Streubel B, Vinatzer U, Willheim M, et al. Novel t(5;9)(q33;q22) fuses *ITK* to *SYK* in unspecified peripheral T-cell lymphoma. Leukemia. 2006;20:313-8. **DOI: 10.1038/sj.leu.2404045**

Swerdlow S, Campo E, Pileri S, et al. The 2016 revision of the World Health Organization classification of lymphoid neoplasms. Blood. 2016;127(20):2375-90. **DOI: 10.1182/blood-2016-01-643569**

Thorns C, Bastian B, Pinkel D, et al. Chromosomal aberrations in angioimmunoblastic T-cell lymphoma and peripheral T-cell lymphoma unspecified: a matrix-based CGH approach. Genes Chromosomes Cancer. 2007;46:37-44. **DOI: 10.1002/gcc.20386**

Van Dongen JJM, Langerak AW, Brüggemann M, et al. Design and standardization of PCR primers and protocols for detection of clonal immunoglobulin and T-cell receptor gene recombinations in suspect lymphoproliferations: report of the BIOMED-2 Concerted Action BMH4-CT98-3936. Leukemia. 2003;17:2257-2317. **DOI: 10.1002/gcc.20386**

Ward PS, Cross JR, Lu C, et al. Identification of additional IDH mutations associated with oncometabolite R(-)-2-hydroxyglutarate production. Oncogene. 2012;31:2491-8. **DOI: 10.1038/onc.2011.416**

Yoo HY, Sung MK, Lee SH, et al. A recurrent inactivating mutation in *RHOA* GTPase in angioimmunoblastic T cell lymphoma. Nat Genet 2014;46:371-5. **DOI: 10.1038/ng.2916**

Rose C Beck

47

B-lymphoblastic leukemia/lymphoma with rearrangement of *KMT2A* (*MLL*)

History A 42-year-old female presented to the emergency room with progressive dyspnea on exertion and shortness of breath over a 4 week period. A CBC was ordered and selected results are shown at right.

A blood smear review and bone marrow biopsy were performed.

Morphology & flow cytometry The blood smear showed 71% blasts which were small in size with high nuclear-cytoplasmic ratios **f47.1**. A bone marrow aspirate smear and core biopsy showed sheets of similar blasts **f47.2**. Flow cytometry demonstrated atypical B lymphoblasts that were negative for CD10 and CD20 and positive for CD19, CD22, CD15, CD34, HLA-DR, and TdT **f47.3**. Based on the morphologic and immunophenotypic findings, a diagnosis of **B-lymphoblastic leukemia/lymphoma** (B-ALL) was rendered, with concern for presence of *KMT2A* (*MLL*) gene rearrangement given the lack of CD10 expression and positivity for CD15 on the blasts.

Genetics/molecular results Chromosome analysis showed: 46,XX,t(4;11)(q21;q23)[12]/46,XX[3] **f47.4**. A B-ALL FISH panel was positive for rearrangement of *KMT2A* (*MLL*) at 11q23 using a break-apart probe **f47.5**. FISH was negative for hyperdiploidy and the recurrent translocations t(12;21) *ETV6-RUNX1* and t(9;22) *BCR-ABL1*.

Based on the genetic findings, a final diagnosis of **B-lymphoblastic leukemia/lymphoma with rearrangement of *KMT2A*** was rendered.

WBC	51.3×10^9/L
RGB	2.12×10^{12}/L
HGB	6.4 g/dL
HCT	19.9%
MCV	94 fL
RDW	17.1%
Platelets	29×10^9/L

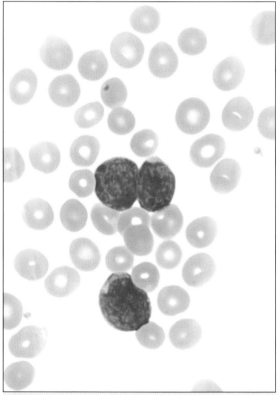

f47.1 Blasts present in blood appear lymphoid, with high nuclear:cytoplasmic ratios & fine chromatin

ISBN 978-089189-6814

47 *B-lymphoblastic leukemia/lymphoma with rearrangement of KMT2A (MLL)*

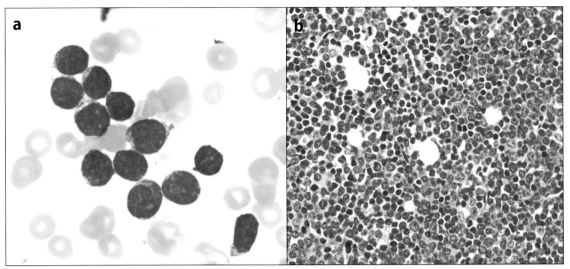

f47.2 Blasts similar to those in the peripheral blood are predominant in **a** the aspirate smear & **b** the core biopsy specimen

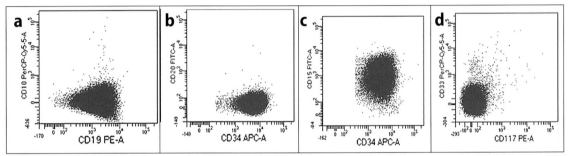

f47.3 Flow cytometry demonstrates B lymphoblasts that **a-b** express CD19 & CD34 but not CD10 or CD20; **c-d** there is atypical expression of CD15 without expression of other myeloid markers including CD33 & CD117

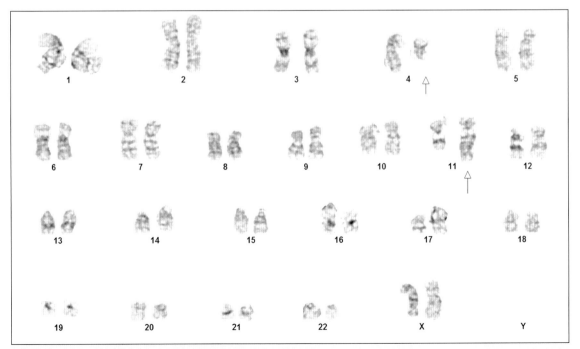

f47.4 Karyotype shows the presence of t(4;11)(q21;q23) (arrows), consistent with *KMT2A-AF4* fusion

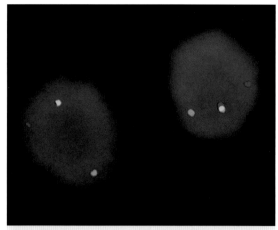

f47.5 FISH using a break-apart probe for *KMT2A* (11q23, yellow) is positive for rearrangement, with production of separate red & green signals

t47.1 Recurrent genetic abnormalities in pediatric B-lymphoblastic leukemia/lymphoma with associated prognosis
(see also **Cases 48-51**)

Genetic finding	Prognosis
t(12;21) *ETV6-RUNX1*	favorable
hyperdiploidy (51-65 chromosomes)	favorable
t(1;19) *TCF3-PBX1*	intermediate
t(9;22) *BCR-ABL1*	unfavorable (historical)*
BCR-ABL1-like genetics	unfavorable
iAMP21	unfavorable
rearrangement of *KMT2A*	unfavorable
hypodiploidy (<46 chromosomes)	unfavorable

*With the advent of tyrosine kinase inhibitor therapy, prognosis for these patients has improved, though high-risk treatment protocols are still required

t47.2 Common *KMT2A* (*MLL*) rearrangements in acute leukemias*

Fusion	Partner gene (former name)	More frequent disease association
t(4;11)(q21;q23)	*AF4 (AFF1)*	infant & adult ALL
t(6;11)(q27;q23)	*AF6 (MLLT4)*	pediatric & adult AML; T-ALL
t(9;11)(p21;q23)	*AF9 (MLLT3)*	infant ALL, pediatric & adult AML
t(10;11)(p12;q23)	*AF10 (MLLT10)*	infant ALL & AML, pediatric & adult AML
t(11;19)(q23;p13.1)	*ELL*	AML, all age groups
t(11;19)(q23;p13.3)	*ENL (MLLT1)*	ALL (especially T-ALL) > AML, all ages

ALL, acute lymphoblastic leukemia; AML, acute myeloid leukemia; T-ALL, T-lymphoblastic leukemia/lymphoma
**Infant is defined as being <1 year of age; pediatric is defined by 1 to 18 years of age*

Discussion B-ALL is characterized by recurrent genetic abnormalities which have significant impact on prognosis **t47.1**. In nonadult B-ALL, a rearrangement involving *KMT2A* (formerly known as *MLL*) is predominantly found in patients younger than 1 year of age (~75% of infant B-ALL cases) and is uncommon in older children; incidence increases again in adult B-ALL (10%-15% of cases). Patients often present with high WBC and may have central nervous system involvement. Although there is no distinct morphology, B-ALL cases with *KMT2A* rearrangement, especially those with t(4;11) *KMT2A-AF4*, have an early, "pro-B" immunophenotype with lack of CD10 and atypical expression of CD15 (as seen in this example case). Thus, flow cytometry can raise suspicion for the presence of *KMT2A* rearrangement.

The *mixed lineage leukemia* (*MLL*) gene, subsequently renamed *lysine methyltransferase 2A* (*KMT2A*), forms oncogenic fusions with many different genes:

>130 unique chromosomal rearrangements have been identified, involving at least 90 distinct partner genes. The most common *KMT2A* fusion is t(4;11)(q21;q23) *KMT2A-AF4*; this and 5 other fusions listed in **t47.2** account for ~90%-95% of all *KMT2A* rearrangements in acute leukemia. *KMT2A* fusions are not specific to B-ALL and are also found in T-ALL, mixed phenotype acute leukemia, acute myeloid leukemia (AML), and therapy-related acute leukemia (see **Case 25**). The KMT2A protein functions to maintain expression of homeobox (*HOX*) genes which drive expansion of early hematopoietic precursor cells; the abnormal fusion proteins act as transcription factors that cause continuous transcription of the *HOX* genes, resulting in uncontrolled stem cell self-renewal. Most *KMT2A* rearrangements are associated with poor prognosis across all acute leukemias, with the exception being t(9;11) *KMT2A-AF9* which carries an intermediate prognosis in AML.

Because of the pronounced diversity of *KMT2A* rearrangements and the fact that some are cryptic or subtle by karyotype, these fusions are typically detected using break-apart FISH probes for the 11q23 region; such probes will indicate whether rearrangement of *KMT2A* has occurred but will not identify the specific gene partner. Dual-fusion FISH probes as well as quantitative polymerase chain reaction (qPCR) assays are available, which detect the most common individual *KMT2A* rearrangements **t47.2**; however, most clinical laboratories do not perform these specific *KMT2A* assays. Karyotype analysis may help to identify the partner if the rearrangement is visible, as in this example case with t(4;11)(q21;q23), indicating *KMT2A-AF4*. Clinically, however, identification of the partner gene is not usually necessary unless follow-up using qPCR for detection of minimal residual disease (MRD) is performed. Recent studies have demonstrated that measurement of MRD has important prognostic implications in both pediatric and adult ALL patients with *KMT2A* rearrangement, indicating that routine use of MRD assays is likely in the near future. Newer NGS-based assays are able to both detect the presence of rearrangement as well as identify the partner gene by using a *KMT2A*-specific primer combined with a random primer, thus amplifying any *KMT2A* rearrangements with subsequent sequencing to identify the partner.

The patient in this case experienced complete remission after induction and consolidation chemotherapy, with no evidence of *KM2TA-AF4* transcripts by qPCR performed on bone marrow 2 and 4 months after diagnosis; she subsequently underwent stem cell transplantation because of her high risk disease.

Diagnostic pearls/pitfalls

– *KMT2A* gene fusions occur across all types of acute leukemia and most of these rearrangements are associated with poor prognosis.

– The t(4;11) *KMT2A-AF4* fusion is the most common *KMT2A* rearrangement in B-ALL and is found in the majority of infant ALL cases.

– *KMT2A* has many possible gene fusion partners which occasionally form cryptic rearrangements (ie, undetectable with conventional karyotyping); therefore, FISH using a break-apart probe for 11q23 is typically recommended for detection.

– Newer assays for detection of *KMT2A* rearrangements include fusion-specific qPCR for the detection of minimal residual disease and NGS-based assays which can identify partner genes by direct sequencing.

Readings

Afrin S, Zhang CRC, Meyer C, et al. Targeted next-generation sequencing for detecting *MLL* gene fusions in leukemia. Mol Cancer Res. 2018;16(2):279-85.
DOI: 10.1158/1541-7786.MCR-17-0569

Esteve J, Giebel S, Labopin M, et al. Allogeneic hematopoietic stem cell transplantation for adult patients with t(4;11)(q21;q23) *KMT2A/AFF1* B-cell precursor acute lymphoblastic leukemia in first complete remission: impact of pretransplant measurable residual disease (MRD) status. An analysis from the Acute Leukemia Working Party of the EBMT [published online ahead of print, 2021 Feb 4]. Leukemia. 2021;10.1038/s41375-021-01135-2. **DOI:10.1038/s41375-021-01135-2**

Gole B, Wiesmüller L. Leukemogenic rearrangements at the mixed lineage leukemia gene (*MLL*)-multiple rather than a single mechanism. Front Cell Dev Biol. 2015;3:41.
DOI: 10.3389/fcell.2015.00041

Meyer C, Burmeister T, Gröger D, et al. The *MLL* recombinome of acute leukemias in 2017. Leukemia. 2018;32(2):273-84.
DOI: 10.1038/leu.2017.213

Moorman AV. The clinical relevance of chromosomal and genomic abnormalities in B-cell precursor acute lymphoblastic leukaemia. Blood Rev. 2012;26(3):123-35.
DOI: 10.1016/j.blre.2012.01.001

Moorman AV. New and emerging prognostic and predictive genetic biomarkers in B-cell precursor acute lymphoblastic leukemia. Haematologica. 2016;101(4):407-16.
DOI: 10.3324/haematol.2015.141101

Sam TN, Kersey JH, Linabery AM, et al. *MLL* gene rearrangements in infant leukemia vary with age at diagnosis and selected demographic factors: a Children's Oncology Group (COG) study. Pediatr Blood Cancer. 2012;58(6):836-9.
DOI: 10.1002/pbc.23274

Stutterheim J, van der Sluis IM, de Lorenzo P, et al. Clinical implications of minimal residual disease detection in infants with *KMT2A*-rearranged acute lymphoblastic leukemia treated on the interfant-06 protocol. J Clin Oncol. 2021;39(6):652-662.
DOI:10.1200/JCO.20.02333

Yokoyama A. Molecular mechanisms of *MLL*-associated leukemia. Int J Hematol. 2015;101(4):352-61.
DOI: 10.1007/s12185-015-1774-4

Howard Meyerson

48

B-lymphoblastic leukemia/lymphoma with t(1;19)(q23;p13.3) *TCF3-PBX1*

History A 12-month-old asymptomatic male was noted incidentally to have leukocytosis on routine peripheral blood counts at his 1-year well-child visit. A repeat CBC and differential was obtained a day later and the results are shown at right.

A bone marrow biopsy with peripheral smear review, as well as flow cytometry and genetic studies, was performed.

Morphology & flow cytometry A peripheral blood smear revealed blasts that were small to medium in size with high nuclear-cytoplasmic ratios, irregular nuclei, and fine chromatin **f48.1**. The bone marrow aspirate demonstrated 65% blasts with morphology similar to that seen in the peripheral blood **f48.2**. The trephine biopsy was 90% cellular with sheets of immature cells consistent with blasts **f48.2**. Flow cytometry revealed a population of blasts that was positive for CD9, CD10 (moderate to bright), CD19, CD22 (dim to moderate), CD38 (moderate to bright), CD45 (dim to negative), HLA-DR, and TDT, and negative for CD13, CD20, CD33, CD34, CD117, and surface light chain **f48.3**. Based on the morphologic and flow cytometry findings, a diagnosis of **B-lymphoblastic leukemia/lymphoma** (**B-ALL**), pending genetic studies, was made.

WBC	37.1×10^9/L
Differential	
Neutrophils	25%
Lymphocytes	47%
Monocytes	3%
Blasts	25%
RBC	3.39×10^{12}/L
HGB	10.2 g/dL
HCT	29.4
MCV	83 fL
RDW	13.2%
Platelets	233×10^9/L

ISBN 978-089189-6814

48 *B-lymphoblastic leukemia/lymphoma with t(1;19)(q23;p13.3) TCF3-PBX1*

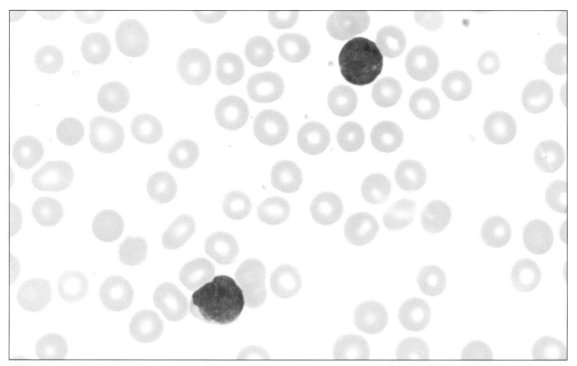

f48.1 Peripheral blood smear demonstrating small to intermediate-sized blasts with high nuclear:cytoplasmic ratio, irregular nuclear contours, fine chromatin & a minimal amount of cytoplasm

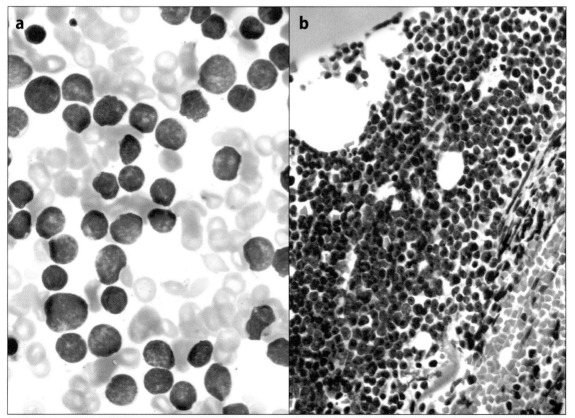

f48.2 **a** Bone marrow aspirate & **b** core biopsy specimens showing numerous blasts similar to those observed in the blood, with loss of normal hematopoiesis

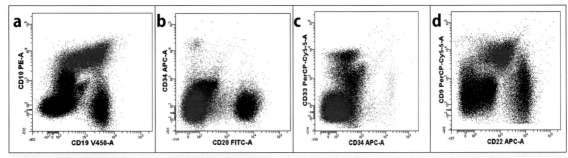

f48.3 Flow cytometry performed on the bone marrow demonstrates a blast population (highlighted in red) that is **a** CD10 and CD19 positive, **b** CD34 and CD20 negative, **c** CD33 negative, and **d** CD22 and CD9 positive

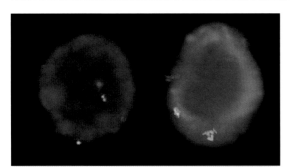

f48.4 Dual-fusion FISH probes for *TCF3* (19p13, green) and *PBX1* (1q23, orange) demonstrating 2 orange, 1 green & 1 yellow signal, consistent with t(1;19)(q23;p13.3) *TCF3-PBX1* with loss of the reciprocal 19p13 region (a typical reciprocal fusion result would demonstrate 1 orange, 1 green, & 2 yellow signals)

Genetics/molecular results Cytogenetics showed 46,XY, der(19)t(1;19)(q23;p13.3) in 3 of 20 metaphases. FISH was positive for *TCF3-PBX1* translocation in 86.8% of 250 interphase cells studied using a dual-fusion probe set **f48.4**. FISH was negative for hyperdiploidy of chromosomes 4, 10 or 17, t(9;22) *BCR-ABL1*, t(12;21) *ETV6-RUNX1*, amplification of *RUNX1* (iAMP21) and *KMT2A* (*MLL*) rearrangement. The genetic findings indicated a final diagnosis of **B-lymphoblastic leukemia/lymphoma with t(1;19)(q23;p13.3)** *TCF3-PBX1*.

Discussion The diagnosis of B-ALL is not especially difficult in this case. However, accurate subclassification requires genetic studies, which revealed a der(19)t(1;19)(q23;p13.3). Based on age alone (12 months) the expected genetic finding in this patient was actually rearrangement of *KMT2A* (*MLL*), t(v:11q23.3), specifically t(4;11), which is the most common recurrent genetic finding in infant (<1 year of age) B-ALL. Notably, however, the immunophenotype of the blasts in this case was atypical for a t(v:11q23.3) translocation, being positive for CD10 and lacking myeloid antigen expression (see also **Case 47**).

Although B-ALL with t(1;19)(q23;p13.3) *TCF3-PBX1* does not demonstrate any specific morphology, the phenotype of the blasts in this B-ALL subtype is rather unique in that the blasts have a more mature pre-B phenotype rather than the typical pro-B phenotype of other B-ALL subtypes. These blasts commonly lack CD34 and demonstrate cytoplasmic IgM expression (however, in some cases cytoplasmic IgM expression is absent, and other B-ALLs subtypes may also demonstrate a pre-B cell phenotype). The myeloid antigens CD13 and CD33 are usually absent in B-ALL with *TCF3-PBX1*, while CD123 is generally weak or not detected, and CD9 is almost always uniformly expressed. Bcl-6 expression (detected by IHC) has been noted in a high percentage of cases and may serve to distinguish B-ALL with *TCF3-PBX1* from other subtypes. Expression of bcl-6, however, in the absence of CD34, may lead to confusion with high-grade B-cell lymphomas of germinal center cell origin. The phenotype in the present case fit well with t(1;19) (q23;p13.3) B-ALL as the cells were negative for CD13, CD33, and CD34 and positive for CD9. Interestingly, a monoclonal antibody is available that detects the *TCF3-PBX1* fusion protein, although it is not routinely used clinically.

The t(1;19)(q23;p13.3) translocation is 1 of 4 common recurring translocations in B-ALL, with the others being t(12;21) *ETV6-RUNX1*, t(9;22) *BCR-ABL1*, and t(v;11) *KMT2A* rearranged. The t(1;19) translocation is less common, observed in approximately 3%-5% of children and 6% of adult cases. As opposed to B-ALL with *ETV6-RUNX1* or *KMT2A* rearrangement, B-ALL with *TCF3-PBX1* does not appear to arise in utero based on Guthrie card studies. In addition, the incidence of B-ALL with *TCF3-PBX1* is uniform throughout childhood and does not show the early childhood peak observed with B-ALL with *ETV6-RUNX1* or hyperdiploidy.

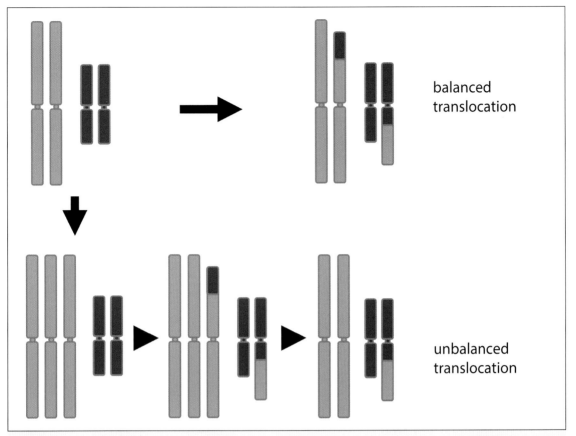

f48.5 Balanced (top) & unbalanced (bottom) translocations observed with the *TCF3-PBX1* fusion resulting from t(1;19)(q23;p13.3). The translocation results in fusion of the long arm of chromosome 1 (blue) with the short arm of chromosome 19 (red) creating a derivative chromosome 19 [der(19)] & derivative chromosome 1 [der(1)]. In the balanced translocation, both derivative chromosomes are present. The unbalanced translocation arises after duplication of 1 of the 2 copies of chromosome 1 (bottom left) & subsequent loss of derivative chromosome 1 after the translocation has occurred (bottom right). This results in triploidy for a portion of the long arm of chromosome 1 & monosomy for a portion of the short arm of chromosome 19

The t(1;19)(q23;p13.3) translocation leads to the fusion of the *TCF3* (formally *E2A*) and *PBX1* genes. In most cases, exons 1-16 in *TCF3* are fused to exons 4-9 in *PBX1*; this fusion is amenable to PCR amplification and detection. However, in some circumstances, the fusion results in the use of an alternative breakpoint in intron 4 of *PBX1*, which is not detectable using the standard primers for t(1;19). At the chromosomal level, the translocation occurs in 2 forms: balanced and unbalanced, with the unbalanced form seen in most cases. In balanced t(1;19), both a der(1) and a der(19) are present along with a normal chromosome 1 and normal chromosome 19, whereas in the unbalanced form, only the der(19) is present along with 2 normal chromosomes 1 and a single normal chromosome 19 **f48.5**. The latter results in partial trisomy for the distal end of the long arm of chromosome 1 (1q23->1qter) and monosomy for the distal end of the short arm of chromosome 19 (19p13.3->19pter). In rare cases,

the 2 structural forms can be present as a mosaic. The unbalanced form appears to originate from an initial trisomy of chromosome 1 followed by acquisition of the t(1;19) and subsequent loss of the derivative chromosome 1.

Rare B-ALLs may have a t(1;19) without fusion of *TCF3* and *PBX1* and should not be misconstrued as B-ALL with (1;19)(q23;p13.3) *TCF3-PBX1*. In addition, *TCF3* fusion with the *HLF* gene on chromosome 17 has been described in B-ALL resulting in a t(17;19)(q21-q22;p13). These very rare B-ALLs are associated with hypercalcemia, coagulopathy, and an extremely poor prognosis.

PBX1 (pre-B-cell leukemia homeobox-1) is an atypical homeodomain transcription factor involved in the activation of a wide array of genes related to development and cell differentiation. *TCF3* encodes

2 proteins, E12 and E47 via alternative splicing, which are basic helix-loop-helix transcription factors that play critical roles in B-cell maturation. The TCF3/PBX1 fusion protein causes constitutive nuclear localization of PBX1, resulting in activation of multiple pathways including those related to Notch, mTOR, JAK/STAT, AuroraB kinase, and the B-cell receptor.

The t(1;19)(q23;p13.3) translocation in children was initially felt to be an unfavorable prognostic factor, particularly for the balanced form; however, more recent studies of patients receiving newer therapeutics indicate that the translocation is now associated with standard risk prognosis in children and adults. However, patients with this translocation do appear to have an increased risk of central nervous system relapse, possibly because of uniquely high surface level expression of the Mer tyrosine kinase on t(1;19)(q23;p13.3) blasts and/or upregulation of PBX1 after interaction with the choroid plexus leading to enhanced cell survival.

Additional cytogenetic abnormalities are observed in ~2/3 of cases with no significant differences between unbalanced and balanced cases. The most common secondary abnormalities result in deletion of *CDKN2A* (34%-42%) on chromosome 9p either via del(9p) or i(9q). These additional cytogenetic aberrations do not impact survival.

The patient in this case was treated using a standard risk Children's Oncology Group protocol and went into remission without evidence of minimal residual disease in a bone marrow biopsy specimen taken on day 29; the patient continues to show no evidence of disease 1 year after diagnosis.

Diagnostic pearls/pitfalls

– B-ALL with t(1;19) *TCF3-PBX1* frequently has a pre-B phenotype lacking CD34 and expressing cytoplasmic IgM. The lymphoblasts in this disease do not have a specific morphologic appearance, and diagnosis requires detection with karyotyping, FISH, or PCR, although PCR may be negative in cases with a variant breakpoint in the *PBX1* gene.
– B-ALL with t(1;19) *TCF3-PBX1* may contain a balanced or unbalanced translocation, both detectable with karyotyping, with no significant outcome differences with current therapies.
– With modern B-ALL chemotherapy regimens, the presence of *TCF3-PBX1* is considered a standard risk cytogenetic feature, although there may be an increased incidence of CNS relapse.

Readings

Alsadeq A, Schewe DM. Acute lymphoblastic leukemia of the central nervous system: on the role of *PBX1*. Haematologica. 2017;102(4):611-3. **DOI: 10.3324/haematol.2017.165142**

Andersen MK, Autio K, Barbany G, et al. Paediatric B-cell precursor acute lymphoblastic leukaemia with t(1;19)(q23;p13): clinical and cytogenetic characteristics of 47 cases from the Nordic countries treated according to NOPHO protocols. Br J Haematol. 2011;155(2):235-43.
DOI: 10.1111/j.1365-2141.2011.08824.x

Blasi F, Bruckmann C, Penkov D, Dardaei L. A tale of *TALE, PREP1, PBX1*, and *MEIS1*: interconnections and competition in cancer. Bioessays. 2017;39(5). **DOI: 10.1002/bies.201600245.**

Burmeister T, Gökbuget N, Schwartz S, et al. Clinical features and prognostic implications of *TCF3-PBX1* and *ETV6-RUNX1* in adult acute lymphoblastic leukemia. Haematologica. 2010;95(2):241-6. **DOI: 10.3324/haematol.2009.011346**

Deucher AM, Qi Z, Yu J, et al. BCL6 expression correlates with the t(1;19) translocation in B-lymphoblastic leukemia. Am J Clin Pathol. 2015;143(4):547-57. **DOI: 10.1309/ AJCPO4U4VYAAOTEL**

Forestier E, Schmiegelow K. The incidence peaks of the childhood acute leukemias reflect specific cytogenetic aberrations. J Pediatr Hematol Oncol. 2006;28(8):486-95.
DOI: 10.1097/01.mph.0000212972.90877.28

Gaynes JS, Jonart LM, Zamora EA, et al. The central nervous system microenvironment influences the leukemia transcriptome and enhances leukemia chemo-resistance. Haematologica. 2017;102(4):e136-9.
DOI: 10.3324/haematol.2016.152926

Inukai T, Hirose K, Inaba T, et al. Hypercalcemia in childhood acute lymphoblastic leukemia: frequent implication of parathyroid hormone-related peptide and *E2A-HLF* from translocation 17;19. Leukemia. 2007;21(2):288-96.
DOI: 10.1038/sj.leu.2404496

Izraeli S, Henn T, Strobl H, et al. Expression of identical *E2A/PBX1* fusion transcripts occurs in both pre-B and early pre-B immunological subtypes of childhood acute lymphoblastic leukemia. Leukemia. 1993;7(12):2054-6. **PMID: 8255105**

Krause S, Pfeiffer C, Strube S, et al. Mer tyrosine kinase promotes the survival of t(1;19)-positive acute lymphoblastic leukemia (ALL) in the central nervous system (CNS). Blood. 2015;125(5):820-30.
DOI: 10.1182/blood-2014-06-583062

Lin CH, Wang Z, Duque-Afonso J, et al. Oligomeric self-association contributes to E2A-PBX1-mediated oncogenesis. Sci Rep. 2019;9(1):4915. **DOI: 10.1038/s41598-019-41393-w**

Malouf C, Ottersbach K. Molecular processes involved in B cell acute lymphoblastic leukaemia. Cell Mol Life Sci. 2018;75(3):417-46.
DOI: 10.1007/s00018-017-2620-z

Mrózek K, Harper DP, Aplan PD. Cytogenetics and molecular genetics of acute lymphoblastic leukemia. Hematol Oncol Clin North Am. 2009;23(5):991-1010.
DOI: 10.1016/j.hoc.2009.07.001

Paulsson K, Horvat A, Fioretos T, et al. Formation of der(19) t(1;19)(q23;p13) in acute lymphoblastic leukemia. Genes Chromosomes Cancer. 2005;42(2):144-8.
DOI: 10.1002/gcc.20133

Pui CH, Raimondi SC, Hancock ML, et al. Immunologic, cytogenetic, and clinical characterization of childhood acute lymphoblastic leukemia with the t(1;19) (q23; p13) or its derivative. J Clin Oncol. 1994;12(12):2601-6.
DOI: 10.1200/JCO.1994.12.12.2601

Sang BC, Shi L, Dias P, et al. Monoclonal antibodies specific to the acute lymphoblastic leukemia t(1;19)-associated E2A/pbx1 chimeric protein: characterization and diagnostic utility. Blood. 1997;89(8):2909-14. **PMID: 9108411**

Tsagarakis NJ, Papadhimitriou SI, Pavlidis D, et al. Flow cytometric predictive scoring systems for common fusions *ETV6/RUNX1, BCR/ABL1, TCF3/PBX1* and rearrangements of the *KMT2A* gene, proposed for the initial cytogenetic approach in cases of B-acute lymphoblastic leukemia. Int J Lab Hematol. 2019;41(3):364-72. **DOI: 10.1111/ijlh.12983**

Wiemels JL, Leonard BC, Wang Y, et al. Site-specific translocation and evidence of postnatal origin of the t(1;19) *E2A-PBX1* fusion in childhood acute lymphoblastic leukemia. Proc Natl Acad Sci U S A. 2002;99(23):15101-6. **DOI: 10.1073/pnas.222481199**

Rose C Beck

49

B-lymphoblastic leukemia/lymphoma with iAMP21

History A 4-year-old female presented with a 2 week history of cervical lymphadenopathy and fevers. A CBC was ordered and results are shown at right.

A peripheral blood smear review was performed.

Morphology & flow cytometry The blood smear showed 25% blasts that appeared lymphoid, with fine chromatin and high nuclear:cytoplasmic ratios **f49.1**. A bone marrow biopsy was performed, and the aspirate smear and core biopsy showed sheets of blasts, which were medium to large in size **f49.2**, similar to those seen in blood. Flow cytometry demonstrated B lymphoblasts that expressed CD10, CD19, CD22, CD34, HLA-DR, and TdT. The morphologic and immunophenotypic findings indicated a diagnosis of **B-lymphoblastic leukemia/lymphoma** (**B-ALL**), with final subclassification pending genetic studies.

WBC	3.1×10^9/L
Differential	
Neutrophils	9%
Lymphocytes	59%
Monocytes	1%
Eosinophils	2%
Metamyelocytes	1%
Myelocytes	3%
Blasts	25%
HGB	10.9 g/dL
Platelets	62×10^9/L

ISBN 978-089189-6814

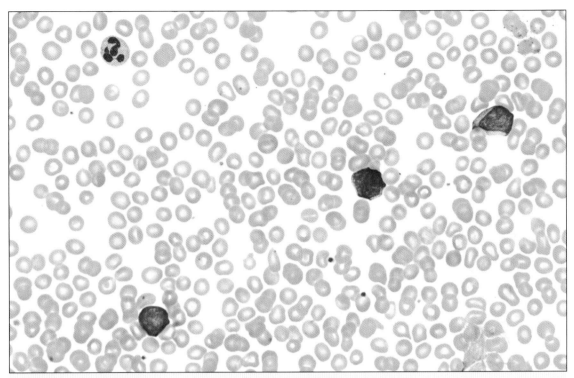

f49.1 Blasts identified in blood appear lymphoid, with a high nuclear:cytoplasmic ratio & fine chromatin

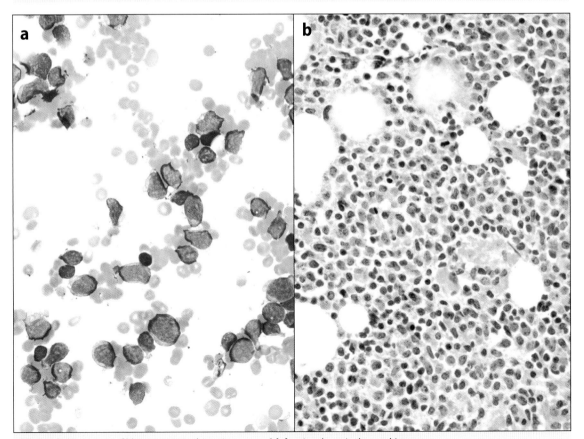

f49.2 **a** Predominance of blasts present in the aspirate smear & **b** forming sheets in the core biopsy

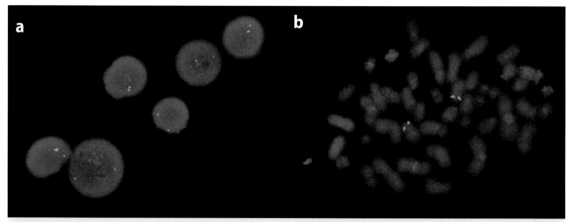

f49.3 Dual-fusion FISH probes for *ETV6* (12p13, green) & *RUNX1* (21q22, orange) do not show an *ETV6-RUNX1* translocation but **a** demonstrate many copies of *RUNX1*, noted to be on the same chromosome by **b** metaphase FISH

Genetics/molecular results A B-ALL FISH panel was negative for hyperdiploidy, rearrangement of 11q23 *KMT2A (MLL)*, and the recurrent translocations t(12;21) *ETV6-RUNX1*, t(9;22) *BCR-ABL1*, and t(1;19) *TCF3-PBX1*. However, multiple copies of the *RUNX1* (21q22) probe were present, notably clustered on one chromosome as seen on metaphase FISH **f49.3**, consistent with intrachromosomal amplification of 21. Karyotype analysis revealed additional material attached to the short arm of chromosome 21: 46,XX,add(21) (p11.2)[12]/46,XX[8].

Based on the genetic findings, a final diagnosis of **B-lymphoblastic leukemia/lymphoma with iAMP21** was rendered.

Discussion Unfavorable genetic risk factors for childhood B-ALL include hypodiploidy (<44 chromosomes), *KM2TA (MLL)* rearrangement, t(9;22)(q34;q11) *BCR-ABL1*, complex karyotype (≥5 chromosomal abnormalities), *BCR-ABL1*-like genetics, and intrachromosomal amplification of 21 (iAMP21) **t49.1**. B-ALL with iAMP21 comprises ~2% of all pediatric B-ALL cases and typically presents with lower WBC counts (median 5×10^9/L) in older children, with median age of 9 years. Cases of pediatric B-ALL with iAMP21 have a high relapse rate with standard-risk chemotherapy and fare significantly better when treated with high-risk regimens; therefore, identification of this particular chromosomal abnormality is essential for appropriate risk stratification.

t49.1 Recurrent genetic abnormalities in pediatric B-lymphoblastic leukemia/lymphoma with associated prognosis

Genetic finding	Prognosis
t(12;21) *ETV6-RUNX1*	favorable
hyperdiploidy (51-65 chromosomes)	favorable
t(1;19) *TCF3-PBX1*	intermediate
t(9;22) *BCR-ABL1*	unfavorable (historical)*
BCR-ABL1-like genetics	unfavorable
iAMP21	unfavorable
rearrangement of *KMT2A*	unfavorable
hypodiploidy (<46 chromosomes)	unfavorable

With the advent of tyrosine kinase inhibitor therapy, prognosis for these patients has improved, though high-risk treatment protocols are still required

The most reliable method for detection of iAMP21 is FISH using a probe for *RUNX1* on 21q22, and iAMP21 is defined by the presence of multiple copies (at least 5) of the *RUNX1* probe within the same cell or ≥3 copies on the same chromosome. Extra copies of *RUNX1* (usually ≤4) resulting from aneuploidy of chromosome 21 (eg, as in hyperdiploid cases) do not constitute iAMP21. Thus, FISH alone is only reliable when metaphase analysis is available to delineate the nature of extra *RUNX1* signals. In the absence of metaphase FISH analysis, additional FISH probes or karyotype analysis should be used to exclude the presence of multiple intact copies of chromosome 21.

iAMP21 is considered a primary cytogenetic abnormality caused by multiple breakage-fusion-bridge cycles in an unstable portion of chromosome 21, resulting in a complex structure with gains, inversions, and deletions. A common region of highest-level amplification has been identified, spanning a 5.1 Mb portion of chromosome 21 and including the *RUNX1* gene, which encodes for the protein, runt-related transcription factor 1 (RUNX1). RUNX1 is part of the core binding factor transcription complex, critical for the normal development of hematopoietic stem cells, and aberrations in this gene are found in both ALL and acute myeloid leukemia (AML). However, the role of amplification of this region in the disease pathogenesis of B-ALL is still unclear; RUNX1 itself has not been implicated since expression levels of RUNX1 in cells with iAMP21 are not elevated. Recent investigation has identified several other candidate genes in the amplified region, which do exhibit RNA overexpression compared to other B-ALL subtypes. Other genetic abnormalities also likely play a role in pathogenesis, since genomic analysis of 94 cases of B-ALL with iAMP21 identified deletions in genes involved in key B-cell pathways such as *IKZF1, CDKN2A/B, PAX5, ETV6, RB1*, and *SH2B3*, as well as *CRLF2* rearrangements (which are also found in *BCR-ABL1*-like B-ALL).

Other chromosomal abnormalities are typically present with iAMP21; in the largest published series of 530 cases, iAMP21 as the sole cytogenetic change was found in only 20%. Often there is loss of the normal chromosome 21 and/or gain of X. iAMP21 appears to be mutually exclusive of *KMT2A* (*MLL*) rearrangements and rearrangements of *TCF3* such as t(1;19) *TCF3-PBX1*. However, rare cases (<1%) do harbor a recurrent translocation such as t(9;22) *BCR-ABL* or are associated with high hyperdiploidy.

The patient in this case suffered multiple relapses and refractory disease, despite intensive therapy including hematopoietic stem cell transplantation, and succumbed to her disease 4 years after initial diagnosis.

Diagnostic pearls/pitfalls

– Intrachromosomal amplification of 21 is defined as the presence of at least 3 *RUNX1* (21q22) signals on the same chromosome 21, as detected on metaphase FISH, and is distinct from multiple FISH probe signals present due to hyperdiploidy.

– Because of a high risk of relapse using standard-risk chemotherapy protocols, identification of iAMP21 in B-ALL patients is critical for appropriate treatment with more intensive regimens.

– Although very rare, other B-ALL-associated translocations can occur with iAMP21 and these cases are also associated with poor prognosis.

Readings

Ivanov Öfverholm I, Zachariadis V, Taylan F, et al. Overexpression of chromatin remodeling and tyrosine kinase genes in iAMP21-positive acute lymphoblastic leukemia. Leuk Lymphoma. 2020; 61(3):604-613. **DOI:10.1080/10428194.2019.1678153**

Baughn LB, Meredith MM, Oseth L, et al. *SH2B3* aberrations enriched in iAMP21 B lymphoblastic leukemia. Cancer Genet. 2018;226-7:30-5. **DOI: 10.1016/j.cancergen.2018.05.004**

Johnson RC, Weinberg OK, Cascio MJ, et al. Cytogenetic variation of B-lymphoblastic leukemia with intrachromosomal amplification of chromosome 21 (iAMP21): a multi-institutional series review. Am J Clin Pathol. 2015;144(1):103-12. **DOI: 10.1309/AJCPLUYF11HQBYRB**

Harrison CJ, Moorman AV, Schwab C, et al; Ponte di Legno International Workshop in Childhood Acute Lymphoblastic Leukemia. An international study of intrachromosomal amplification of chromosome 21 (iAMP21): cytogenetic characterization and outcome. Leukemia. 2014;28(5):1015-21. **DOI: 10.1038/leu.2013.317**

Heerema NA, Carroll AJ, Devidas M, et al. Intrachromosomal amplification of chromosome 21 is associated with inferior outcomes in children with acute lymphoblastic leukemia treated in contemporary standard-risk children's oncology group studies: a report from the children's oncology group. J Clin Oncol. 2013;31(27):3397-402. **DOI: 10.1200/JCO.2013.49.1308**

Rand V, Parker H, Russell LJ, et al. Genomic characterization implicates iAMP21 as a likely primary genetic event in childhood B-cell precursor acute lymphoblastic leukemia. Blood. 2011;117(25):6848-55. **DOI: 10.1200/JCO.2013.49.1308**

Robinson HM, Harrison CJ, Moorman AV, et al. Intrachromosomal amplification of chromosome 21 (iAMP21) may arise from a breakage-fusion-bridge cycle. Genes Chromosomes Cancer. 2007;46(4):318-26. **DOI: 10.1002/gcc.20412**

Megan O Nakashima & Erika M Moore

50

B-lymphoblastic leukemia/lymphoma with t(9;22)(q34.1;q11.2) *BCR-ABL1*

History A 22-year-old woman who was previously healthy presented to her primary care physician with increasing fatigue. CBC results are shown at right.

WBC	9.4×10^9/L
HGB	8.2 g/dL
HCT	25.2%
MCV	94 fL
Platelets	70×10^9/L

Review of the peripheral blood smear demonstrated circulating blasts, which prompted a bone marrow biopsy.

Morphology & flow cytometry The blood smear showed anemia and thrombocytopenia as well as circulating blasts (42%) with variable morphology; some were small with scant cytoplasm and inconspicuous nucleoli **f50.1**, while others were intermediate-sized to large with moderate cytoplasm and prominent nucleoli. The cytoplasm did not show Auer rods.

The cellular bone marrow aspirate smears showed 70% blasts, some with azurophilic granules. Erythropoiesis and granulopoiesis were markedly decreased. The trephine core and clot sections were nearly 100% cellular due to the presence of many mononuclear cells consistent with blasts **f50.2**. Trilineage hematopoiesis was markedly reduced.

Flow cytometry showed 65% atypical B lymphoblasts that were positive for CD34, CD10 (bright), CD13 (heterogeneous), CD33 (partial), CD15 (partial dim), CD7 (partial), and CD19 **f50.3**; the blasts were also positive for TdT and negative for myeloperoxidase. CD34 IHC was also performed and confirmed the blasts accounted for 60%-70% of cellularity. Based on the morphologic and flow cytometry findings, a diagnosis of **B-lymphoblastic leukemia/lymphoma** was rendered, with final classification pending genetic studies.

Genetics/molecular results A B-ALL FISH panel was negative for t(12;21) *ETV6-RUNX1*, *KMT2A* (*MLL*) rearrangement, t(1;19) *TCF3-PBX1*, and hyperdiploidy of chromosomes 4, 10, and 17, but positive for t(9;22) *BCR-ABL1* using dual-fusion probes **f50.4a**. The t(9;22)(q34.1;q11.2) was detected by karyotype analysis, which also showed monosomy 7 and inversion duplication within the long arm of chromosome 8 at breakpoints q13 and q24.1 **f50.4b**. Based on the genetic findings, a final diagnosis of **B-lymphoblastic leukemia/lymphoma with t(9;22)(q34.1;q11.2)** *BCR-ABL1* was rendered.

Discussion The t(9;22)(q34.1;q11.2) translocation resulting in the Philadelphia chromosome is present in ~25% of adult B-ALL and 2%-4% of pediatric cases. Such cases are referred to as Philadelphia chromosome-positive B-ALL (Ph+ B-ALL). The clinical presentation and morphology are similar to other B-ALLs, although extramedullary disease is less common. By immunophenotyping, the lymphoblasts in Ph+ B-ALL are typically positive for CD10, CD19, and TdT, with frequent expression of the myeloid antigens CD13 and CD33, as seen in this case. Blasts may also express CD25 (~50%) or CD66c (~80%).

ISBN 978-089189-6814   ©2021 ASCP

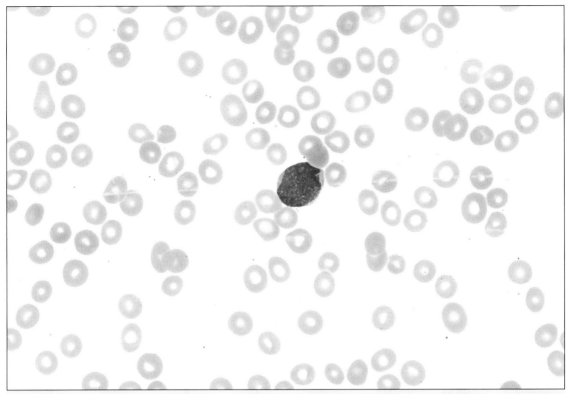

f50.1 Peripheral blood smear showing a circulating blast in a background of anemia & thrombocytopenia

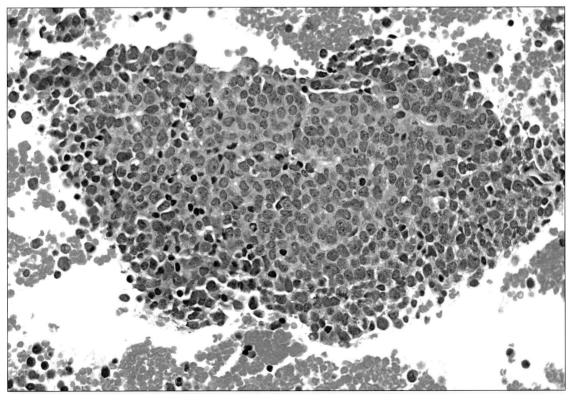

f50.2 The clot section contains sheets of mononuclear cells with fine chromatin & small nucleoli; residual hematopoiesis is virtually absent

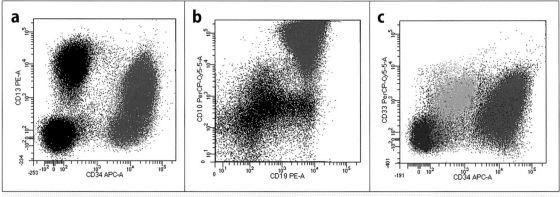

f50.3 Flow cytometry performed on the bone marrow demonstrates a CD34-positive blast population (highlighted in purple) with **a** heterogeneous CD13 expression, **b** bright CD10 & CD19 expression, & **c** partial CD33 expression; monocytes (green) & lymphocytes (red) are shown for comparison in **c**

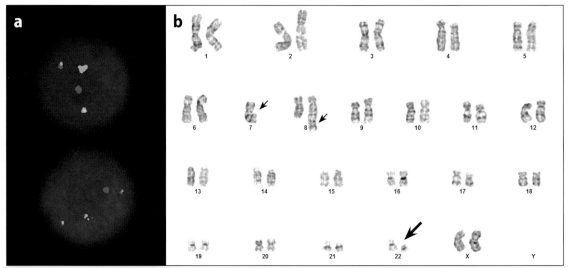

f50.4 a FISH using dual-fusion probes shows reciprocal translocation between *ABL1* at 9q34 (orange) & *BCR* at 22q11 (green); **b** karyotype analysis demonstrates the Philadelphia chromosome (large arrow) as well as monosomy 7 & an inversion duplication in the long arm of chromosome 8 (small arrows)

The translocation results in the same gene fusion seen in chronic myeloid leukemia (CML), with *BCR* fused to the tyrosine kinase gene *ABL1*. The same breakpoints are also used; adult cases are split approximately equally between the minor breakpoint (producing the p190 protein) and the major one (producing p210), while most childhood cases have the p190 fusion protein (see **Case 1** for detailed discussion of these breakpoints). As in CML, quantitative assessment of these transcripts by qRT-PCR can be used to assess treatment response and monitor disease. Also similar to CML, cases of Ph+ B-ALL can harbor the *ABL1* T315I kinase domain mutation that confers resistance to tyrosine kinase inhibitors (TKIs). Interestingly, deep sequencing has shown that resistance mutations are present at low levels even at onset of disease, so currently there is no consensus on when to test for these mutations.

Historically, cases of Ph+ B-ALL carried the worst prognosis among B-ALL cytogenetic subtypes. The development of TKIs has greatly affected prognosis in these patients. TKIs are now used in frontline therapy in conjunction with standard chemotherapeutic drugs and may alleviate a requirement for allogeneic stem cell transplantation. With these newer regimens, overall survival of patients with Ph+ B-ALL may approach those with more favorable risk B-ALL. Cases with the T315I mutation, which are resistant to frontline TKIs, may respond to the newer generation inhibitor, ponatinib.

Studies using high-resolution SNP arrays have identified deletions in the *IKZF1* (IKAROS zinc finger protein 1) gene in 75% of pediatric and 91% of adult Ph+ B-ALL cases. Interestingly, these are not found in chronic phase CML but are present in some cases of CML with B-lymphoid blast crisis. *IKZF1* deletions or mutations are also highly enriched in Ph-like (or *BCR-ABL1*-like) B-ALL (see **Case 51**) vs other B-ALL subtypes and are an independent risk factor for poor prognosis. IKAROS family proteins are key transcriptional regulators in B-lymphoid development; they act as tumor suppressors that bind DNA directly through a zinc-finger domain. Normal IKZF1 promotes B-cell differentiation, but in mutated cases there is decreased activity either due to reduced expression or expression of dominant-negative isoforms. Decreased tumor suppressor activity of IKZF1 supports leukemogenesis via multiple pathways. There is increased expression of signal transducers cKIT, FLT3, and IL7R, which drive early lymphoid development, and cell proliferation is encouraged via increased expression of THY1, BCL6 and cMYC, with decreased expression of CDKN1A/2A. The leukemic cells also have a growth advantage because of increased expression of cell surface receptors such as CD34 and CD43. Decreased IKZF1 activity also confers a metabolic advantage, increasing proteins involved in glucose transportation and metabolism. In addition to their role in leukemogenesis, aberrations in *IKZF1* are also associated with resistance to TKI therapy; this is thought to be related to decreased expression of adhesion molecules and expression/activity of the adhesion regulator FAK, although the exact mechanism has not yet been determined. Additional studies have confirmed the adverse prognostic significance of this lesion, especially accompanied by mutations in *CDKN2A/B* and/or *PAX5*. Structural lesions resulting in loss of the short arm of chromosome 9 also confer a worse prognosis in Ph+ B-ALL, while high hyperdiploidy may be protective.

Current research is ongoing to determine the importance of minimal residual disease and best methods for detection in Ph+ B-ALL. Molecular methods include qRT-PCR detection of the *BCR-ABL1* transcript or NGS assays that identify and follow disease-specific immunoglobulin gene rearrangements. Flow cytometry is also often used and comprehensive immunophenotyping in general will remain important in this disease as antibodies and cellular therapies targeted against B-cell antigens are added to current treatment regimens.

Diagnostic pearls/pitfalls

- B-lymphoblastic leukemia/lymphoma with t(9;22)(q34.1;q11.2) *BCR-ABL1* is a distinct cytogenetic subtype of B-ALL, which comprises roughly 25% of adult B-ALL, but <5% of pediatric cases.
- Although there is no unique morphology for Ph+ B-ALL, the blasts in this disorder typically have expression of the myeloid antigens CD13 and CD33. CD25 may also be expressed.
- The *BCR-ABL1* fusion is a targetable genetic alteration and outcomes are greatly improved with tyrosine kinase inhibitor therapy, so all new cases of B-ALL should be tested for this translocation.
- The presence of *BCR-ABL1* allows for the use of qRT-PCR for monitoring of minimal residual disease.
- Deletions or mutations in *IKZF1* are highly prevalent in *BCR-ABL1*-positive B-ALL and contribute both to disease pathogenesis and resistance to therapy.

Readings

Fedullo AL, Messina M, Elia L, et al. Prognostic implications of additional genomic lesions in adult Philadelphia chromosome-positive acute lymphoblastic leukemia. Haematologica. 2019;104(2):312-8. **DOI: 10.3324/haematol.2018.196055**

Fielding AK. 2019. Curing Ph+ ALL: assessing the relative contributions of chemotherapy, TKIs, and allogeneic stem cell transplant. Hematology. 2019(1):24-29. **DOI: 10.1182/hematology.2019000010**

Hrusak O, Porwitt-MacDonald A. Antigen expression patterns reflecting genotype of acute leukemias. Leukemia. 2002;16(7):1233-58. **DOI: 10.1038/sj.leu.2402504**

Marke R, van Leeuwen FN, Scheijen B. The many faces of *IKZF1* in B-cell precursor acute lymphoblastic leukemia. Haematologica. 2018;103(4):565-74. **DOI: 10.3324/haematol.2017.185603**

Mullighan CG, Miller CB, Radtke I, et al. *BCR-ABL1* lymphoblastic leukaemia is characterized by the deletion of Ikaros. Nature. 2008;453(7191):110-4. **DOI: 10.1038/nature06866.**

Mulligan CG, Su X, Zhang J, et al. Deletion of *IKZF1* and prognosis in acute lymphoblastic leukemia. N Engl J Med. 2009;360(5):470-80. **DOI: 10.1056/NEJMoa0808253**

Schultz KR, Carroll A, Heerema NA, et al. Long-term follow-up of imatinib in pediatric Philadelphia chromosome-positive acute lymphoblastic leukemia: Children's Oncology Group study AALL0031. Leukemia. 2014;28(7):1467-71. **DOI: 10.1038/leu.2014.30**

Yilmaz M, Kantarjian H, Ravandi-Kashani F, et al. Philadelphia chromosome-positive acute lymphoblastic leukemia in adults: current treatments and future perspectives. Clin Adv Hematol Oncol. 2018;16(3):216-23. **PMID: 29742077**

Christopher Ryder

51

B-lymphoblastic leukemia/lymphoma *BCR-ABL1*-like, with *P2YR8-CRLF2*

History A 4-year-old female with no pertinent medical history presented with fever, body aches, and lower extremity petechiae. Physical examination also revealed cervical lymphadenopathy and splenomegaly. Selected CBC results are shown at right. A peripheral blood smear was performed.

Morphology & flow cytometry The blood smear showed thrombocytopenia, normocytic anemia with circulating nucleated red blood cells, and marked leukocytosis consisting predominantly of intermediate-sized to large blasts with irregular nuclear contours, finely dispersed chromatin, inconspicuous nucleoli, and a minimal amount of cytoplasm **f51.1**. A bone marrow biopsy was performed, and the aspirate smears demonstrated approximately 90% blasts; the core biopsy was essentially 100% cellular with sheets of blasts and minimal residual hematopoiesis **f51.2**.

Flow cytometry performed on the peripheral blood revealed 88% blasts that were positive for CD45 (dim), CD34, HLA-DR, CD10 (moderate to bright), CD19, CD20 (dim partial), CD22, TdT (partial), CD9, and CD38 (moderate), and negative for CD117, CD13, CD15, CD33, and surface light chain **f51.3**. Additional flow cytometric studies demonstrated partial expression of cytokine receptor-like factor 2 (CRLF2; see Discussion). Immunohistochemistry was not performed. The overall findings supported a **diagnosis of B-lymphoblastic leukemia/lymphoma** (**B-ALL**), with final WHO classification pending results of genetic testing.

Genetics/molecular results Cytogenetic evaluation produced 10 interpretable metaphase cells. The karyotype was as follows: 46,XX,dic(9;20) (p13.2;q11.2),+21[5]/47,idem,+20[3]/46,XX[2]

WBC	139.4 × 10⁹/L
Differential	
Neutrophils	2%
Lymphocytes	6%
Blasts	92%
HGB	6.2 g/dL
Platelets	22 × 10⁹/L

f51.4. Initial FISH studies identified deletion of 9p21 and gain of 21q22 and were negative for t(1;19) *TCF3-PBX*, t(9;22) *BCR-ABL1*, t(12;21) *ETV6-RUNX1*, *KMT2A* (*MLL*) rearrangement, and hyperdiploidy of chromosomes 4, 10, or 17. Following the karyotype results, confirmatory FISH studies using centromeric probes for chromosomes 9 and 20 confirmed fusion of the 2 centromeric probe signals consistent with dic(9;20) **f51.5**.

Because no defining cytogenetic aberration was found by karyotype or standard B-ALL FISH, a portion of the bone marrow aspirate was sent for Philadelphia (Ph)-like B-ALL testing. A low-density array (LDA) for gene expression was positive for a Ph-like gene signature with high CRLF2 expression, consistent with the CRLF2 positivity observed by flow cytometry. Subsequent testing identified a *P2YR8-CRLF2* fusion transcript. Based on these results, mutation analysis of *JAK1*, *JAK2*, and *IL7R* was performed and a pathogenic variant in *JAK2* (p.Arg683Ser) and a likely pathogenic variant in *IL7R* (c.730-731insTGTGCCTAA p.Leu243_Thr244insMetCysLeu) were detected. The combined morphologic and genetic findings established a final diagnosis of **B-lymphoblastic leukemia/lymphoma, *BCR-ABL1*-like**.

ISBN 978-089189-6814

51 *B-lymphoblastic leukemia/lymphoma BCR-ABL1-like, with P2YR8-CRLF2*

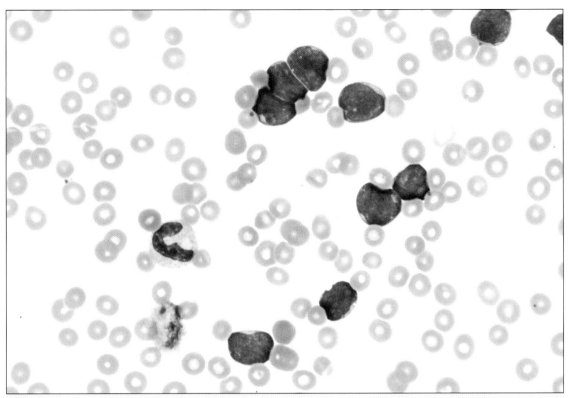

f51.1 The peripheral blood demonstrates many intermediate-sized to large blasts with irregular nuclear contours, fine chromatin & a minimal amount of cytoplasm

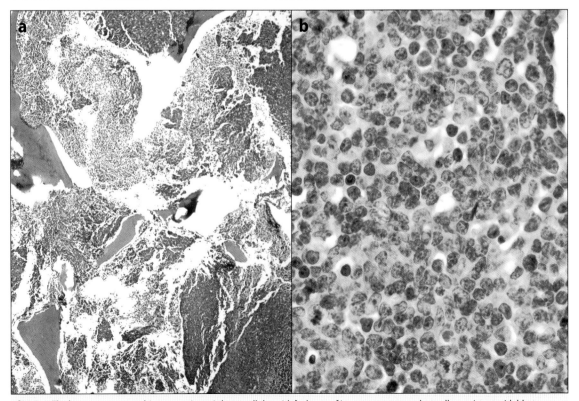

f51.2 **a** The bone marrow core biopsy specimen is hypercellular with **b** sheets of immature mononuclear cells consistent with blasts

51 *B-lymphoblastic leukemia/lymphoma BCR-ABL1-like, with P2YR8-CRLF2*

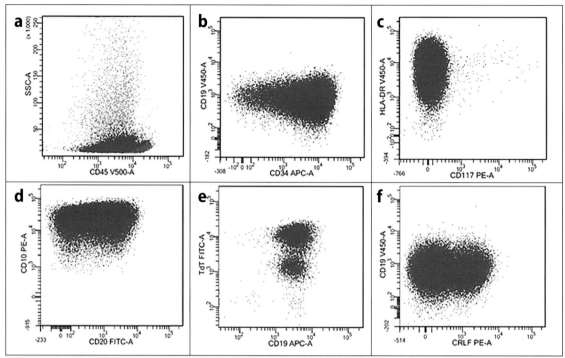

f51.3 Flow cytometry demonstrates a blast population (highlighted in purple) that is **a** CD45 dim to negative, **b** CD34 mostly positive, CD19 positive, **c** HLA-DR positive, CD117 negative, **d** CD10 moderate to bright, CD20 (partial), **e** TdT (partial), and **f** with partial expression of CRLF2

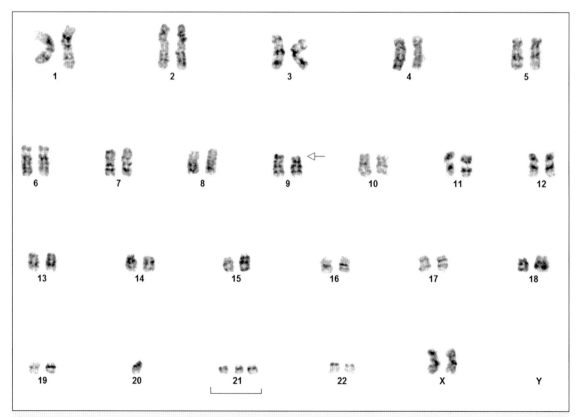

f51.4 Karyotype demonstrating deletion of 9p (arrow) as a result of dic(9;20), as well as gain of 21 (bracket)

ISBN 978-089189-6814

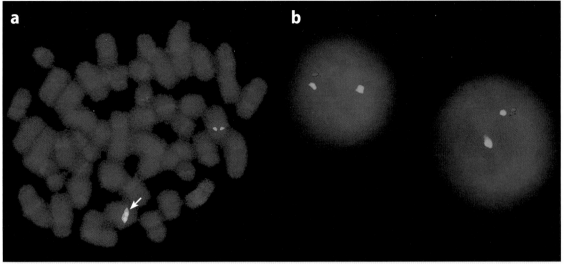

f51.5 **a** FISH using *CEP9* (centromere 9, green) & *CEP20* (centromere 20, orange) shows fusion of both CEPs producing 1 yellow signal (arrow), consistent with a dicentric t(9;20); **b** FISH for *CDKN2A* on 9p (orange) shows loss of 1 9p signal

Discussion *BCR-ABL1*-like (or Ph-like) B-ALL is a provisional entity according to the 2017 WHO classification of hematologic neoplasms. This distinction stems from its unique genetics, poor prognosis, and emerging potential for targeted therapies. Like *BCR-ABL1*-positive B-ALL (**Case 50**), this leukemia is driven by constitutive activation of oncogenic kinase signaling. However, in contrast with *BCR-ABL1*-positive disease, there is marked genetic heterogeneity among driver translocations/mutations in *BCR-ABL1*-like B-ALL. Its initial identification stemmed from the work of separate collaborative efforts, including a Dutch group attempting to predictively classify genetically defined subsets of B-ALL based on gene expression profiling and a separate group seeking to better understand the biology of a specific group of *BCR-ABL1*-negative B-ALL cases with poor outcomes. The 2 groups generated distinct, nonoverlapping gene sets capable of detecting cases lacking *BCR-ABL1* but with a similar gene expression profile (GEP). The latter work, by members of the Children's Oncology Group (COG), has led to subsequent refinement to a limited gene expression panel (the LDA used in the clinical vignette), now used to prioritize B-ALL cases in which additional genetic testing is likely to uncover driver mutations/translocations associated with the *BCR-ABL1*-like gene signature. It is important to be aware that the different strategies to identify *BCR-ABL1*-like B-ALL show only modest concordance; those cases identified by the COG approach are termed "Ph-like" and those cases identified by the Dutch group algorithm are termed "*BCR-ABL1*-like." The moniker

"*BCR-ABL1*-like B-ALL" will be used in the remainder of this chapter, as this is the nomenclature adopted by the WHO classification.

Clinically, *BCR-ABL1*-like B-ALL manifests similarly to most B-ALLs, albeit with a notable propensity for high WBC counts at presentation. It accounts for ~10% of B-ALL cases among young children and increases in frequency to ~25% of young adult and adult cases, though it may be lower among older individuals. In addition, the disease shows a male predominance (1.5-2:1 male-female ratio among children and adults and as high as 4:1 among young adults). There is also an increased predisposition for *BCR-ABL1*-like B-ALL among persons of Hispanic and Native American descent, which has been attributed to a single nucleotide polymorphism in *GATA*3 that is prevalent among these populations.

The typical immunophenotypes of *BCR-ABL1*-like B-ALL include CD19 and CD10 positivity, or so-called "common" acute lymphoblastic leukemia (ALL); no specific immunophenotype for *BCR-ABL1*-like B-ALL has been reported. Studies have shown a nearly perfect correlation between surface CRLF2 protein expression on flow cytometry and presence of a *CRLF2* rearrangement detected by FISH. Because of its strong predictive value, some algorithms promote universal assessment of CRLF 2 expression by flow cytometry in new B-ALL cases. In contrast, high gene expression identified by array does not share the same level of correlation with *CRLF2* rearrangements.

Normally, heterodimerization of CRLF2 with IL7Rα (gene product of *IL7R*) produces the thymic stromal lymphopoetin receptor, which signals via the JAK/STAT pathway and has known roles in lymphoid development. Two major recurrent rearrangements involving CRLF2 are seen in *BCR-ABL1*-like B-ALL, (resulting from interstitial deletion at chromosome Xp22.3/Yp11.3) and *IGH-CRLF2*, each of which leads to high surface expression of the receptor. Both are typically cryptic on karyotype analysis, as occurred in this case, with the former often requiring RT-PCR and the latter detectable by FISH studies. These 2 rearrangements show demographic variability, with the *P2YR8* partner being more common in younger patients and *IGH* rearrangement more common in adult, Hispanic, and Native American populations. Rarely, *CRLF2* rearrangements are found in B-ALL cases lacking a *BCR-ABL1*-like GEP signature. Both rearrangements of *CLRF2* and CRLF2 overexpression by flow cytometry had been established as negative prognostic markers before the recognition of the *BCR-ABL1*-like category of B-ALL.

Although *CRLF2* rearrangements are identified in roughly half of *BCR-ABL1*-like B-ALLs, other, nearly mutually exclusive cytogenetic abnormalities associated with this entity include activating translocations involving *EPOR,* tyrosine kinases of the *ABL* and *JAK* families, and several other kinases. Many of these translocations can involve multiple translocation partners. In addition to structural changes that activate kinase pathways, several genes that function within the same pathways are recurrently mutated in *BCR-ABL1*-like B-ALL. These include activating mutations in *JAK1, JAK2, IL7R,* and Ras pathway genes and loss-of-function mutations in negative regulators of JAK/STAT signaling **t51.1**. In this example case, reflex NGS testing identified *JAK2* and *IL7R* mutations in addition to the *P2YR8-CRLF2* translocation. The *JAK2* mutation occurred within the pseudokinase domain at codon R683, the most commonly mutated site for *JAK2* in *BCR-ABL1*-like B-ALL (as opposed to the V617F mutation characteristic of myeloproliferative neoplasms). Of note, *JAK2* and/or *JAK1* mutations co-occur in around half of *CRLF2*-rearranged B-ALLs. Currently, clinical trials are underway to determine the therapeutic efficacy of targeting pathways activated by these oncogenic events, specifically with ABL or JAK kinase inhibitors as an adjunct to standard risk-adjusted therapy.

t51.1 Recurrent genetic drivers in *BCR-ABL1*-like B-ALL*

Alteration subtype	Frequency (%)
ABL class	9-17
CRLF2 translocations	40-60
JAK2/EPOR	10-15
Other JAK/STAT	5-14
Other kinase	3-5
Ras pathway	2-6
Unknown	8-15

* Alterations include translocations or mutations

In addition to genetic activation of oncogenic kinase signaling, other genetic alterations are enriched in *BCR ABL1*-like B-ALL. Among these are mutation and/or deletion of genes encoding lymphoid transcription factors, such as *IKZF1, PAX5* and *EBF1*. In this specific case, cytogenetic abnormalities identified included gain of chromosome 21 and dic(9;20) resulting in del(9p); these abnormalities are associated with *BCR-ABL1*-like disease. Deletions encompassing the *CDKN2A* gene on chromosome 9p21 are among the most common abnormalities in B-ALL, occurring in up to 40% of cases, and are not specific for *BCR-ABL1*-like B-ALL. Existing literature contains conflicting results regarding the prognostic importance of *CDKN2A* deletion, likely because of its prevalence across multiple genetic risk subtypes. In some instances, chromosome 9p21 is lost as a result of the translocation producing a dic(9;20). This recurrent abnormality occurs in up to 5% of B-ALL cases, carries negative prognostic impact, and is enriched in *BCR-ABL1*-like B-ALL. Finally, both trisomy and intrachromosomal amplification of chromosome 21 are associated with genetic abnormalities seen in *BCR-ABL1*-like B-ALL. Down syndrome (constitutional trisomy 21)-associated ALL also has a high rate of *CRLF2* rearrangement and *JAK2* mutation (genetic features of *BCR-ABL1*-like disease). These correlations suggest cooperativity of *BCR-ABL1*-like driver mutations with genes on chromosome 21 and/or loss of lymphoid transcription factors in leukemogenesis.

In summary, *BCR-ABL1*-like (or "Ph-like") B-ALL represents a genetically diverse group of leukemias driven by activated kinase signaling. It bears similarities to *BCR-ABL1*-positive B-ALL, including a similar GEP, increased frequency with age, and poor prognosis. Ongoing clinical trials are examining the potential of incorporating targeted kinase inhibitors into treatment protocols for patients with this disease. Positive results from these trials will further reinforce the need to clinically identify this heterogeneous subset of B-ALL cases to ensure optimal care for affected patients.

Diagnostic pearls/pitfalls

– Recognition of *BCR-ABL1*-like B-ALL is important for risk stratification and the potential for kinase targeting therapy.

– *BCR-ABL1*-like B-ALL is not associated with a distinctive immunophenotype or histology; however, surface CRLF2 expression may be detected with flow cytometry and is associated with the presence of a *CRLF2* fusion, the most common recurring translocation in *BCR-ABL1*-like B-ALL. The most frequent *CRLF2* fusions are typically cryptic on karyotype and require directed (FISH or RT-PCR) methods for detection.

– Comprehensive *BCR-ABL1*-like/Ph-like testing should be performed on new B-ALL cases lacking recurrent genetic abnormalities as defined by the WHO classification. Notably, Ph-like LDA screening assay may be positive in B-ALL cases with *BCR-ABL1* or *ETV6-RUNX*1 translocations.

– At present there is no standard method for detecting *BCR-ABL1*-like B-ALL, and diagnosis typically relies on FISH and/or molecular assays to detect both fusions and mutations of recurrently involved genes.

Readings

Boer JM, Marchante JR, Evans WE, et al. *BCR-ABL1*-like cases in pediatric acute lymphoblastic leukemia: a comparison between DCOG/Erasmus MC and COG/St. Jude signatures. Haematologica. 2015;100:e354-7.
DOI: 10.3324/haematol.2015.124941

Den Boer ML, Van Slegtenhorst M, De Menezes RX, et al. A subtype of childhood acute lymphoblastic leukaemia with poor treatment outcome: a genome-wide classification study. Lancet Oncol. 2009;10:125-34. **DOI: 10.1016/S1470-2045(08)70339-5**

Harvey RC, Mulligan CG, Chen IM, et al. Rearrangement of CRLF2 is associated with mutation of *JAK* kinases, alteration of *IKZF1*, Hispanic/Latino ethnicity, and a poor outcome in pediatric B-progenitor acute lymphoblastic leukemia. Blood. 2010a;115:5312-21. **DOI: 10.1182/blood-2009-09-245944**

Harvey RC, Mulligan CG, Wang X, et al. Identification of novel cluster groups in pediatric high-risk B-precursor acute lymphoblastic leukemia with gene expression profiling: correlation with genome-wide DNA copy number alterations, clinical characteristics, and outcome. Blood. 2010b;116:4874-84. **DOI: 10.1182/blood-2009-08-239681**

Harvey RC, Tasian SK. Clinical diagnostics and treatment strategies for Philadelphia chromosome-like acute lymphoblastic leukemia. Blood Advances. 2020;4:218-228.
DOI: 10.1182/bloodadvances.2019000163

Herold T, Baldus CD, Gokbuget N. Ph-like acute lymphoblastic leukemia in older adults. N Engl J Med. 2014;371:2235.
DOI: 10.1056/NEJMc1412123#SA1

Jain N, Roberts KG, Jabbour E, et al. Ph-like acute lymphoblastic leukemia: a high-risk subtype in adults. Blood. 2017;129:572-81.
DOI: 10.1182/blood-2016-07-726588

Konoplev S, Lu X, Konopleva M, et al. *CRLF2*-positive B-cell acute lymphoblastic leukemia in adult patients: a single-institution experience. Am J Clin Pathol. 2017;147:357-63.
DOI: 10.1093/ajcp/aqx005

Mulligan CG, Su X, Zhang J, et al; Children's Oncology Group. Deletion of *IKZF1* and prognosis in acute lymphoblastic leukemia. N Engl J Med. 2009;360:470-80.
DOI: 10.1056/NEJMoa0808253

Reshmi SC, Harvey RC, Roberts KG, et al. Targetable kinase gene fusions in high-risk B-ALL: a study from the Children's Oncology Group. Blood. 2017;129:3352-61.
DOI: 10.1182/blood-2016-12-758979

Roberts KG, Gu Z, Payne-Turner D, et al. High frequency and poor outcome of Philadelphia chromosome-like acute lymphoblastic leukemia in adults. J Clin Oncol. 2017;35:394-401.
DOI: 10.1200/JCO.2016.69.0073

Roberts KG, Li Y, Payne-Turner D, et al. Targetable kinase-activating lesions in Ph-like acute lymphoblastic leukemia. N Engl J Med. 2014;371:1005-15. **DOI: 10.1056/NEJMoa1403088**

Tasian SK, Loh ML, Hunger SP. Philadelphia chromosome-like acute lymphoblastic leukemia. Blood. 2017;130:2064-72.
DOI: 10.1182/blood-2017-06-743252

Tran TH, Loh ML. Ph-like acute lymphoblastic leukemia. Hematology Am Soc Hematol Educ Program. 2016;2016:561-6.
DOI: 10.1182/asheducation-2016.1.561.

Van Der Veer A, Waanders E, Pieters R, et al. Independent prognostic value of *BCR-ABL1*-like signature and *IKZF1* deletion, but not high *CRLF2* expression, in children with B-cell precursor ALL. Blood. 2013;122:2622-9.
DOI: 10.1182/blood-2012-10-462358

Yoda A, Yoda Y, Chiaretti S, et al. Functional screening identifies *CRLF2* in precursor B-cell acute lymphoblastic leukemia. Proc Natl Acad Sci U S A. 2010;107:252-7.
DOI: 10.1073/pnas.0911726107

Zachariadis V, Gauffin F, Kuchinskaya E, et al; Swedish Cytogenetic Leukemia Study Group. The frequency and prognostic impact of dic(9;20)(p13.2;q11.2) in childhood B-cell precursor acute lymphoblastic leukemia: results from the NOPHO ALL-2000 trial. Leukemia. 2011;25:622-8. **DOI: 10.1038/leu.2010.318**

Zachariadis V, Schoumans J, Barbany G, et al. Homozygous deletions of *CDKN2A* are present in all dic(9;20)(p13.2;q11.2)-positive B-cell precursor acute lymphoblastic leukaemias and may be important for leukaemic transformation. Br J Haematol. 2012;159:488-91. **DOI: 10.1111/bjh.12051**

Rose C Beck

52

Early T-cell precursor lymphoblastic leukemia with t(10;11)(p12;q14) *MLLT10-PICALM*

History A 24-year-old male presented to his primary care physician for follow-up of continued low back pain, now accompanied by fatigue and weakness. Selected CBC results are shown at right.

A peripheral blood smear was performed.

Morphology & flow cytometry The blood smear showed leukocytosis composed of large atypical cells resembling blasts but having coarse chromatin **f52.1**. These cells were originally reported in the WBC differential as atypical lymphocytes but were later re-classified as blasts. A bone marrow biopsy showed sheets of the atypical cells in the aspirate smear and the core biopsy specimen **f52.2**.

By flow cytometry, the atypical cells were positive for CD34, CD33, CD117 (dim partial), CD4 (dim partial), and CD7 (strong), and negative for HLA-DR, CD1a, CD2, CD3, CD5, CD8, CD56, and B-cell and monocytic markers **f52.3**. Despite the presence of strong CD33 and dim CD117 which suggested myeloid blasts, the strong, uniform expression of CD7 raised the possibility of T-cell lineage. Cytoplasmic markers performed by flow cytometry demonstrated the presence of cCD3 **f52.3f** but absence of TdT and myeloperoxidase (MPO), consistent with T-lymphoblasts. Based on the morphologic and immunophenotypic findings, including absence of MPO expression, a diagnosis of **T-lymphoblastic leukemia/lymphoma, early T-cell precursor type**, was made.

WBC	132.1×10^9/L
Differential	
Neutrophils	4%
Lymphocytes	6%
Monocytes	1%
Eosinophils	1%
Atypical lymphocytes	88%
HGB	10.0 g/dL
MCV	89 fL
Platelets	56×10^9/L

Genetics/molecular results The karyotype was complex, with abnormal metaphases having 49-50 chromosomes. The abnormalities included additional material on 7q36, deletion of 11q23, additional material on 12p13, and additional material on 10p11.2. FISH was negative for 11q23 (*KMT2A*) rearrangement but did show the presence of t(10;11)(p12;q14) *MLLT10-PICALM* fusion **f52.4**.

ISBN 978-089189-6814 ©2021 ASCP

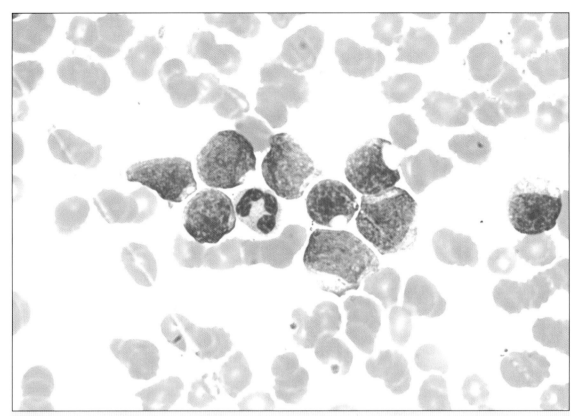

f52.1 Atypical blast-like cells are present in peripheral blood

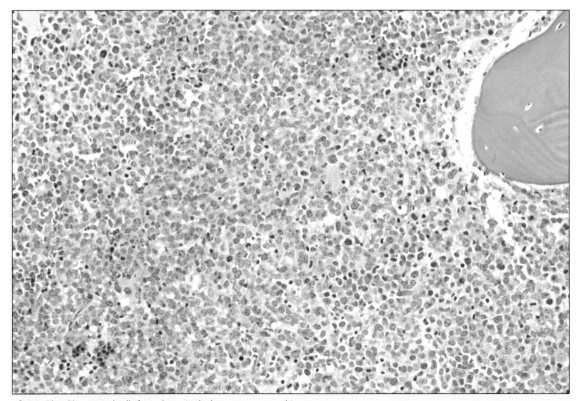

f52.2 Blast-like atypical cells form sheets in the bone marrow core biopsy

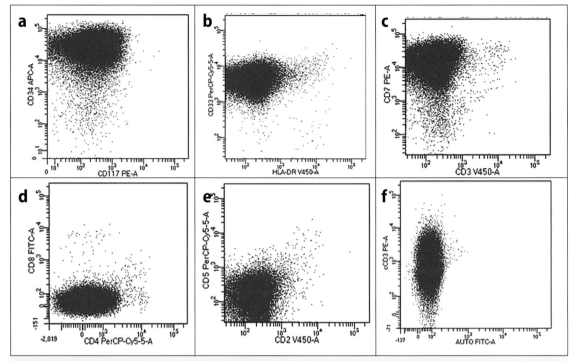

f52.3 Flow cytometry demonstrates an atypical blast population that is **a** CD34+, CD117+, **b** CD33+ (strong uniform), HLA-DR–, **c** CD7+ (strong), surface CD3–, **d** CD4+ (dim), CD8–, **e** CD2–, and CD5– but positive for **f** cytoplasmic CD3, confirming T-cell lineage

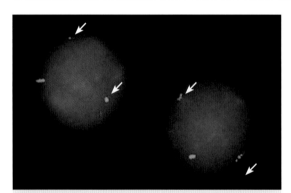

f52.4 Dual-fusion probes for *MLLT10* (10p12, red) & *PICALM* (11q14, green) indicate the presence of *MLLT10-PICALM* fusion (arrows) in the bone marrow aspirate cells (image courtesy of Dr Rhett Ketterling, Mayo Clinic)

Discussion Early T-cell precursor lymphoblastic leukemia (ETP-ALL) is a recently recognized subtype of T-lymphoblastic leukemia/lymphoma (T-ALL) in which the blasts arise from a very early T-lymphoid progenitor that has retained multilineage differentiation potential. Cases of ETP-ALL were originally identified based on having a gene expression profile similar to that of normal early T-cell precursors, and this gene expression profile in T-ALL correlated with a distinctive immunophenotype that is now used to define ETP-ALL. The blasts of ETP-ALL are typically positive for CD7 and by definition

are negative for CD1a and CD8 and positive for at least one of the following myeloid/stem markers in ≥25% of blasts: CD34, CD117, HLA-DR, CD13, CD33, CD11b, or CD65. CD5 is usually negative or weakly expressed by <75% of the blasts. Surface CD3 is usually negative, although cytoplasmic CD3 by definition is expressed. In a series of 33 adult cases, ~2/3 of cases expressed TdT, while CD10 was found in only 2 cases. Due to the frequent presence of early stem cell and myeloid markers, cases of ETP may be misdiagnosed as acute myeloid leukemia (AML) or mixed phenotype acute leukemia. Although blasts in AML not uncommonly express partial CD7, the presence of strong uniform CD7 expression in any blast population should prompt for evaluation of T-cell lineage via expression of cytoplasmic CD3 (assessed with flow cytometry or immunohistochemistry).

ETP-ALL accounts for 10%-15% of childhood T-ALL cases and 15%-20% of adult T-ALL cases. Pediatric patients diagnosed with ETP-ALL are usually older and have high white blood cell counts as well as increased incidence of extramedullary disease. Initial studies in pediatric cases of ETP-ALL indicated increased incidence of residual disease after induction therapy as well as poorer prognosis, as compared to other T-ALL cases. Despite a confirmed higher incidence of initially refractory disease, however, a recent analysis of

1,144 pediatric T-ALL cases demonstrated no significant difference in event-free or overall survival for ETP T-ALL versus other types of T-ALL. The prognostic effect of ETP phenotype in adult cases is still controversial.

Molecular studies of ETP-ALL indicate that the mutational profile of the blasts shares similarity to that of AML, with activating mutations in cytokine receptor and RAS pathway genes (eg, *NRAS, KRAS, FLT3, IL7R, JAK3, JAK1, SH2B3, BRAF*), inactivation of genes involved in hematopoietic development (eg, *GATA3, ETV6, RUNX1, IKZF1, EP300*), and alterations in histone-modifying genes (eg, *EZH2, EED, SUZ12, SETD2*). Mutations in genes commonly seen in other types of T-ALL, such as *NOTCH1* and *CDKN1/2,* are less common in ETP-ALL. In addition, the gene expression profile of ETP-ALL shares more similarities with that of hematopoietic stem cells and myeloid progenitors. These findings indicate that ETP-ALL is biologically distinct from non-ETP-ALL and may respond to AML-type therapies.

At the chromosomal level, occasional cases harbor recurrent translocations such as t(10;11)(p12;q14) *MLLT10-PICALM*. The t(10;11) *MLLT10-PICALM* fusion is a rarer translocation found in acute leukemias of myeloid or lymphoid phenotype. It is the most frequent recurrent translocation in T-ALL, present in 5%-10% of cases, and appears to have prognostic significance particularly in ETP-ALL, where it is associated with decreased overall survival. The *MLLT10-PICALM* fusion is readily detectable by FISH as demonstrated in this case.

Due to the often poor response of ETP-ALL patients to standard chemotherapy induction regimens, newer and more targeted agents are being investigated and include tyrosine kinase inhibitors (for rare cases harboring kinase gene fusions), targeted antibody therapy (eg, gemtuzumab ozogamicin, which binds CD33), and venetoclax (inhibitor of bcl-2 proteins and the anti-apoptosis pathway).

This patient initially received ALL-type therapy with vincristine and daunorubicin; however the day 28 bone marrow biopsy showed induction failure with 30% blasts. He was then treated with AML-type therapy (including high dose cytarabine) and successfully achieved remission, followed shortly by allogeneic stem cell transplant. Consistent with the aggressive nature of his leukemia, he suffered relapse and died 3 years after transplant.

Diagnostic pearls/pitfalls

– ETP-ALL blasts have a specific immunophenotype defined as CD1a negative, cytoplasmic CD3 positive, CD5 negative (or weak positive in <75% of blasts), CD7 positive, CD8 negative, and positivity for at least 1 of the following: CD34, CD117, HLA-DR, CD13, CD33, CD11b, or CD65 (in at least 25% of blasts).

– Due to the lack of surface T-cell markers, ETP-ALL may be misdiagnosed as AML or mixed phenotype acute leukemia (MPAL) with T/myeloid differentiation, and careful and thorough immunophenotyping is necessary to distinguish these disorders. According to current WHO criteria, the presence of both cCD3 and MPO in the blast population warrants a diagnosis of MPAL.

– Recurrent translocations such as t(10;11) *MLLT10-PICALM* may be found in ETP-ALL and may adversely affect prognosis.

Readings

Ben Abdelali R, Asnafi V, Petit A, et al. The prognosis of *CALM-AF10*-positive adult T-cell acute lymphoblastic leukemias depends on the stage of maturation arrest. Haematologica. 2013;98(11):1711-7. **DOI: 10.3324/haematol.2013.086082**

Burns MA, Place AE, Stevenson KE, et al. Identification of prognostic factors in childhood T-cell acute lymphoblastic leukemia: Results from DFCI ALL Consortium Protocols 05-001 and 11-001 [published correction appears in Pediatr Blood Cancer. 2021 Mar;68(3):e28885]. Pediatr Blood Cancer. 2021;68(1):e28719. **DOI:10.1002/pbc.28719**

Castaneda Puglianini O, Papadantonakis N. Early precursor T-cell acute lymphoblastic leukemia: current paradigms and evolving concepts. Ther Adv Hematol. 2020;11:2040620720929475. Published 2020 Jul 16. **DOI:10.1177/2040620720929475**

Coustan-Smith E, Mullighan CG, Onciu M, et al. Early T-cell precursor leukaemia: a subtype of very high-risk acute lymphoblastic leukaemia. Lancet Oncol. 2009;10(2):147-56. **DOI: 10.1016/S1470-2045(08)70314-0**

Khogeer H, Rahman H, Jain N, et al. Early T precursor acute lymphoblastic leukaemia/lymphoma shows differential immunophenotypic characteristics including frequent CD33 expression and in vitro response to targeted CD33 therapy. Br J Haematol. 2019;186(4):538-48. **DOI: 10.1111/bjh.15960**

Lo Nigro L, Mirabile E, Tumino M, et al. Detection of *PICALM-MLLT10* (*CALM-AF10*) and outcome in children with T-lineage acute lymphoblastic leukemia. Leukemia. 2013;27(12):2419-21. **DOI: 10.1038/leu.2013.149**

Vadillo E, Dorantes-Acosta E, Pelayo R, Schnoor M. T cell acute lymphoblastic leukemia (T-ALL): new insights into the cellular origins and infiltration mechanisms common and unique among hematologic malignancies. Blood Rev. 2018;32(1):36-51. **DOI: 10.1016/j.blre.2017.08.006**

Zhang J, Ding L, Holmfeldt L, et al. The genetic basis of early T-cell precursor acute lymphoblastic leukaemia. Nature. 2012;481(7380):157-63. **DOI: 10.1038/nature10725**

Erika M Moore

53

Mixed phenotype acute leukemia with t(9;22)(q34.1;q11.2) *BCR-ABL1*

History A 15-year-old male presented with petechiae and was evaluated by his primary care physician. CBC results are shown at right. A peripheral smear review was performed.

Morphology & flow cytometry The peripheral smear demonstrated marked leukocytosis composed of numerous variably sized blasts, a left-shifted myeloid series, atypical and immature monocytes, and dysplastic hypogranular and/or hypolobated neutrophils **f53.1**. A bone marrow biopsy showed 100% cellularity, with sheets of immature mononuclear cells consistent with blasts. Background trilineage hematopoiesis was present but markedly decreased. A cytochemical stain for myeloperoxidase (MPO) demonstrated staining in ~5%-10% of the blasts, and a stain for nonspecific esterase (NSE) showed weak positivity in ~5% of the blasts **f53.2**. Immunostains performed on the core biopsy specimen showed increased monocytic cells that were positive for lysozyme and negative for MPO.

Flow cytometric studies demonstrated a large B-lymphoblast population with the following immunophenotype: CD19 dim, CD10 partial positive, CD20 negative, CD34 positive, TdT positive, CD38 positive, CD45 dim, HLA-DR positive, CD13 dim, and CD117 positive **f53.3**. In addition, a second atypical, monocytic population was seen, with aberrant partial loss of CD4, HLA-DR and CD14. Based on the morphologic findings, an initial diagnosis of **mixed phenotype acute leukemia, B/myeloid type**, was rendered.

Genetics/molecular results FISH demonstrated the presence of t(9;22)(q34.1;q11.2) *BCR-ABL1* **f53.4** and karyotype analysis showed a complex karyotype: 46,XY,ins(1;?)(q21q25;?)[9]/46,idem,der(9)add(9)

WBC	339.4 × 10⁹/L
Differential	
Neutrophils	9%
Lymphocytes	13%
Monocytes	16%
Eosinophils	4%
Basophils	1%
Metamyelocytes	2%
Myelocytes	4%
Blasts	51%
RBC	2.32 × 10¹²/L
HGB	6.6 g/dL
HCT	20.6%
MCV	89 fL
RDW	16.5%
Platelets	41 × 10⁹/L

(p21)del(9)(q12q21)[9]/46,XY[2], indicating a cryptic *BCR-ABL1* fusion. qPCR studies for *BCR-ABL1* were positive for the major breakpoint.

Based on the overall findings, a final diagnosis of **mixed phenotype acute leukemia with t(9;22)(q34.1;q11.2) *BCR-ABL1*** was rendered.

Discussion Acute leukemias of ambiguous lineage include leukemias that have an undifferentiated or stem cell blast phenotype (acute undifferentiated leukemia) as well as leukemias that express antigens from multiple lineages, otherwise known as mixed phenotype acute leukemia (MPAL) **t53.1**. Historically, several names have been used to describe the latter, including biphenotypic and bilineal acute leukemia. Typically,

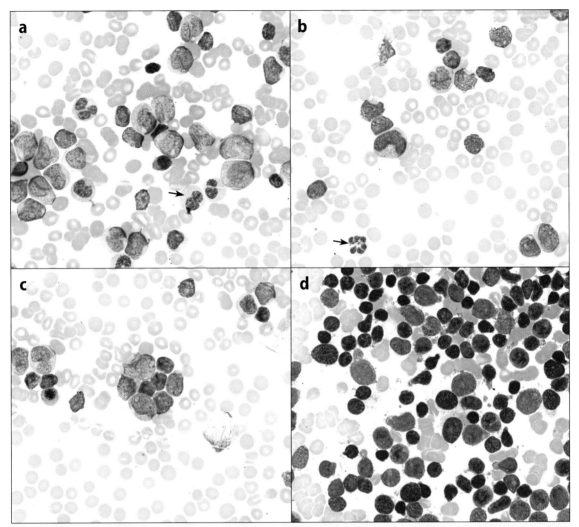

f53.1 **a-c** Peripheral blood demonstrating variably sized blasts, left shift & dysplastic neutrophils (denoted by arrows); **d** the bone marrow aspirate smear contains a predominance of blasts in a range of sizes & morphology, consistent with a mixed population of lymphoid & myeloid blasts

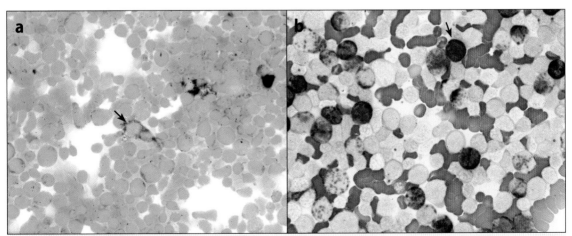

f53.2 Cytochemical staining for **a** nonspecific esterase (NSE) & **b** myeloperoxidase (MPO) each demonstrate positivity in a small subset of the blasts (denoted by arrows)

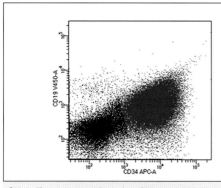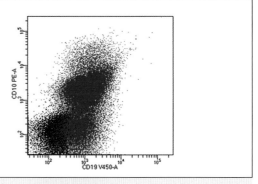

f53.3 Flow cytometry (gated on CD34+ events) demonstrating a B-lymphoblast population (highlighted in red) with dim CD19 & partial CD10 expression; an atypical monocytic population was also present on flow cytometry (not shown)

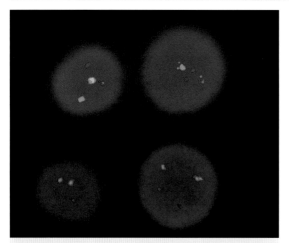

f53.4 Dual-color, dual-fusion probes for *BCR* (22q11, green) and *ABL1* (9q34, orange) demonstrating 2 intact *ABL1* signals, 1 *BCR* signal & 1 fusion signal, confirming the presence of the *BCR-ABL1* fusion as well as loss of the *BCR* hybridization site that is translocated to the abnormal chromosome 9

t53.1 Subtypes of mixed phenotype acute leukemia (MPAL) & their frequencies

MPAL Type	Frequency
MPAL, B/myeloid	~60%
MPAL, T/myeloid	~35%
MPAL, B/T or B/T/myeloid	<5%, extremely rare, case reports
MPAL with t(9;22) (q34.1;q11.2) *BCR-ABL1*	15%-20%, more common in adults, usually B/myeloid
MPAL with t(v;11q23.3) *KMT2A*-rearranged	10%, more common in infants, usually B/myeloid

t53.2 Criteria for lineage assessment in mixed phenotype acute leukemia

Myeloid lineage	myeloperoxidase (using flow cytometry, immunohistochemistry, or cytochemistry)
	monocytic differentiation (≥2 of the following: non-specific esterase, CD11c, CD14, CD64, lysozyme)
B-cell lineage	strong CD19 with ≥1 strongly expressed: CD79a, cytoplasmic CD22, CD10
	Weak CD19 with ≥2 strong expressed: CD79a, cytoplasmic CD22, CD10
T-cell lineage	cytoplasmic CD3 (using flow cytometry with antibodies to CD3 ε chain)
	surface CD3

the term biphenotypic was used to describe a leukemic blast population that simultaneously expressed antigens of 2 different lineages, while bilineal referred to an acute leukemia composed of 2 distinct blast populations of different lineages. Both types of cases are now classified as MPAL, and individual cases of MPAL may also exhibit both biphenotypic and bilineal features. In order to assign lineage of blasts, the 2017 WHO classification of hematologic neoplasms designates specific antigens to be lineage-defining **t53.2**. Although not part of the strict lineage-defining criteria, additional antigens used for lineage assessment include Pax5 for B-cell lineage, CD36 for monocytic lineage, and CD117, CD13, and CD33 for myeloid differentiation. Flow cytometry is the recommended method for antigen assessment but immunohistochemical and cytochemical stains can also be used, when applicable.

This group of disorders is very uncommon, with B/myeloid MPAL occurring most often, followed by T/myeloid. Extremely rare cases of B/T MPAL and B/T/myeloid MPAL have also been reported. There is no official minimum percentage of blasts required to express cross-lineage antigens when diagnosing MPAL, which can be problematic. This is exacerbated by the fact that rarely MPO can non-specifically stain typical B-lymphoblasts or even be weakly positive in some cases of B-lymphoblastic leukemia/lymphoma (B-ALL) by flow cytometry. In these cases, cytochemical expression

ISBN 978-089189-6814   ©2021 ASCP

of MPO or the presence of additional markers for myeloid differentiation described herein can help in more confidently establishing a diagnosis of B/myeloid MPAL. This diagnosis should not be made if known recurrent cytogenetic abnormalities in acute myeloid leukemia (AML) are detected. This prevents a misdiagnosis of MPAL in the context of some acute leukemias that are known to express antigens of a differing lineage, such as AML with t(8;21) in which the myeloblasts often express CD19 and Pax5 (see **Case 19**). In addition, it is not uncommon for B-ALL blasts to express myeloid antigens such as CD13 and/or CD33, especially in B-ALL with *BCR-ABL1* (see **Case 50**); these cases should not be classified as MPAL.

Many cases of MPAL have a normal karyotype but 2 cytogenetic abnormalities occur frequently enough to have their own diagnostic category: MPAL with t(9;22) (q34.1;q11.2) *BCR-ABL1* and MPAL with t(v;11q23.3) *KMT2A*-rearranged. *BCR-ABL1* is the most common recurrent genetic abnormality seen in MPAL, accounting for ~15%-20% of cases and is more frequent in adults. The p190 (minor) fusion is the more common *BCR-ABL1* transcript found in these cases and the presence of a p210 (major) transcript warrants evaluation for chronic myeloid leukemia (CML) in blast crisis (which would not be considered MPAL). In this example case, a p210 fusion was identified but there was no clinical evidence for prior CML. MPAL with *KMT2A* (*MLL*) rearrangement is less common, comprising ~10% of all MPAL cases, and occurs most often in children, especially infants. These leukemias may be challenging to distinguish from other acute leukemias having the same gene fusions; in these cases, careful attention to immunophenotyping is critical. NGS assessment of MPAL cases has also been performed in some studies and identified mutations in genes involved in both lymphoid and myeloid leukemias, such as *IKZF1*, *EZH2*, *ASXL*, *ETV6*, *NOTCH1*, *IDH1*, *CEBPA*, *TP53*, *RUNX1*, and *TET2*, among others. Larger studies, however, are needed to assess the prognostic value of these mutations.

Acute leukemias of ambiguous lineage overall tend to have a poor prognosis, but data are limited due to the rarity of these cases. As MPALs are clinically and immunophenotypically heterogeneous, ideal treatment strategies are uncertain; however, several studies have shown better outcome with ALL-type therapy than AML-directed or combination ALL/AML-directed therapy. Consequently, a lymphoblastic leukemia-type induction chemotherapy protocol is most favored. Subsequent allogeneic stem cell transplantation may also

be advantageous in some patient populations. In MPAL with t(9;22) *BCR-ABL1*, addition of a tyrosine kinase inhibitor (TKI) may also improve outcome.

This patient went into remission following standard-risk B-ALL therapy combined with a TKI. He received an allogeneic stem cell transplant shortly thereafter and remains free of disease at the time of this writing.

Diagnostic pearls/pitfalls

– Diagnosis of MPAL requires accurate determination of lineage using thorough immunophenotyping and in some cases, cytochemical stains.

– Some AMLs, such as AML with t(8;21), characteristically express B-cell markers, but should not be diagnosed as MPAL.

– MPO may be weakly positive or show non-specific staining by flow cytometry in typical B-ALL, and therefore, additional confirmation of myeloid antigen expression is recommended in such cases before making a diagnosis of MPAL.

– MPAL shares recurrent genetic abnormalities with other acute leukemias, and careful lineage determination is essential for correct diagnosis, when these translocations are present.

– Most studies suggest that ALL-like induction chemotherapy is the best treatment strategy for MPAL.

Readings

Alexander TB, Gu Z, Iacobucci I, et al. The genetic basis and cell of origin of mixed phenotype acute leukaemia. Nature. 2018;562:373-9. **DOI: 10.1038/s41586-018-0436-0**

Khan M, Siddiqi R, Naqvi K. An update on classification, genetics, and clinical approach to mixed phenotype acute leukemia (MPAL). Ann Hematol. 2018;97:945-53. **DOI: 10.1007/s00277-018-3297-6**

Matutes E, Pickl WF, Van't Veer M, et al. Mixed-phenotype acute leukemia: clinical and laboratory features and outcome in 100 patients defined according to the WHO 2008 classification. Blood 2011;117:3163-71. **DOI: 10.1182/blood-2010-10-314682**

Porwit A, Béné MC. Multiparameter flow cytometry applications in the diagnosis of mixed phenotype acute leukemia. Cytometry Part B. 2019;96B:183-94. **DOI: 10.1002/cyto.b.21783**

Orgel E, Alexander, TB, Wood BL, Kahwash SB, et al. Mixed-phenotype acute leukemia: a cohort and consensus research strategy from the Children's Oncology Group Acute Leukemia of Ambiguous Lineage Task Force. Cancer. 2020;126:593-601. **DOI: 10.1002/cncr.32552**

Swerdlow SH, Campo E, Harris NL, et al. World Health Organization Classification of Tumours of Haematopoietic and Lymphoid Tissues. 4th ed. Lyon, France: IARC Press; 2017. **ISBN: 9789283244943**

Yan L, Ping N, Zhu M, et al. Clinical, immunophenotypic, cytogenetic, and molecular genetic features in 117 adult patients with mixed-phenotype acute leukemia defined by WHO-2008 classification. Haematologica. 2012; 97:1708-12. **DOI: 10.3324/haematol.2012.064485**

Catherine K Gestrich, Priya Nirmalanantham & Rose C Beck

54

Histiocytic sarcoma arising from a monocytic neoplasm in bone marrow, with mutations in *KRAS, SRSF2 & TET2*

History A 74-year-old male with a past medical history of prostate cancer and leukocytosis presented with recurrent falls, fever, flu-like symptoms, and generalized weakness. A CBC was ordered and results are shown at right. A blood smear review and bone marrow biopsy were performed.

Morphology & flow cytometry The peripheral blood smear demonstrated a leukocytosis with a mild left shift, dysplastic neutrophils, and absolute monocytosis **f54.1**. The monocytes were predominantly mature and included occasional atypical monocytes with more deeply basophilic cytoplasm and/or abnormal lobation. The bone marrow aspirate smear showed granulocytic hyperplasia, increased monocytes, and many large, atypical mononuclear cells with basophilic cytoplasm and convoluted nuclei **f54.2a**. These cells were morphologically consistent with atypical histiocytes and were positive for non-specific esterase cytochemical stain **f54.2b inset**. The aspirate smear also demonstrated hemophagocytosis by both normal and malignant histiocytes **f54.2b**. The core biopsy showed a hypercellular bone marrow with focal sheets of the atypical histiocytes **f54.3**; interstitial infiltration by the atypical histiocytes was also present. Extensive immunohistochemical profiling demonstrated the atypical histiocytes to be positive for CD68, CD4, lysozyme, and CD33 **f54.4**, and negative for stem

WBC	30.3×10^9/L
Differential	
Neutrophils	53%
Lymphocytes	13%
Monocytes	31%
Eosinophils	4%
Metamyelocytes	2%
Myelocytes	1%
RBC	2.79×10^{12}/L
HGB	9.1 g/dL
HCT	26.9%
MCV	96 fL
RDW	17.2%
Platelets	35×10^9/L

cell markers (CD34, CD117, TdT), dendritic cell markers (S100, CD1a, langerin, CD123), and other markers including myeloperoxidase, CD15, CD30, cytokeratins, and those for lymphoid lineage. An immunohistochemical stain for *BRAF* V600E was also negative. Flow cytometry did not detect the atypical histiocytes but did demonstrate some phenotypic atypia including decreased CD177 expression on neutrophils and monocytes with decreased CD15 **f54.5**.

ISBN 978-089189-6814

54 *Histiocytic sarcoma arising from a monocytic neoplasm in bone marrow, with mutations in KRAS, SRSF2 & TET2*

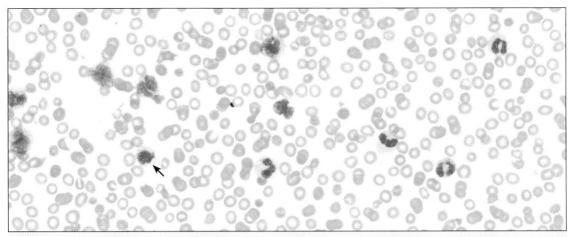

f54.1 Peripheral blood showing leukocytosis with increased monocytes, granulocytic left shift & few dysplastic neutrophils (arrow)

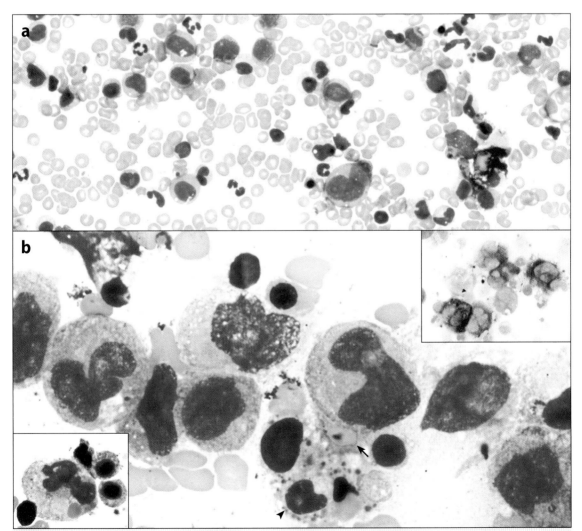

f54.2 The aspirate smear shows **a** granulocytic hyperplasia including hypogranular neutrophils, increased monocytic cells & large atypical cells with convoluted nuclei; **b** the large atypical cells are consistent with atypical histiocytes that demonstrate occasional hemophagocytosis (arrow & lower inset) & are positive for nonspecific esterase cytochemical stain (without fluoride; upper inset); cytophagocytosis by a normal histiocyte is also present (arrowhead)

54 *Histiocytic sarcoma arising from a monocytic neoplasm in bone marrow, with mutations in KRAS, SRSF2 & TET2*

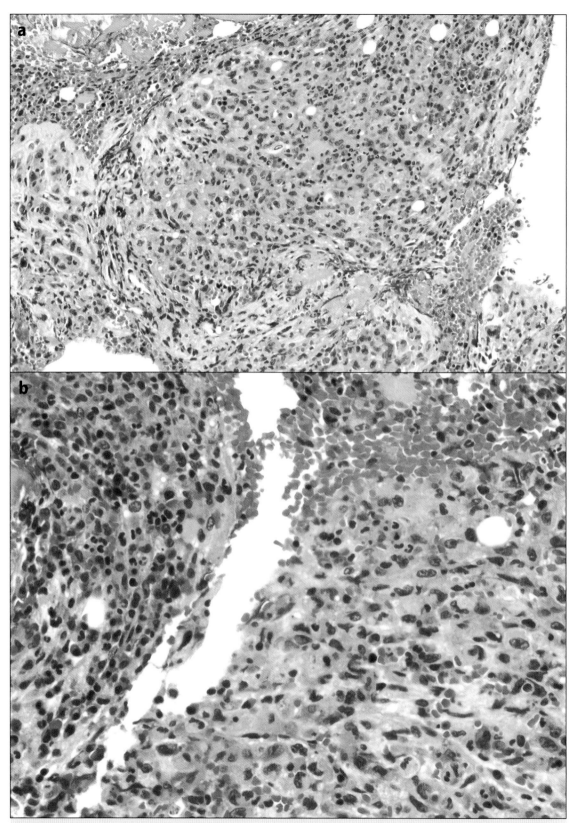

f54.3 H&E stained sections of the bone marrow core biopsy at **a** lower & **b** higher magnification show sheets of the atypical histiocytes adjacent to & compressing residual hematopoietic marrow

ISBN 978-089189-6814   ©2021 ASCP

54 *Histiocytic sarcoma arising from a monocytic neoplasm in bone marrow, with mutations in KRAS, SRSF2 & TET2*

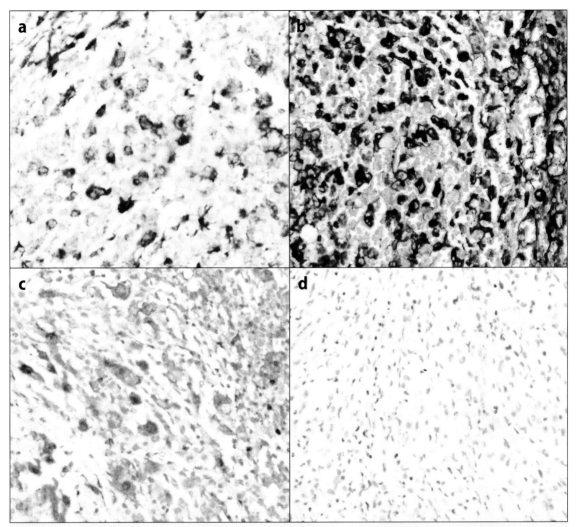

f54.4 Immunohistochemistry performed on the core biopsy demonstrates the atypical histiocytes are positive for **a** CD68, **b** lysozyme & **c** CD4, but **d** negative for CD1a

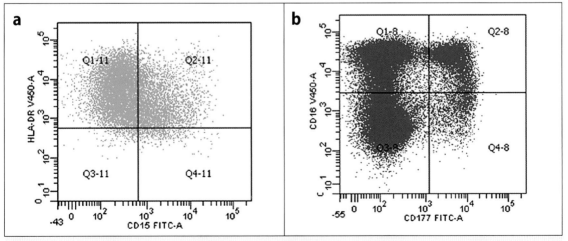

f54.5 Flow cytometry did not detect the atypical histiocytes but did show evidence of myelodysplasia, with **a** decreased CD15 expression by monocytes (gated by CD45/side scatter, highlighted in green) & **b** decreased CD177 expression by neutrophils (gated by CD45/side scatter, highlighted in purple)

The patient had no clinical or radiologic evidence of lymphoma. A CBC performed 20 months prior to the bone marrow biopsy was notable for anemia and thrombocytopenia, normal WBC, and mild absolute monocytosis. Therefore, the presence of a prior undiagnosed myeloid neoplasm such as chronic myelomonocytic leukemia (CMML) was suspected.

Based on the morphologic and immunophenotypic findings of the blood and bone marrow biopsy, as well as review of clinical and radiologic results, a diagnosis of **histiocytic sarcoma arising from a monocytic neoplasm** (favor CMML), was rendered.

Genetics/molecular results Chromosome analysis was performed and revealed a normal male karyotype. A FISH panel was negative for recurrent translocations associated with acute myeloid leukemia (AML). A targeted myeloid NGS panel showed the following alterations: *SRSF2* p.P95H (VAF 47%), *TET2* p.C1811* (VAF 51%), *TET2* splice site variant (c.3595-1G>A; VAF 50%), and *KRAS* p.K117N (VAF 6%), while additional testing was negative for *BRAF* V600E.

Discussion Histiocytes normally reside in bone marrow (BM) and comprise ~10% of the marrow microenvironment. Histologically, they are typically inconspicuous and may be seen in close approximation with maturing erythroid precursors. The vast majority of histiocytic proliferations in BM are reactive and occur in a variety of inflammatory, infectious, hemophagocytic, storage disorder, or neoplastic conditions. Malignant histiocytic proliferations involving BM are rare and generally include Langerhans cell histiocytosis (LCH), extracutaneous juvenile xanthogranuloma (JXG), Erdheim-Chester disease (ECD), and histiocytic sarcoma (HS). Genomic studies have shown that as a group, these neoplasms are associated with mutations in the RAS/RAF/MAPK intracellular signaling pathway.

LCH is characterized by proliferation of characteristic Langerhans-type cells having abundant eosinophilic cytoplasm and grooved ("coffee bean") nuclei; these cells express CD1a and CD207. Extracutaneous JXG and ECD are commonly disseminated at presentation, often involving BM, and morphologically demonstrate Touton-type giant cells and/or foamy histiocytes. ECD and LCH in particular are associated with *BRAF* V600E in ~50% of cases, with mutations in *MAP2K1* and other RAS/RAF/MAPK genes occurring in *BRAF* wild-type cases.

HS is most commonly seen in adults, predominantly males. Presenting symptoms often include fever, weight loss, hepatosplenomegaly, and pancytopenia. HS may involve BM but most often presents in extranodal soft tissue sites; primary BM presentation of HS is extremely rare. Histologically, compared to normal histiocytes, HS cells are typically larger, with a higher N:C ratio and indented or convoluted nuclei. Cellular atypia may be mild to significant and the chromatin is usually vesicular. In addition, hemophagocytosis and focal areas of spindling in H&E-stained sections may be seen. The diagnosis of HS requires expression of histiocytic markers such as CD4, CD68, CD163, and lysozyme. HS cells should be negative for myeloid lineage and T and B cell markers, although aberrant expression of CD56 has been observed, similar to the aberrant CD56 expression that can be seen in monocytic leukemias. A minority of cases have minimal or partial expression of S100, and CD1a should be mostly negative. Recent genomic studies of HS demonstrate the presence of activating mutations in RAS/RAF/MAPK pathway genes in the majority (57-100%) of cases, although in contrast to LCH and ECD, *BRAF* V600E occurs in a minority (~10% in one cohort of 21 cases, although studies vary widely).

HS may be associated in the same patient with other hematopoietic neoplasms, such as T- or B-acute lymphoblastic leukemia and follicular lymphoma, or found in association with mediastinal germ cell tumors. Interestingly, cases of HS arising after a lymphoid neoplasm (so called "secondary HS") may demonstrate clonal rearrangement of T- or B-cell receptor genes identical to the initial neoplasm, indicating transdifferentiation of the neoplastic stem cell. As noted, it is extremely rare for HS to have primary presentation in the BM, and when this occurs, the lesion may occur in conjunction with a myeloid neoplasm, most typically of monocytic lineage such as the presumed CMML seen in this case; concurrent AML has also been described. In this patient, the presence of mutations in *SRSF2* and *TET2* as well as historical CBC showing cytopenias with absolute monocytosis, all suggested the presence of underlying CMML (see **Case 12**). The much lower VAF of the *KRAS* mutation suggested clonal evolution, which may have corresponded to the neoplastic histiocytes, although this was not directly proven. The histologic findings in the aspirate smear and core biopsy of this case suggested the malignant histiocytes were derived from the same abnormal stem cell clone as the CMML cells, but this could not be definitely demonstrated without the use of microdissection or cell sorting techniques. An association of LCH and ECD with clonally-related circulating monocytes, as well as concurrent myeloid neoplasms (especially those with monocytic differentiation), has been well-documented in the literature, suggesting the cell of origin for these histiocytic neoplasms to be a myeloid precursor in BM.

HS is an aggressive neoplasm with poor prognosis that is unresponsive to most therapies. No standard treatment protocols exist and in cases with an associated neoplasm, initial therapy may be directed at that neoplasm. Most patients do not survive >2 years following diagnosis. The identification of recurrent activating mutations in the RAS/RAF/MAPK pathway has led to the possibility of targeted therapy for these patients, including MEK inhibitors; limited anecdotal evidence supports further investigation of these compounds.

True to the nature of the disease, the patient in this case expired within 1 week of diagnosis.

Diagnostic pearls/pitfalls

- Malignant histiocytoses involving bone marrow include LCH, JXG, ECD, and more rarely, HS. These neoplasms may occur in conjunction with a clonally-related myeloid neoplasm with monocytic differentiation. In addition, HS in particular may also arise from a clonally-related lymphoid neoplasm.
- Mutations in the RAS/RAF/MAPK pathway play a key role in the pathogenesis of malignant histiocytoses. Detection of these mutations may aid in diagnosis and indicate potential targeted therapeutic options.
- HS can be distinguished from other malignant histiocytoses using careful immunophenotyping and morphologic analysis. HS cells should express histiocytic markers such as CD4, CD68, CD163, and lysozyme, without predominant expression of S100 or CD1a.
- Regardless of the site of involvement, HS is an aggressive neoplasm with a poor prognosis.

Readings

Badalian-Very G, Vergilio JA, Degar BA, et al. Recurrent *BRAF* mutations in Langerhans cell histiocytosis. Blood. 2010;116(11):1919-1923. **DOI: 10.1182/blood-2010-04-279083**

Diamond EL, Durham BH, Haroche J, et al. Diverse and targetable kinase alterations drive histiocytic neoplasms. Cancer Discov. 2016;6(2):154-165. **DOI: 10.1158/2159-8290.CD-15-0913**

Durham BH, Roos-Weil D, Baillou C, et al. Functional evidence for derivation of systemic histiocytic neoplasms from hematopoietic stem/progenitor cells. Blood. 2017;130(2):176-180. **DOI: 10.1182/blood-2016-12-757377**

Egan C, Lack J, Skarshaug S, et al. The mutational landscape of histiocytic sarcoma associated with lymphoid malignancy. Mod Pathol. 2021;34(2):336-347. **DOI: 10.1038/s41379-020-00673-x**

Egan C, Nicolae A, Lack J, et al. Genomic profiling of primary histiocytic sarcoma reveals 2 molecular subgroups. Haematologica. 2020;105(4):951-960. **DOI: 10.3324/haematol.2019.230375**

Emile JF, Abla O, Fraitag S, et al. Revised classification of histiocytoses and neoplasms of the macrophage-dendritic cell lineages. Blood. 2016;127(22):2672-2681. **DOI: 10.1182/blood-2016-01-690636**

Haroche J, Charlotte F, Arnaud L, et al. High prevalence of *BRAF* V600E mutations in Erdheim-Chester disease but not in other non-Langerhans cell histiocytoses. Blood. 2012;120(13):2700-2703. **DOI: 10.1182/blood-2012-05-430140**

Hornick JL, Jaffe ES, Fletcher CD. Extranodal histiocytic sarcoma: clinicopathologic analysis of 14 cases of a rare epithelioid malignancy. Am J Surg Pathol. 2004;28(9):1133-1144. **DOI: 10.1097/01.pas.0000131541.95394.23**

Mitani S, Kaneko H, Imada K. Bone marrow infiltration of histiocytic sarcoma. Blood Res. 2018 Sep;53(3):185. **DOI: 10.5045/br.2018.53.3.185**

Mori M, Matsushita A, Takiuchi Y, et al. Histiocytic sarcoma and underlying chronic myelomonocytic leukemia: a proposal for the developmental classification of histiocytic sarcoma. Int J Hematol. 2010 Jul;92(1):168-73. **DOI: 10.1007/s12185-010-0603-z**

Shanmugam V, Griffin GK, Jacobsen ED, et al. Identification of diverse activating mutations of the *RAS-MAPK* pathway in histiocytic sarcoma. Mod Pathol. 2019 Jun;32(6):830-843. **DOI: 10.1038/s41379-018-0200-x**

Swerdlow, SH, Campo, E, Harris, et al (Eds). WHO Classification of Tumours of Haematopoietic and Lymphoid Tissues (Revised 4th edition). IARC: Lyon 2017. **ISBN: 978-9283224310**

Tzankov A, Kremer M, Leguit R, et al. Histiocytic cell neoplasms involving the bone marrow: summary of the workshop cases submitted to the 18th Meeting of the European Association for Haematopathology (EAHP) organized by the European Bone Marrow Working Group, Basel 2016. Ann Hematol. 2018 Nov;97(11):2117-2128. **DOI: 10.1007/s00277-018-3436-0**

Self-Study

Q Questions

Myeloid neoplasms (questions 1-20)

1. Which of the following is true of FISH assay detection of the Philadelphia chromosome, t(9;22) *BCR-ABL1*?
   A. FISH can detect virtually all variants of *BCR-ABL1* fusion, including 3-way translocations.
   B. FISH has a lower threshold of detection than most quantitative PCR assays.
   C. FISH can distinguish between the minor and major breakpoints of BCR.
   D. FISH is typically used to monitor for molecular remission.
   E. FISH can be performed only with break-apart FISH probes.

2. Which of the following statements regarding *BCR-ABL1* breakpoints is correct?
   A. The "major" breakpoint produces a protein with molecular weight of 190 kd.
   B. The "micro" breakpoint produces a protein with molecular weight of 210 kd.
   C. The "minor" breakpoint is the most frequent form found in chronic myeloid leukemia (CML).
   D. The "micro" breakpoint is associated with a neutrophilic form of CML.
   E. The "major", "minor", and "micro" breakpoints are the only fusion forms which have been described for CML.

3. The most common driver mutations found in essential thrombocytosis (ET) occur in which of the following genes?
   A. *JAK2, DNMT3A, TET2*
   B. *JAK2, CALR, MPL*
   C. *JAK2, CALR, SF3B1*
   D. *JAK2, CALR, SETBP1*
   E. *JAK2, MPL, ABL1*

4. In contrast to the eosinophils found in idiopathic hypereosinophilic syndrome, the eosinophils present in chronic eosinophilic leukemia (CEL) typically are:
   A. less likely to be dysplastic.
   B. the result of a clonally expanded population.
   C. associated with chronic myeloid leukemia (CML).
   D. a sign of a lymphoid neoplasm such as Hodgkin lymphoma.
   E. always accompanied by increased mast cells in the bone marrow.

5. Which of the following gene function groups is NOT associated with mutations typically found in myeloid neoplasms?
   A. Epigenetic regulation
   B. Transcription factors
   C. Spliceosome complex
   D. Cohesins
   E. Cytoskeleton complex

6. Among hematologic neoplasms, mutations in spliceosome complex genes such as *SF3B1*, *SRSF2, U2AF1*, and *ZRSR2*, are most commonly found in which of the following?
   A. Chronic myeloid leukemia
   B. T-cell lymphoma
   C. Hodgkin lymphoma
   D. Myelodysplastic syndromes
   E. Myeloproliferative neoplasms

ISBN 978-089189-6814 ©2021 ASCP

7. A myeloid neoplasm characterized by thrombocytosis, hypercellular bone marrow, atypical, enlarged megakaryocytes, and dyserythropoiesis including ring sideroblasts is most likely to have which of the following molecular profiles?
   A. Mutation in *JAK2* only
   B. Mutation in *DNMT3A* only
   C. Mutations in *JAK2* and *TET2*
   D. Mutations in *JAK2* and *CALR*
   E. Mutations in *JAK2* and *SF3B1*

8. Several myeloid neoplasms are characterized by granulocytic leukocytosis in peripheral blood. Match the characteristic genetic finding with the appropriate granulocytic neoplasm.

Chronic myeloid leukemia	Often has concurrent *TET2* & *SRSF2* mutations
Chronic neutrophilic leukemia	Always has t(9;22) *BCR-ABL1*
Atypical chronic myeloid leukemia	~30% of cases have *SETBP1* mutation
Chronic myelomonocytic leukemia	Majority of cases have *CSF3R* mutation

9. Recognition of mutations occurring in clonal hematopoiesis of indeterminate potential (CHIP) is important because:
   A. the presence of a mutation indicates necessity for stem cell transplant if malignancy develops.
   B. the presence of a mutation is highly correlated with the presence of cytopenia.
   C. patients with CHIP have increased risk of developing hematologic malignancy.
   D. patients with CHIP have increased risk of obesity.
   E. CHIP mutations are identical to those found in myeloid malignancy but are not diagnostic by themselves.
   F. A, B, and C
   G. C and E
   H. all of the above

10. The presence of ring sideroblasts may be associated with all of the following conditions except:
    A. Antibiotic use
    B. Vitamin B_{12} deficiency
    C. Myelodysplastic syndrome
    D. Copper deficiency
    E. Chronic myelomonocytic leukemia

11. Which **3** of the following cytogenetic abnormalities are diagnostic for myelodysplastic syndrome, when found in a patient with cytopenias?
    A. deletion 5q
    B. deletion 7q
    C. trisomy 8
    D. deletion 17p
    E. deletion 20q
    F. loss of Y

12. Assessing for the presence of *SF3B1* mutation is important in the evaluation of myelodysplastic syndrome (MDS) for which of the following **2** reasons?
    A. *SF3B1* mutation in MDS portends a worse prognosis.
    B. In the presence of *SF3B1* mutation, only 5% ring sideroblasts (RS) are necessary to diagnosis MDS with RS.
    C. Cases with RS and *SF3B1* mutation have a better prognosis.
    D. *SF3B1* mutation in MDS is associated with increased blast percentage.
    E. *SF3B1* mutation in MDS is associated with concurrent *TP53* mutations.

13. Among the myeloid/lymphoid neoplasms presenting with eosinophilia and a specific gene rearrangement, cases with rearranged *FGFR1* differ from those having rearrangements of *PDGFRA* and *PDGFRB* because:
    A. cases with *FGFR1* rearrangement are more likely to present as Hodgkin lymphoma.
    B. cases with *FGFR1* rearrangement must be detected by FISH rather than karyotype, due to a typically cryptic rearrangement.
    C. cases with *FGFR1* rearrangement can be monitored by quantitative PCR.
    D. cases with *FGFR1* rearrangement have significantly better prognosis.
    E. cases with *FGFR1* rearrangement do not have significant response to tyrosine kinase inhibitor therapy.

14. In acute myeloid leukemia (AML) with mutated *RUNX1*, the blast morphology is most typically:
    A. undifferentiated
    B. with many Auer rods
    C. with monocytic features
    D. with erythroid features
    E. with megakaryocytic features

15. Which of the following genetic findings is diagnostic for acute myeloid leukemia (AML), regardless of the actual blast percentage in blood or bone marrow?
    A. t(9;22) *BCR-ABL1*
    B. t(6;9) *DEK-CAN*
    C. inv(3) *GATA, MECOM*
    D. t(8;21) *RUNX1-RUNX1T1*
    E. t(9;11) *KMT2A-MLLT3*

16. A bone marrow biopsy shows 25% blasts with monocytic differentiation, in a background of significant dyserythropoiesis and dysgranulopoiesis. The karyotype is normal and both mutated *NPM1* and *FLT3-ITD* are identified. This neoplasm should be classified as:
    A. AML with myelodysplasia-related changes.
    B. AML with mutated *NPM1*.
    C. AML with mutated *FLT3*.
    D. therapy-related myeloid neoplasm.
    E. AML, not otherwise specified.

17. Which of the following statements regarding AML with biallelic *CEBPA* mutations is true?
    A. Most cases have the same molecular variant present on the N-terminus of both *CEBPA* alleles.
    B. Almost all cases have monocytic differentiation.
    C. Assays for evaluating mutations in *CEBPA* often use Sanger sequencing.
    D. Most cases have complex karyotype including deletion of 9q.
    E. The occurrence of *FLT3-ITD* in AML is mutually exclusive with biallelic *CEBPA* mutations.

18. Megakaryocytic differentiation of blasts in acute leukemia is associated with which **3** of the following conditions?
    A. AML with t(1;22) *RBM15-MKL1*
    B. AML with inv(16) *CBFB-MYH11*
    C. Down syndrome
    D. blasts having a phenotype that includes bright CD56 with lack of HLA-DR and CD45
    E. blasts having a phenotype that includes bright CD71 with lack of CD34 and CD33

19. Therapy-related myeloid neoplasm (TRMN) occurring after alkylating agent therapy is characterized by which **3** of the following?
    A. latency of 1-2 years
    B. latency of 2-5 years
    C. recurrent genetic translocations, especially *KMT2A* rearrangement
    D. complex karyotype
    E. mutations in *TP53*
    F. mutations in *DNMT3A*

20. A myeloid neoplasm associated with a germline mutation should be suspected when:
    A. a younger patient presents with myelodysplastic syndrome.
    B. a younger patient presents with *CALR*-mutated myeloproliferative neoplasm.
    C. there is a family history of hereditary spherocytosis.
    D. a myeloid neoplasm demonstrates *GATA2* mutation, regardless of variant allele frequency.
    E. a lymphoid neoplasm occurs with elevated levels of hemoglobin F.

ISBN 978-089189-6814 ©2021 ASCP

Lymphoid neoplasms (questions 21-40)

21. Which of the following is not associated with a poor prognosis in chronic lymphocytic leukemia/small lymphocytic lymphoma (CLL/SLL)?
    A. CD49d positivity
    B. loss of 17p
    C. *NOTCH1* mutation
    D. mutated immunoglobulin heavy chain variable region
    E. ZAP70 positivity

22. Hairy cell leukemia is associated with all of the following features except:
    A. splenomegaly
    B. monocytosis
    C. CD11c expression
    D. bone marrow fibrosis
    E. *BRAF* V600E mutation

23. A 70-year-old man presents with a leukocytosis, WBC 120×10^9/L. Flow cytometry studies demonstrate a T-cell population which is positive for CD2, surface CD3, CD4, CD5, CD7, and TCR α/β. Cytogenetic studies demonstrated t(14;14)(q11;q32). What is the most likely diagnosis?
    A. T-cell large granular lymphocytic leukemia
    B. T-lymphoblastic leukemia/lymphoma
    C. ALK-negative anaplastic large cell lymphoma
    D. angioimmunoblastic T-cell lymphoma
    E. T-cell prolymphocytic leukemia

24. Which of the following is true regarding differentiating between a diagnosis of T-cell large granular lymphocytic leukemia (T-LGL leukemia) and hepatosplenic T-cell lymphoma (HSTCL)?
    A. *STAT3* mutations are found in T-LGL leukemia but not in HSTCL.
    B. HSTCL is of TCR γ/δ origin while T-LGL leukemia is of TCR α/β origin.
    C. Isochromsome 7q is found in HSTCL but not in T-LGL leukemia.
    D. Perforin is positive in HSTCL and negative in T-LGL leukemia.
    E. Loss of CD5 expression is seen in HSTCL but not in T-LGL leukemia.

25. Which of the following regarding *BCR-ABL1*-like B-lymphoblastic leukemia/lymphoma (B-ALL) is true?
    A. A t(9;22)(q34.1;q11.2) is typically present.
    B. *CRLF2* translocations are common.
    C. The B lymphoblasts typically have CD13 and/or CD33 myeloid antigen expression.
    D. Multiple copies of *BCR* are present, often on the same chromosome.
    E. It has a favorable prognosis.

26. All of the following genetic alterations have been identified in follicular lymphoma and follicular lymphoma variants EXCEPT:
    A. deletion of 1p36 locus
    B. t(14;18)(q32;q21)
    C. *BCL6* rearrangement
    D. *MAP2K1* mutations
    E. amplification of 9p24.1

27. Which of the following cytogenetic findings is compatible with a diagnosis of B-lymphoblastic leukemia/lymphoma with iAMP21?
    A. rearrangement of chromosome 21 by karyotype
    B. 3 copies of the *RUNX1* probe within the same chromosome by metaphase FISH
    C. extra copies of the entire chromosome 21 (>3 copies) by karyotype
    D. 4 copies of the *RUNX1* probe within the same cell by metaphase FISH
    E. 6 copies of *RUNX1* probe within the same cell by interphase FISH

28. Which of the following regarding early T-cell precursor T-lymphoblastic leukemia/lymphoma (ETP-ALL) is correct?
    A. Blasts are generally negative for cytoplasmic CD3.
    B. It has a worse prognosis in children compared to other T-ALL subtypes.
    C. It may be positive for both cytoplasmic CD3 and MPO.
    D. The most frequently detected translocation, t(10;11)(p12;q14), is not identifiable by FISH.
    E. Gene expression profiling demonstrates more similarities with acute myeloid leukemia than with other T-ALL.

29. Which of the following B-cell lymphomas is least likely to be positive for CD5?
    A. follicular lymphoma
    B. mantle cell lymphoma
    C. chronic lymphocytic leukemia/small lymphocytic lymphoma
    D. splenic marginal zone lymphoma
    E. lymphoplasmacytic lymphoma

30. Mutations in all of the following genes have been described in mantle cell lymphoma except
    A. *TP53*
    B. *MYD88*
    C. *NOTCH2*
    D. *ATM*
    E. *MLL2*

31. Which of the following statements about high grade B-cell lymphoma is correct?
    A. MYC protein expression of >40% in the neoplastic B cells is predictive of a *MYC* gene rearrangement.
    B. Having a MYC gene rearrangement is diagnostic of a high grade B-cell lymphoma.
    C. Co-expression of MYC and BCL2 protein by immunohistochemistry is diagnostic of a high grade B-cell lymphoma.
    D. Using a break-apart FISH probe for the *MYC* gene should detect all *MYC* gene rearrangements.
    E. Most high grade B-cell lymphomas with *MYC* and *BCL2* and/or *BCL6* gene rearrangements are of germinal center origin.

32. Which of the following cytogenetic abnormalities is considered high risk in plasma cell myeloma?
    A. *IGH/MAF* rearrangement
    B. hyperdiploidy
    C. *CCND1/IGH* rearrangement
    D. *FGFR3/IGH* rearrangement
    E. deletion of chromosome 13

33. Which of the following is true regarding site-specific cytogenetic abnormalities in extranodal marginal zone lymphoma of mucosa-associated lymphoid tissue (MALT lymphoma)?
    A. t(14;18)(q32;q21) *IGH-MALT1* is often found in thyroid MALT lymphomas.
    B. t(14;18)(q32;q21) *IGH-MALT1* is the most frequently detected translocation in gastric MALT lymphomas.
    C. t(11;18)(q21;q21) *BIRC3-MALT1* is frequently identified in intestinal MALT lymphomas.
    D. t(3;14)(p13;q32) *IGH-FOXP1* is commonly detected in lung MALT lymphomas.
    E. t(1;14)(p22;q32) *IGH-BCL10* is often seen in MALT lymphomas of the ocular adnexa.

34. Which of the following statements is true regarding anaplastic large cell lymphoma (ALCL)?
    A. *DUSP22* rearrangements in systemic ALK-negative ALCL are associated with a worse prognosis.
    B. ALK translocations are commonly identified in breast implant-associated ALCL.
    C. TP63 rearrangements in systemic ALK-positive ALCL are associated with a worse prognosis.
    D. *DUSP22* rearrangements in primary cutaneous ALCL is associated with a favorable prognosis.
    E. t(2;5)(p23;q35) is the most common translocation in systemic ALK-positive ALCL.

35. Which of the following statements is true regarding lymphoplasmacytic lymphoma (LPL)?
    A. *MYD88* L265P mutations are specific for lymphoplasmacytic lymphoma
    B. *MYD88* and *CXCR4* mutations are mutually exclusive
    C. *MYD88* non-mutated LPL have a better clinical outcome than *MYD88* mutated LPL
    D. Somatic *CXCR4* mutations identified in LPL are identical to the germline *CXCR4* mutations associated with WHIM syndrome
    E. *MYD88* mutations are not typically identified in IgM monoclonal gammopathy of uncertain significance (MGUS)

36. All of the following are correct regarding B-lymphoblastic leukemia/lymphoma with t(9;22)(q34.1;q112); *BCR-ABL1* (Ph+ B-ALL) except:
    A. Most adult cases have the p190 fusion protein.
    B. Deletions in *IKZF1* are common.
    C. Loss of 9p confers a worse prognosis.
    D. Cases with *T315I* mutations are resistant to first-line tyrosine kinase inhibitors.
    E. The *BCR-ABL1* breakpoints are identical to those in chronic myeloid leukemia.

37. Which of the following is true regarding angioimmunoblastic T-cell lymphoma (AITL)?
    A. Loss of 13q can help differentiate AITL from peripheral T-cell lymphoma, not otherwise specified.
    B. *ITK-SYK* rearrangements are more common than *CTLA2-CD28* rearrangements in AITL.
    C. *RHOA* mutations are thought to be driver mutations in AITL.
    D. *IDH2* p.R172 hotspot mutations are observed in ~75% of AITL.
    E. Clonal T-cell receptor gene rearrangements are only present in ~50% of AITL.

38. Which of the following is true regarding pediatric-type follicular lymphoma and adult-type follicular lymphoma?
    A. Pediatric-type follicular lymphomas have a similar prognosis to grade 3B adult-type follicular lymphomas.
    B. *BCL2* rearrangements are common in adult-type follicular lymphoma while BCL6 rearrangements are common in pediatric-type follicular lymphoma.
    C. *KMT2D* mutations are more often identified in pediatric-type follicular lymphoma than in adult-type follicular lymphoma.
    D. Pediatric-type follicular lymphoma is much more frequent in men whereas adult-type follicular lymphoma occurs equally in men and women.
    E. By definition, pediatric-type follicular lymphoma can only be diagnosed in patients <30 years of age.

39. All of the following are true regarding B-lymphoblastic leukemia/lymphoma with t(v;11q23.3); *KMT2A*-rearranged except:
    A. The t(6;11)(q27;q23) rearrangement with AF6 as the *KMT2A* fusion partner is the most commonly detected rearrangement
    B. The lymphoblasts may express myeloid antigen CD15
    C. It is the most common type of B-lymphoblastic leukemia/lymphoma in children younger than 1
    D. A break-apart FISH probe for the 11q23 region is the best way to detect a rearrangement
    E. *KMT2A* rearrangements are not specific to B-lymphoblastic leukemia/lymphoma

40. Which of the following is true regarding the genetic features of primary mediastinal large B-cell lymphoma (PMBL)?
    A. It has a distinct genetic profile from classic Hodgkin lymphoma
    B. BCL2 and BCL6 rearrangements are frequently identified
    C. Amplifications of 9p24.1 are found in approximately 20% of PMBL
    D. Loss of 2p16 is a common abnormality in PMBL
    E. *CIITA* rearrangements are often identified

E

Self-Study

Explanations & case references

Myeloid neoplasms (questions 1-20)

1. **Answer** A. Although FISH for *BCR-ABL1* is not as sensitive as qPCR, it will detect virtually all variant translocations, as opposed to PCR which is limited by the primer sets used. FISH cannot distinguish between the different BCR breakpoints, however, and cannot be used to monitor for molecular remission. Most typical *BCR-ABL1* FISH assays use dual-fusion probes. See **Case 1**.

2. **Answer** D. The major, minor, and micro breakpoints are the 3 predominant forms described for *BCR-ABL1* fusion, producing proteins with molecular weights of 210, 190, and 230 kd, respectively. The major breakpoint occurs in the vast majority of CML cases, while the minor is typically found in de novo B-lymphoblastic leukemia. The rare micro breakpoint is associated with thrombocytosis and neutrophilic leukocytosis of mostly mature neutrophils. It is important to note that other rare breakpoints may occur, and these may not be detectable by PCR methods, depending on the probe set(s) used. See **Case 1**.

3. **Answer** B. Mutations in *JAK2*, *CALR*, and *MPL* all have the same downstream effect of increased signaling via the JAK/STAT pathway, resulting in unchecked cellular proliferation. Mutations in *DNMT3A* and *TET2* are associated with age-related clonal hematopoiesis and may also occur in patients with ET, but are not considered the main drivers of disease. Mutations in *SF3B1* and *SETBP1* are more commonly found in myelodysplastic neoplasms, while mutations in *ABL1* are not characteristic of myeloid neoplasms in general. See **Case 3**.

4. **Answer** B. Eosinophil dysplasia occurs in both reactive and malignant conditions, but is more likely to be seen in the clonal neoplastic eosinophils of CEL. Malignant T cell proliferations, Hodgkin lymphoma, and systemic mastocytosis may all be associated with an increase in benign eosinophils, while the eosinophilia present in CML is derived from the neoplastic stem cell clone. See **Case 5**.

5. **Answer** E. As opposed to the other functional groups listed, mutations in genes related to the cytoskeleton are not typically found in myeloid neoplasms and are instead related to hereditary red cell membrane disorders. See **Case 8**.

6. **Answer** D. Mutations in spliceosome genes tend to characterize myelodysplastic syndromes or MDS/MPN overlap neoplasms such as chronic myelomonocytic leukemia. Among lymphoid neoplasms, mutations in *SF3B1* are found in chronic lymphocytic leukemia, but not typically in T-cell or Hodgkin lymphoma. Myeloproliferative neoplasms typically have genetic aberrations in signaling pathways involving kinases. See **Cases 8, 10 & 12**.

7. **Answer** E. The neoplasm described is consistent with myelodysplastic/myeloproliferative neoplasm with ring sideroblasts and thrombocytosis, which has both dysplastic and proliferative features by morphology and by molecular findings. Approximately 60% of cases will have mutations in both *JAK2* and *SF3B1*; rarely mutations in both *CALR* and *SF3B1* are identified. See **Case 15.**

ISBN 978-089189-6814 ©2021 ASCP

8. **Answer** Chronic myeloid leukemia is defined by the presence of *BCR-ABL1*, while chronic neutrophilic leukemia is characterized by *CSF3R* mutations in most cases. Of the 2 MDS/MPN overlap neoplasms, atypical chronic myeloid leukemia is associated with *SETBP1* mutations, although these are not specific for this disorder, while the combination of *TET2* and *SRSF2* mutations is often seen in chronic myelomonocytic leukemia. See **Cases 1, 4, 12 & 14**.

9. **Answer** G. Individuals with CHIP have an increased risk for developing hematologic malignancy as well as increased risk of cardiovascular disease (not obesity, per se). By definition, CHIP occurs in the absence of known hematologic abnormality, while the term "clonal cytopenia of undetermined significance" (CCUS) is used when a clonal lesion is found in the presence of unexplained cytopenia, but without diagnostic evidence for myelodysplastic syndrome. The presence of CHIP mutations does not by itself indicate malignancy. See **Cases 7 & 17**.

10. **Answer** B. The presence of ring sideroblasts indicates dyserythropoiesis but is not specific for malignancy. Benign conditions which can cause ring sideroblasts include antibiotics such as isoniazid, copper deficiency, zinc toxicity, and hemoglobinopathies. Among myeloid neoplasms, the presence of *SF3B1* mutations is highly associated with ring sideroblasts, not just in myelodysplastic syndrome but also MDS/MPN overlap neoplasms such as chronic myelomonocytic leukemia. See **Cases 10 & 15**.

11. **Answer** A, B, and D. The remaining abnormalities are indicative of clonal hematopoiesis but may be found in individuals without evidence of hematologic disease. Loss of Y especially is an age-related phenomenon. See **Case 8**.

12. **Answer** B and C. *SF3B1* mutation in myeloid neoplasms is highly correlative with the presence of ring sideroblasts. It is important to recognize MDS with RS because these patients have relatively favorable prognosis compared to other MDS subtypes. A diagnosis of MDS with RS requires at least 15% RS (out of erythroid precursors) unless an *SF3B1* mutation is present, in which case at least 5% RS should be present. See **Case 10**.

13. **Answer** E. This group of disorders most commonly presents as a myeloid neoplasm, although some can also present as lymphoblastic leukemia/lymphoma. Rearrangements of *PDGFRA* (not *FGFR1*) are typically cryptic by conventional karyotyping, and only cases having rearranged *PDGFRA* or *PDGFRB* have been shown to respond significantly to imatinib therapy. See **Case 16**.

14. **Answer** A. Although there is no single specific blast morphology for AML having *RUNX1* mutation (**Case 23**), many cases will have undifferentiated, small blasts exhibiting high nuclear to cytoplasmic ratios. The presence of many Auer rods is typical of acute promyelocytic leukemia (**Case 20**), while monocytic differentiation is often found in AML with mutated *NPM1* (**Case 21**), AML with *KMT2A* (*MLL*) rearrangement (**Case 25**), and AML with inv(16). Cases of pure erythroleukemia often have mutation in *TP53*, while megakaryocytic blasts are associated with rarer genetic abnormalities. See **Cases 27 & 28**.

15. **Answer** D. According to 2017 WHO criteria, the presence of t(15;17) *PML-RARA*, t(8;21) *RUNX1-RUNX1T1*, or inv(16) *CBFB* rearrangement is diagnostic for AML regardless of blast count in blood or bone marrow, and such cases should be treated with appropriate AML therapy. Note that inv(3) may also be found in myelodysplastic syndrome, and t(9;11) also occurs in acute lymphoblastic leukemia. See **Cases 19 & 20**.

16. **Answer** B. In the 2017 WHO classification of hematopoietic neoplasms, AML with mutated *NPM1* is a distinct entity, with favorable prognosis if the karyotype is normal and if present, *FLT3-ITD* has a variant allelic ratio <0.5. The presence of background dysplasia does not preclude a diagnosis of AML with mutated *NPM1*, so long as an MDS-associated karyotype abnormality is not present. See **Case 21**.

17. **Answer** C. Cases of AML with biallelic *CEBPA* mutations have a characteristic mutation pattern, with one allele having an N-terminal mutation and the other with a C-terminal mutation. The gene is typically analyzed in part using Sanger sequencing, as it has a high GC content which may interfere with assays using NGS. These cases typically have morphologic features of AML with or without maturation; cases with monocytic differentiation are more rare. The karyotype is typically normal, although a subset demonstrate deletion of 9q, and co-occuring *FLT3-ITD* occurs in a minority of cases. See **Case 22**.

18. **Answer** A, C, D. AML with t(1;22) *RBM15-MKL1* and AML associated with Down syndrome typically demonstrate megakaryocytic differentiation, as do rare cases of AML having a unique immunophenotype including bright CD56 and lack of HLA-DR and CD45 (the "RAM" phenotype). AML with inv(16) classically presents with myelomonocytic differentiation, and the phenotype in choice E is non-specific but could be seen with erythroleukemia. See **Cases 27 & 28**.

19. **Answer** B, D, and E are all characteristics of TRMN related to alkylating agents. A shorter latency period (1-2 years) and recurrent genetic translocations are typical of TRMN occurring after topoisomerase inhibitor therapy. Mutations in *DNMT3A* are associated with aging and are more commonly found in de novo myeloid neoplasms. See **Case 26**.

20. **Answer** A. Myeloid neoplasms associated with a germline mutation most typically manifest as MDS, MDS/MPN, or AML in younger patients, although some patients present at older ages. Any diagnosis of MDS in a child or young adult should prompt evaluation for a germline mutation. These disorders are typically characterized by heterozygous mutations, resulting in variant allele frequencies at approximately 50% since all cells in the sample have one copy of the mutated gene. Juvenile myelomonocytic leukemia (JMML) is an MDS/MPN overlap neoplasm occurring in children and is rarely associated with congenital mutation in *RAS* or *PTPN11* genes; affected patients often have elevated levels of hemoglobin F. See **Case 11**.

ISBN 978-089189-6814   ©2021 ASCP

Lymphoid neoplasms (questions 21-40)

21. **Answer** D. A mutated immunoglobulin heavy chain variable region (*IGHV*), defined as <98% homology with the germline *IGHV* sequence, is associated with a favorable prognosis in CLL/SLL. Unmutated *IGHV* CLL/SLL has a poorer prognosis and CD49d, ZAP70, and CD38 positivity are all associated with an unmutated *IGHV* as well as independent high risk factors. Loss of 17p, the locus containing *TP53*, as well as *TP53* mutations, are also associated with an adverse prognosis as are *NOTCH1* mutations. See **Case 29**.

22. **Answer** B. Hairy cell leukemia (HCL) is typically associated with monocytopenia at presentation, not monocytosis. Most patients have splenomegaly due to splenic infiltration and significant bone marrow fibrosis resulting in a "dry tap" when attempting bone marrow aspiration. HCL cells characteristically express CD11c, CD25, CD103, and CD123, and although *BRAF* V600E mutation is not specific for HCL, it is present in almost 100% of cases. See **Case 31**.

23. **Answer** E. Patients with T-cell prolymphocytic leukemia (T-PLL) typically present with a very high white blood cell count. T-PLL cells usually do not demonstrate significant T-cell antigen loss, even of CD7, which is often decreased or lost in other T-cell lymphoproliferative disorders. Rearrangements of chromosome 14 involving the *TRA*, *TCL1A* and *TCL1B* genes are characteristic in T-PLL, typically resulting in an inv(14)(q11q32) or t(14;14)(q11;q32). Less commonly, t(x;14)(q28;q11) is seen. A t(14;14)(q11;q32) is not associated with any of the other listed T-cell lymphoproliferative disorders. See **Case 43**.

24. **Answer** C. Isochromsome 7q is identified in approximately 50% of HSTCL but is not a feature of T-LGL leukemia. *STAT3* mutations, although more common in T-LGL leukemia, are also present in approximately 10% of HSTCL. While most cases of HSTCL are of TCR γ/δ origin and most cases of T-LGL leukemia are of TCR α/β origin, HSTCL can arise from TCR α/β cells and T-LGL leukemia can arise from TCR γ/δ cells. Perforin is typically negative in HSTCL and positive in T-LGL leukemia. Loss of CD5 expression can be seen in both T-LGL leukemia and HSTCL. See **Cases 42 & 44**.

25. **Answer** B. Although many different rearrangements and gene mutations are present in *BCR-ABL1*-like B-ALL, over half exhibit *CRLF2* translocations. *BCR/ABL1* translocations t(9;22)(q34.1;q11.2) are present in *BCR-ABL1* positive B-ALL, but not in *BCR-ABL1*-like B-ALL. CD13 and/or CD33 antigen expression is common in *BCR-ABL1* positive B-ALL but is not a feature of *BCR-ABL1*-like B-ALL. Additional copies of the *BCR* gene are not a feature of *BCR-ABL1*-like B-ALL. *BCR-ABL1*-like B-ALL tends to have a poor prognosis. See **Cases 50 & 51**.

26. **Answer** E. Amplification of 9p24.1 is a common abnormality in primary mediastinal large B-cell lymphoma and in classic Hodgkin lymphoma but is not a feature of follicular lymphoma. t(14;18)(q32;q21) *IGH-BCL2* is the most common genetic abnormality detected in adult-type follicular lymphoma, particularly low grade follicular lymphomas (grade 1-2). This rearrangement is typically absent in primary cutaneous follicle center lymphoma and pediatric-type follicular lymphoma. Grade 3B adult-type follicular lymphomas also often lack *IGH/BCL2* rearrangements. Deletion of 1p36 is often associated with a diffuse variant of follicular lymphoma that generally expresses CD10 and CD23 and lacks an *IGH/BCL2* rearrangement; however, 1p36 abnormalities have also been reported in pediatric and standard, adult-type follicular lymphomas. *BCL6* rearrangements are absent in pediatric-type follicular lymphomas but occur in 5%-15% of cases of adult-type follicular lymphoma. *MAP2K1* is frequently mutated in follicular lymphoma. See **Cases 33, 34, 39 & 40**.

27. **Answer** B. B-lymphoblastic leukemia/lymphoma (B-ALL) with intrachromosomal amplification of 21 (iAMP21) is typically detected via metaphase FISH using a *RUNX1* probe and should demonstrate at least 3 copies on a single abnormal chromosome or at least 5 copies within a single cell. Extra copies of the *RUNX1* probe due to extra copies of chromosome 21 are not diagnostic of B-ALL with iAMP21. Chromosome 21 is not rearranged in B-ALL with iAMP21. While 6 copies of *RUNX1* within the same cell (choice E) could be compatible with B-ALL with iAMP21, metaphase FISH is needed to exclude the possibility that the extra copies of *RUNX1* are simply due to extra copies of chromosome 21. See **Case 49**.

28. **Answer** E. Early T-cell precursor T-lymphoblastic leukemia/lymphoma has a typical immunophenotype: CD7 positive, CD1a and CD8 negative, and positive for at least one of the following markers: CD34, CD117, HLA-DR, CD13, CD33, CD11b, or CD65. Blasts also usually express cytoplasmic CD3. An acute leukemia which expresses both MPO and cytoplasmic CD3 should be diagnosed as T/myeloid mixed-phenotype acute leukemia, not ETP-ALL. Although initially the prognosis of ETP-ALL was thought to be worse in children than other types of T-ALL, subsequent larger studies have not shown a statistically significant difference in outcome. The most frequently detected translocation in ETP-ALL is t(10;11)(p12;q14); however, this is detectable by FISH. Gene expression profiling in ETP-ALL has demonstrated findings distinct from other T-ALL with overexpression of genes that are typically associated with myeloid or stem cells. See **Case 52**.

29. **Answer** A. While chronic lymphocytic leukemia/small lymphocytic lymphoma and mantle cell lymphoma have a prototypic CD5 positive B-cell immunophenotype, CD5 expression is also present in other B-cell lymphomas including up to a quarter of splenic marginal zone lymphomas, up to 43% of lymphoplasmacytic lymphomas, and diffuse large B-cell lymphoma. Follicular lymphoma can very rarely express CD5, particularly in the floral variant, but is the least likely to be positive of all the choices. See **Cases 29, 32, 33, 35, and 36**.

30. **Answer** B. *MYD88* L265P mutations are most commonly seen in lymphoplasmacytic lymphoma, a subset of diffuse large B-cell lymphomas, and in rare marginal zone lymphomas but have not been described in mantle cell lymphoma. See **Cases 32 & 35**.

31. **Answer** E. There are 2 official categories of high grade B-cell lymphoma in the 2017 World Health Organization classification including high grade B-cell lymphoma, not otherwise specified (HGBL, NOS) and high grade B-cell lymphoma (HGBL) with MYC and BCL2 and/or BCL6 rearrangements. While the latter is defined primarily by cytogenetic aberrations, the former category is diagnosed mostly by morphology. HGBL, NOS is a diagnosis that should be used sparingly in cases of B-cell lymphoma with features intermediate between Burkitt lymphoma and diffuse large B-cell lymphoma or in large B-cell lymphomas with a blastoid-type appearance. MYC protein expression levels by immunohistochemistry is not a reliable predictor of a *MYC* rearrangement. *MYC* gene rearrangement alone is not diagnostic of a high grade B-cell lymphoma. An additional *BCL2* and/or *BCL6* rearrangement must also be present for a diagnosis of HGBL with *MYC* and *BCL2* and/or *BCL6* rearrangements or the morphologic/immunophenotypic features must meet criteria for HGBCL, NOS. Co-expression of MYC and BCL2 protein by immunohistochemistry is not diagnostic of a high grade B-cell lymphoma; instead, it denotes a "double expressor" large B-cell lymphoma, which independently confers a poor prognosis. A break-apart FISH probe for MYC will miss a small percentage of *MYC* rearrangements. A dual-color, dual-fusion probe for *MYC/IGH* should be used in addition to a *MYC* break-apart probe in order to detect all MYC rearrangements. The vast majority of HGBL with *MYC* and *BCL2* and/or *BCL6* rearrangements are of germinal center origin. See **Case 38**.

32. **Answer** A. Of this list, only *IGH/MAF* rearrangements confer a high risk. *IGH/MAFB* rearrangements, deletion(17p), and a high risk gene expression signature are also considered high risk abnormalities. Deletion of chromosome 13 and *FGFR3/IGH* rearrangements, along with hypodiploidy, are considered intermediate risk. Hyperdiploidy and *CCND1/IGH* rearrangements are considered standard risk, along with *CCND3/IGH1* rearrangements and all other abnormalities. See **Case 41**.

33. **Answer** C. The t(11;18)(q21;q21) *BIRC3-MALT1* translocation is detected most often in MALT lymphomas of the intestine and lung and is also the most frequently identified translocation in gastric MALT lymphomas. The t(14;18)(q32;q21) *IGH-MALT1* translocation has been reported in MALT lymphomas of the stomach, ocular adnexa, salivary gland, lung, and skin but not in the intestine or thyroid. The t(3;14)(p13;q32) *IGH-FOXP1* translocation has been described in MALT lymphomas of the ocular adnexa, skin, and thyroid but not of the stomach, intestine, salivary gland, or lung. The t(1;14)(p22;q32) *IGH-BCL10* translocation may be identified in the intestine, salivary gland, or lung, but not in the stomach, ocular adnexa, skin, or thyroid. See **Case 37**.

34. **Answer** E. Systemic ALK-negative ALCL in general has a worse prognosis than systemic ALK positive ALCL; however, ALK-negative ALCL cases with a DUSP22 rearrangement have been shown to have improved survival, similar to that of ALK-positive ALCL. ALK translocations are absent in breast implant-

associated ALCL. TP63 rearrangements are typically detected in ALK-negative ALCL, not ALK-positive ALCL, and are associated with an aggressive disease course. ALK-negative and ALK-positive ALCL are morphologically similar but clinically distinct with differing prognostic implications. The t(2;5)(p23;q35) rearrangement is the most common ALK rearrangement in systemic ALK-positive ALCL and is present in ~80% of cases. See **Case 45**.

35. **Answer** D. Somatic *CXCR4* mutations identified in LPL are identical to germline mutations found in WHIM (warts, hypogammaglobulinemia, infections, myelokathexis) syndrome. *MYD88* L265P mutations are found in >90% of LPL cases but are not specific and can also be seen in a subset of other small B-cell lymphomas, including some splenic marginal zone lymphomas, as well as in diffuse large B-cell lymphoma. *CXCR4* mutations occur almost exclusively in *MYD88* mutated LPL and are often subclonal in nature. The rare cases of LPL that lack *MYD88* mutations are reported to have a worse clinical outcome than *MYD88* mutated LPL. *MYD88* L265P mutations can be identified in approximately half of IgM MGUS cases. See **Case 35**.

36. **Answer** A. Most pediatric Ph+ B-ALL cases harbor the p190 fusion protein while approximately half of the adult cases have the p190 fusion protein and half have the p210 fusion protein. Deletions in *IKZF1* are identified in ~75% of pediatric cases and 91% of adult Ph+ B-ALL cases. Structural changes to chromosome 9 which result in loss of the short arm (9p) confer a worse prognosis in Ph+ B-ALL. Ph+ B-ALL with mutations in *T315I* are resistant to frontline tyrosine kinase inhibitors (TKI) including imatinib, but may be responsive to newer generation TKI therapy, such as ponatinib. The *BCR-ABL1* breakpoints present in Ph+ B-ALL are identical to those in chronic myeloid leukemia. See **Cases 1 & 50**.

37. **Answer** C. Loss of 13q is a common cytogenetic abnormality in AITL but is not specific and can also be seen in peripheral T-cell lymphoma, not otherwise specified. *ITK-SYK* and *CTLA4-CD28* rearrangements are both present in AITL but *ITK-SYK* rearrangements are less common than *CTLA4-CD28* rearrangements, with a frequency of approximately 18% and 58%, respectively. *IDH2* p.R172 mutations are present in AITL at a frequency of ~45%, not 75%. Clonal T-cell receptor gene rearrangements are present in >95% of AITL. See **Case 46**.

38. **Answer** D. While pediatric-type follicular lymphomas have a similar morphology to grade 3B adult-type follicular lymphoma, they have a much better prognosis as they are often localized, and surgery alone can be curative although systemic therapy may also be administered. While *BCL2* rearrangements are common in adult-type follicular lymphomas (present in >80%), *BCL6* rearrangements occur in a minority of adult-type follicular lymphomas but are not present in pediatric-type follicular lymphomas. *KMT2D* mutations are reported in pediatric-type follicular lymphoma (frequency of 0-15%) but are much more common in adult-type follicular lymphoma (frequency of 50%-80%). Although the vast majority of pediatric-type follicular lymphomas occur in patients <30 years old, it is rarely seen in older individuals (including **Case 34**). See **Cases 33 & 34**.

39. **Answer** A. The most common partner gene is AF4 on chromosome 4q21 [t(4;11)(q21;q23)]. *KMT2A* rearrangements are not specific to B-ALL and are also found in acute myeloid leukemia (AML) and T-lymphoblastic leukemia/lymphoma (T-ALL). The t(6;11)(q27;q23) rearrangement is primarily seen in pediatric and adult AML as well as in some T-ALL. The lymphoblasts in *KMT2A*-rearranged B-ALL typically lack CD10 and express myeloid antigen CD15. *KMT2A*-rearranged B-ALL is the most common type of B-lymphoblastic leukemia/lymphoma and most common leukemia overall, in children younger than 1. Because more than 100 different unique translocations have been described in *KMT2A*-rearranged B-ALL (and some may be cryptic by karyotype), the best method for detection is a break-apart FISH probe for the 11q23 region. See **Case 47**.

40. **Answer** E. There is significant genetic overlap between PMBL and classic Hodgkin lymphoma (CHL) based on gene expression profiling studies. Both can exhibit amplifications of 9p241 and 2p16 as well as mutations in the JAK/STAT and NF-κB pathways. *BCL2*, *BCL6*, and *MYC* rearrangements are common in diffuse large B-cell lymphoma, not otherwise specified but are very infrequent in PMBL. Amplifications of 9p24.1 are present in ~50%-70% of PMBL, not 20%. Gains of 2p16, not loss, are a common abnormality in PMBL. *CIITA* rearrangements, often with *PDL1* or *PDL2*, are common and have been reported in up to half of PMBL. See **Case 39**.

Amelia Nakanishi & Shashirekha Shetty

A

Overview of genetic & molecular testing methodologies used in the evaluation of hematologic disorders

Introduction

Genetic testing is integral to the practice of hematopathology and the classification of myeloid and lymphoid disorders. The current WHO classification of hematologic neoplasms relies heavily on molecular and genetic findings. Cytogenetic testing examines chromosomal changes, while molecular testing analyzes lesions at the DNA level. Together, these techniques play an important roles in diagnosis, prognosis, treatment, and residual disease detection. This appendix summarizes current molecular and cytogenetic methodologies used for the evaluation of hematologic disease, including the advantages and limitations associated with each assay, and their interpretational challenges.

Routine tests performed in the cytogenetics laboratory for hematological conditions include:

1. Conventional cytogenetics, also known as karyotyping or chromosome analysis
2. Fluorescence in situ hybridization (FISH)
3. Chromosomal microarray (CMA) or single nucleotide polymorphism (SNP) karyotyping or molecular karyotyping

Routine tests performed in the molecular laboratory for hematological conditions include:
1. Polymerase chain reaction (PCR) for single or panel gene analysis
2. Sequencing by the Sanger method or by high throughput, next generation sequencing (NGS)
3. Clonality assessment for T and B cells

Specimen considerations

Specimen considerations are critical for the success of any genetic testing. Cytogenetic studies, such as chromosome analysis and metaphase FISH, require fresh, viable tissue for cell culturing and harvesting. Fresh tissue is typically sourced from bone marrow aspirates, peripheral blood, or portions of lymph node/tissue biopsies. Peripheral fluids such as pleural and ascitic effusions, or cerebrospinal fluid, may also be used. If fresh tissue is not available, FISH can be performed on uncultured or non-dividing cells or from formalin-fixed tissue embedded in paraffin (FFPE). To facilitate a successful culture and harvest, it is important that specimens are collected under sterile conditions into an appropriate medium (eg, sodium heparin medium, Hanks balanced salt solution, or sterile saline) and maintained at ambient temperature during transport and storage. Sodium heparin is the preferred anticoagulant, because other anticoagulants may interfere with cell viability. It is important to note that multiple pre-analytical factors, such as anticoagulants, temperature, and transit time, may interfere with the viability of the cells and compromise results.

For molecular testing or CMA, bone marrow aspirates and peripheral blood specimens can be collected in ethylenediaminetetraacetic acid (EDTA) and refrigerated prior to DNA extraction. DNA can also be extracted from fresh or FFPE tissue.

For RNA-based tests, especially those examining gene expression or fusion genes, it is imperative that the RNA is stabilized to prevent degradation after collection. Bone marrow and blood specimens can be collected in EDTA and ideally should be processed within 24 hours

ISBN 978-089189-6814

of collection. To improve RNA stability, the specimen can be transported in preservative reagents (such as Sigma's RNA*later*®). Like DNA, RNA can be extracted from fresh or FFPE tissue although quality is lost after processing and fixation. The most amenable tissue fixative for nucleic acid testing is 10% buffered neutral formalin, which is the least damaging to tissue and does not contain heavy metals, such as zinc or mercury, which may interfere with later PCR reactions.

Chromosome analysis

Chromosome analysis provides a "gross examination" of all the chromosomes and is the gold standard of cytogenetic testing. It is used to detect aneuploidies, rearrangements, and ≥5-10 megabase (Mb)-sized gains and losses. Notably, chromosome analysis lacks the resolution to demonstrate changes smaller than 3-5 Mb, and when present, such changes are referred to as being *cryptic* and must be detected by other methods such as FISH or microarray. A major advantage of chromosome analysis is the ability to detect clonal changes and discern individual clones. Since the chromosome architecture is intact, chromosome analysis also aids in the identification of apparently balanced chromosomal rearrangements that cannot be elucidated via other techniques such as CMA.

As mentioned above, chromosome analysis requires fresh, viable tumor cells that can be cultured and harvested. Hypocellular, small or necrotic samples of tumor or samples exposed to fixatives are the most common causes of culture failure. Tumors with high proliferation indices are easily cultured, whereas tumors with low mitotic indices, such as mature lymphoid neoplasms, often require chemical or mitogen stimulation. The cultures are maintained for 1-3 days to accumulate and synchronize cell cycles, before being arrested in metaphase with colcemid (a mitotic spindle inhibitor that keeps sister chromatids together). The cells are then exposed to a hypotonic solution to make them swell, separating chromosomes within the nuclei for clear visualization. Finally, the cells are fixed with a solution such as Carnoy fixative, which is a 3:1 methanol to glacial acetic acid mixture.

After fixation, the cells are pretreated with trypsin and stained with Giemsa to reveal predictable banding patterns that are unique to each chromosome. The mechanism of G-banding is not fully understood. One explanation is this: chromatin is packaged differently based on how frequently genes need to be accessed

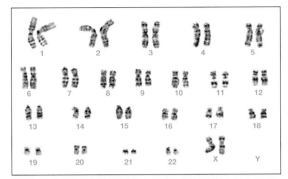

fA.1 A normal female (46,XX) karyogram using Giemsa banding

for transcription; the lighter staining euchromatin is loosely wrapped and bound to fewer proteins compared to the tightly wrapped, protein dense genes of the darker heterochromatin. Treating cells with trypsin, a proteolytic agent that removes some of the proteins binding chromatin, increases the contrast between euchromatin and heterochromatin. After staining with Giemsa, heterochromatin appears dark because it retains more stained proteins than euchromatin; the resultant alternating dark and pale stained regions are called *bands;* normal banding patterns in humans are elaborated in the International Standard Cytogenetic Nomenclature, 2016. Using a microscope, a highly trained individual can then sort the pairs of chromosomes by their banding patterns, and produce an image known as a *karyogram* (commonly referred to as a *karyotype*). The metaphases of twenty cells are examined, which allows for detection of a clone present in greater than or equal to 14% of cells with a 95% confidence interval. A thirty cell count can detect a clone present in greater than or equal to 10% of cells with a 95% confidence interval. A normal female karyogram is shown in **fA.1**.

Fluorescence in situ hybridization (FISH)

FISH uses targeted single strand DNA (ssDNA) probes to reveal chromosomal gains/losses and rearrangements, including deletions or amplifications. In the diagnostic setting, there are 4 commonly used types of FISH probes for evaluating hematologic malignancies: centromere, locus-specific, fusion, and break-apart. Regardless of probe type, the basic FISH technique is performed as follows: the target DNA and the probe are denatured, the fluorescently labelled probe is hybridized to target DNA, excess probe is washed off, and the cells are examined with a fluorescent microscope that excites the probes. Since the fluorescent signals will quench with time, images are recorded electronically to

A Overview of genetic & molecular testing methodologies used in the evaluation of hematologic disorders

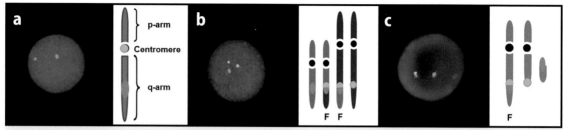

fA.2 FISH strategies to detect different types of chromosome abnormalities in hematological malignancies
a CEP for the chromosome 7 centromere in green and probe for 7q in red, indicating a normal signal pattern with 2 of each signal. The chromosome 7 ideogram is pictured to the right
b Dual-color, dual-fusion probe set to detect *PML-RARA* rearrangement shows 1 red, 1 green & 2 fusions (yellow signals), consistent with t(15;17) and its reciprocal fusion (the normal pattern for a dual fusion probe set is 2 each of red & green signals)
c Break-apart probes revealing the *KMT2A (MLL)* rearrangement, with 1 intact yellow signal & 1 yellow split into separate red & green signals (the normal pattern for a break-apart probe is 2 yellow signals)

document signal patterns. Most FISH probes are labeled with red/orange or green fluorochromes; aqua may also be used for a third color. Typically, 200 random nuclei per probe are examined, which imparts a sensitivity and specificity of detection >95%.

Probes are designed to attach to specific targets measuring thousands of base pairs in length, which allows FISH to detect cryptic abnormalities, but also implies that FISH will miss abnormalities that are <30-70 kb, or very small abnormalities within an otherwise intact target. Unlike conventional chromosome analysis, FISH is not limited to cultured cells and can be performed on fresh, frozen, or FFPE tissues, or alcohol-fixed cytology specimens. Since FISH probes are designed to attach to very specific stretches of DNA, FISH is generally used to confirm suspected diagnostic abnormalities and makes for a poor screening tool. Before PCR became widely available, FISH had been used to monitor minimal residual disease (MRD), but PCR is faster and more sensitive for MRD detection (see below), unless the aberration is rare or overly complex.

Details of specific types of FISH probes

Centromere enumeration probes (CEPs) Detect the presence of a centromere of a chromosome by targeting the highly repetitive sequences of DNA surrounding them **fA.2a**. CEPs are often used as a control probe to differentiate between deletion of a portion of chromosome (eg, 5q) and monosomy, in which the entire chromosome including the centromere is lost.

Locus-specific probes (non-centromeric) Bind to a particular region of a chromosome that is not the centromere. This type of probe is used to determine how

many copies of a gene or locus are present within the sample.

Dual-fusion probes Detect the presence of a particular fusion or gene rearrangement; these are commonly used in diseases with recurrent translocations such as *BCR-ABL1* found in chronic myeloid leukemia. This type of probe relies on the fact that a yellow color is seen when red and green signals are in close proximity. In the absence of the specific fusion, the red and green signals remain distinct, but in the presence of the fusion, a yellow signal appears. In the case of a balanced reciprocal translocation, 2 yellow signals will be produced from the equal exchange between 2 different chromosomes **fA.2b**.

Break-apart probes Bind to opposing sides of known chromosome breakpoints and used especially for the detection of gene fusions when a gene is prone to unpredictable rearrangement with multiple partners (such as *KMT2A* [*MLL*]). Rather than using multiple fusion probes, it is often more efficient to examine whether the gene of interest is intact on its native chromosome. The expected normal pattern of a break-apart probe is *opposite* that of a dual fusion probe. In the absence of rearrangement, 2 yellow signals are present from the proximity of 2 red and 2 green signals; the expected abnormal is to have 1 intact yellow signal, 1 red, and 1 green signal, ie, the yellow signal is "broken" apart **fA.2c**.

Chromosomal microarray (CMA)/molecular karyotyping

CMA is a DNA-based technique used to detect copy number changes. CMA requires fragmentation of the sample DNA, precluding structural evaluation of the chromosomes. The gains and losses seen on

ISBN 978-089189-6814

A *Overview of genetic & molecular testing methodologies used in the evaluation of hematologic disorders*

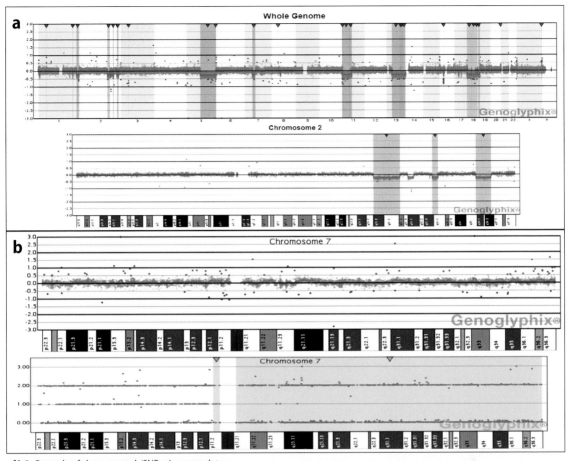

fA.3 Example of chromosomal /SNP microarray data
a CMA/SNP array showing loss of binding of patient DNA (purple regions), consistent with deletion or loss of a chromosome segment; this example represents a chromothripsis event on chromosome 2, with loss of multiple chromosome 2 areas seen in the bottom panel;
b CMA demonstrating loss of heterozygosity (LOH) from uniparental disomy; the top image represents the copy number track showing there are 2 copies of chromosome 7; the bottom image represents SNP marker analysis, with the shaded green region indicating loss of heterozygosity for the long arm of chromosome 7

microarray correlate to trisomies, monosomies, and partial gains/losses visualized directly with chromosome analysis. CMA with SNP markers can also be used to detect allelic imbalances that result in loss of heterozygosity (LOH). However, microarrays do not detect balanced rearrangements as the chromosome structure is fragmented, unlike in conventional karyotyping.

A commonly used type of CMA is the SNP cytogenomic microarray (also known as SNP karyotyping or SNP array). Microarray chips are composed of hundreds of thousands to millions of DNA probes that are complementary to regions of interest in the genome. To perform this technique, the sample DNA is fragmented, labeled, and hybridized to the array. Special software merges information on the address of each probe position and the address of each probe in

the genome, then aligns the probes in chromosomal order to provide information on copy number changes **fA.3a** and LOH **fA.3b**.

CMA has many technical advantages over conventional cytogenetics and FISH, including improved resolution, LOH assessment, and amenability to automation. In addition, array-based karyotyping is able to identify aberrations present at below the resolution of standard FISH or chromosome analysis. The number of probes varies between platforms, ranging between 800,000 to over 2,000,000 genetic markers for a resolution of 10-20 kb, which is comparable to the size of an average gene. This is at least a 1,000-fold increase in resolution compared to conventional cytogenetics, and depending on the coverage, may even aid in the precise identification of pathologic gene abnormalities. Microarray conveniently uses both fresh and FFPE

A *Overview of genetic & molecular testing methodologies used in the evaluation of hematologic disorders*

tissues. SNP arrays in particular are excellent for the assessment of LOH, which is commonly acquired in both hematologic and solid tumors; LOH cannot be detected by comparative genomic hybridization array (a previous version of microarray using a reference DNA sample rather than SNPs), FISH, or conventional cytogenetics. Additionally, compared to conventional cytogenetics, CMA is less time consuming to perform due to its multiplexing and automatization potential.

Polymerase chain reaction (PCR)

PCR is a revolutionary method of rapid DNA replication and is the basis of most modern diagnostic molecular testing. In PCR, specific primers are added to patient DNA to isolate a region of interest, and a thermostable DNA polymerase amplifies it exponentially. DNA procured from fresh tissue is the best specimen for PCR and can be stored indefinitely at –70°C. DNA from tissues preserved with non-crosslinking fixatives, such as ethanol, are also acceptable; DNA from FFPE tissues can be treated with heat and proteinases to reverse some of the crosslinking that would otherwise sterically hinder the polymerase. Very little intact DNA can be recovered from other, more permanent preparations, such as Carnoy fixative.

The patient DNA serves as the template, and the DNA sequence of interest is targeted using oligonucleotide primers that hybridize to the 5' and 3' ends of the target. Added to this is a pooled mixture of deoxynucleotide triphosphates (dATP, dCTP, dGTP, and dTTP) and a thermostable DNA polymerase (eg, Taq polymerase). To amplify the target DNA, these elements are then subjected to timed cycles at different temperatures until the reagents are exhausted and a maximum amount of product is replicated. The first step of the cycle is to denature the double stranded template DNA by heating it to 95°C so that it separates into single strands. Next, the reaction is cooled to allow primer annealing to the exposed target template. Then the reaction is heated to 70°C -75°C for optimal DNA polymerase activity, and the primed DNA strands are replicated by incorporation of dNTPs. Typically, the thermal cycling is repeated forty times, with newly synthesized strands serving as template strands for each subsequent reaction, until amplified products (amplicons) predominate and the reagents are exhausted. The background starting DNA is diluted out by the amplicons. In traditional or end point PCR, these end point products can be quantified by banding on a gel.

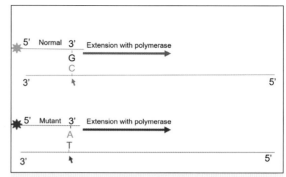

fA.4 Diagrammatic representation of allele-specific PCR, which generates allele-specific amplicons to differentiate normal and variant genotypes. The diagram illustrates an example of a C>T variant. The 3' end of the primer must perfectly match the template for amplification to occur due to stringent binding conditions. The variant-specific probe (labeled red) will not bind adequately to the normal allele (labeled blue) & vice versa

The rate of product synthesis and reaction efficiency follow a predictable plot that can be divided into 3 phases with unique kinetics: exponential, linear, and plateau. In the exponential phase, there are more components than products. These favorable kinetics facilitate ideal doubling. In the linear phase, the reaction rate slows because fewer components are available and products may start to degrade. In the plateau phase, the reaction stops because there are no more components and some products have degraded. End point PCR is less accurate than assays specifically designed for quantitation (see below), because it measures end point products (after all cycles are completed) including those generated under less than favorable kinetics. Qualitative testing for *JAK2 V617F* mutation is an example of an end point PCR assay.

Specialized PCR techniques

Allele-specific PCR (AS-PCR) evaluates a specific mutation. This method allows direct detection of any single base point mutation or single nucleotide polymorphism. Normal and mutant probes that differ by as little as a single base pair are hybridized to sample DNA under stringent conditions, which means that a perfect match must be present for primer binding and subsequent amplification to occur **fA.4**.

Reverse transcriptase PCR (RT-PCR) uses RNA as the starting material, with generation of complementary DNA (cDNA) from RNA prior to amplification. Note in this book, "RT-PCR" refers to "reverse transcriptase PCR" as opposed to "real time PCR" (which is synonymous with quantitative PCR). RT-

ISBN 978-089189-6814

A *Overview of genetic & molecular testing methodologies used in the evaluation of hematologic disorders*

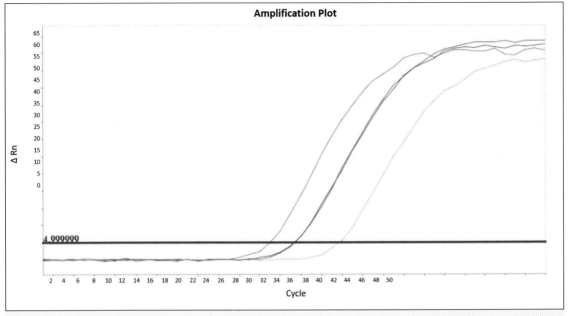

Amplification Plot

fA.5 DNA amplification plot generated using quantitative (or "real-time") PCR. Each curve represents a single sample; the samples in this figure are a dilution series of a target DNA sequence. Fluorescent probes are used such that relative fluorescence is accumulated with each PCR cycle (ie, in *real time*) as the sample amplifies. The exponential portion of each curve represents the region of optimal amplification (and therefore quantitation), while the upper plateau represents exhaustion of reagents. This technique allows for a quantitative measurement of synthesized target DNA in each PCR cycle when compared to a known quantity (standard control)

PCR uses a reverse transcriptase and random primers to convert RNA sequences from the patient sample into cDNA. cDNA is efficient in the identification of gene fusions, because cDNA lacks the intronic regions present at most rearrangement breakpoints in genomic DNA; these intronic regions also interfere with the detection of rearrangements by other methods such as microarray. The use of RNA as starting material also enhances sensitivity, because multiple transcribed copies of the sequence of interest will be present in a cell, vs the maximum of 2 copies in genomic DNA. After the generation of cDNA, amplification is performed with specific primers and the amplicons are used in a subsequent quantitative or qualitative PCR assay. As an example, RT-PCR is often used in combination with subsequent qPCR for quantitation of fusion products, such as *BCR-ABL1*. Qualitatively, RT-PCR can also be used to detect point mutations in the ABL1 kinase domain, where RT-PCR is first used to amplify *BCR-ABL* transcripts and the kinase domain for bidirectional sequence analysis. RT-PCR can also be used to evaluate gene expression profiles, by amplifying all cellular RNA, or gene expression patterns, by targeting a limited number of cDNAs with specific primers. As an example, limited gene expression arrays are used clinically by some academic institutions to classify diffuse large B-cell lymphoma by cell of origin.

Quantitative PCR (qPCR) allows for accurate calculation of the amount of starting template DNA or RNA. qPCR is most often used to quantify minimal residual disease (eg, detection of low-level *BCR-ABL1* transcripts). In qPCR, primers are labeled with fluorescent dyes that emit a signal as amplification occurs. Specialized thermocyclers detect these fluorescent signals (which reflects the amount of double-stranded DNA present) in each reaction well as they accumulate in real time. This signal is plotted in relative fluorescent units to the cycle number by thermocycler software. qPCR data are calculated from cycle threshold (Ct) values measured from amplification curves. The presence of contaminants may decrease the efficiency of the reaction by interfering with Taq polymerase activity or primer binding, thus causing artifactual results. Samples with high levels of impurities and low target concentrations are the least interpretable by qPCR because they cannot be adequately diluted to eliminate the effect of contamination on data quality **fA.5**.

Digital droplet PCR (ddPCR) or emulsion PCR is a highly sensitive quantification method. ddPCR enables precise and accurate quantitation of target DNA molecules by diluting and partitioning the sample into many compartments that each contain an average of 1 DNA molecule. Automated partitioning can be

A *Overview of genetic & molecular testing methodologies used in the evaluation of hematologic disorders*

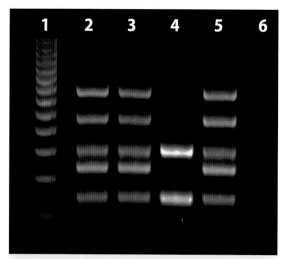

fA.6 PCR products visualized using gel electrophoresis; lane 1 contains DNA fragments of known sizes, which serve as *molecular weight markers* or a *ladder* for accurate sizing of DNA fragments in other lanes; lanes 2 & 3 are patient specimens, lane 4 is a positive abnormal control, & lane 5 is a normal test control, while lane 6 is a no template or blank control; patient 2 & patient 3 show a normal result

Detection & analysis of PCR products

Downstream detection of PCR products can be done in several ways, with gel electrophoresis being the most common visualization method. This involves separating nucleic acid fragments in a solid phase with an electric current, then staining the nucleic acids with an intercalating dye, such as ethidium bromide. The stained fragments are detected using a UV light source and imaging system **fA.6**. Other methods for product detection include capillary electrophoresis, Southern blot, and direct sequencing.

In summary, these and other variations in PCR protocols and methods of detection allow for a wide array of molecular assays that are routinely used for the diagnosis and monitoring of hematologic disease. Although the mechanism of PCR is essentially unchanged, novel methods of PCR-based testing continue to advance our ability to understand and evaluate these complex neoplasms.

Sanger sequencing

Sanger sequencing was the first method of DNA sequencing widely used clinically and is still used today for cost-effective sequencing of short stretches of DNA in small batches. The Sanger method directly determines each base in sequence using a chain termination strategy that involves synthesis of DNA complementary to the target strand with oligonucleotide primers and random incorporation of ddNTPs, which lack a 3' hydroxyl group. DNA polymerase can incorporate the ddNTPs at their 5' end, but without a 3' OH, a subsequent phosphodiester bond cannot form and the chain is terminated.

In the traditional Sanger method, a separate reaction occurs for each base, A, C, T, and G, with high levels of conventional dNTPs and low levels of analog ddNTPs to facilitate competition that results in sporadic, but specific chain termination. This results in production of a variety of DNA strand lengths that share the same 5' sequencing primer. The different DNA strands are then sorted by size on a gel and their linear pattern reveals the sequence. In the automated Sanger method, the ddNTPs are labelled with different fluorescent dyes and all reactions occur together at the same time; the resulting fragments are organized by size in a single gel lane, and as they migrate, the dyes are activated by a stationary laser. The fluorescence emissions are recorded by a detector and converted to an inferred base

attained by creating "water-in-oil" emulsion (emulsion-based ddPCR) or using a chip with a microchannel (microfluidics-based ddPCR). In emulsion-based ddPCR, a droplet generator partitions samples into ~20,000 individual, nanoliter-sized aqueous-droplet compartments containing PCR reagents and 1 (or possibly no) DNA molecule; the droplets are cycled to end point, with separate PCR reactions occurring within each compartment. After amplification, the reader analyzes each compartment using a dual color fluorescence detection system, counting individual compartments (droplets) in single file as positive or negative for the target sequence. Using Poisson statistics, which rely on the random distribution of target sequences across compartments of the same volume, the sample's starting amount of target DNA can be inferred from the observed distribution. This concentration is determined from the number of positive droplets out of the total droplets, rather than being inferred from a curve such as in qPCR. ddPCR works well in the presence of inhibitory contaminants and is currently the most accurate quantitative PCR method.

ISBN 978-089189-6814

A *Overview of genetic & molecular testing methodologies used in the evaluation of hematologic disorders*

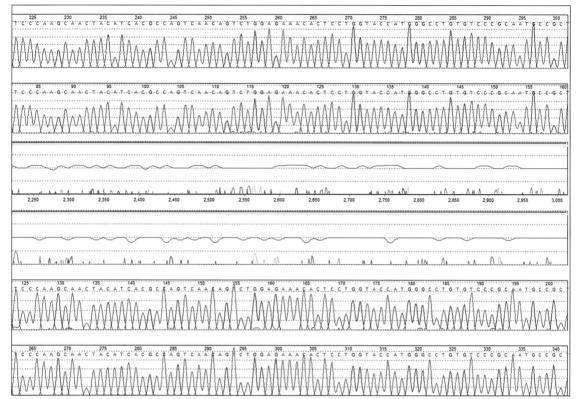

fA.7 Result of automated Sanger sequencing. An electropherogram from a PCR product is shown. The sequencing reaction includes target DNA & DNA polymerase with high levels of normal dNTPs & low levels of analog ddNTPs, which are fluorescently labeled. When a ddNTP is randomly incorporated, the polymerase stops ("chain termination"). When individual synthesized products are aligned by size, the resultant fluorescent signals at the end of each product then indicate the target sequence. Each peak in the electropherogram represents a single nucleotide in the DNA sequence, with each nucleotide represented by a different color; A is green, T is red, C is blue, and G is black

sequence **fA.7**. Sanger sequencing is the gold standard for confirming variations in the genome; however, its lower sensitivity requires at least 15%-20% variant DNA to be present within a sample, making it less desirable for testing of disease having clonal heterogeneity such as malignancy.

Next generation sequencing (NGS)

In contrast to the linear strategy of Sanger sequencing, NGS or massively parallel sequencing, refers to the sequencing of many shorter segments of target DNA simultaneously, with subsequent use of sophisticated informatics algorithms to reconstruct the original template from amplified, overlapping sequences. This technique allows for the sequencing of millions of fragments simultaneously with a typical limit of detection of 1% variant sequence out of total amplified sequences (also known as "reads"), and also allows for analysis of multiple genes in 1 reaction with the construction of large multi-gene panels. So-called

"targeted" panels analyze only "hotspots" (disease-related regions) of a gene rather than the entire gene sequence. There are multiple commercialized NGS platforms (eg, Illumina, Ion Torrent) that vary in their exact technique and instrumentation but follow the same general workflow of target preparation, target amplification, sequencing, and data imaging with bioinformatics.

Regardless of the platform used, the first step in NGS is to create a collection of DNA sequences termed a library, and to prepare them for sequencing. Library preparation starts with long pieces of isolated genomic DNA that are then broken into smaller pieces with blunted ends to be fitted with adapters. Adapters are known DNA oligonucleotide sequences that serve as primer-binding sites as well as include a barcode sequence that is unique to each patient. Because multiple patient libraries can be sequenced simultaneously ("multiplexing"), the DNA barcode is

A *Overview of genetic & molecular testing methodologies used in the evaluation of hematologic disorders*

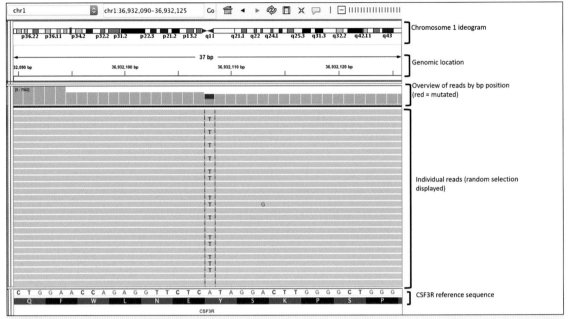

fA.8 Example of analyzed NGS data for CSF3R p.Y787* (c.2361T>A), detected at 50% variant allele frequency & resulting in a premature stop codon (TAA; see also **Case 4**). Data were analyzed & sorted using Integrated Genomics Viewer software (used throughout this book). The reference amino acid & nucleotide sequences are shown at the bottom. Each horizontal gray bar in the main area of the figure represents a single read (individual sequence resultant from the amplification reaction). Individual nucleotide changes throughout the reads are shown as colored base letters & will often represent background "noise". However, a recurring mutation is present, colored in red and outlined in brackets; the reverse strand is shown, so the mutation appears in this view as A>T

necessary as a label that assigns amplification products to individual patients.

After library preparation, the samples can undergo either whole exome sequencing directly, or more practically, target enrichment, which increases efficiency and sensitivity by isolating the genes/gene segments of interest. There are several methods used for target enrichment, each with its own applications and limitations, including hybrid capture and amplicon sequencing. Most clinical laboratories are interested in interrogating regions with pathologic or therapeutic significance and proceed with target enrichment accordingly.

The enriched library is then amplified by PCR and sequenced using the chemistries specific to each platform. After the parallel sequencing reactions occur, the millions of sequence reads generated are read and sorted by specialized software, which also aligns reads to a genomic reference sequence in a binary format that allows for storing and analyzing the data in a "BAM" file **fA.8**. During the amplification reaction, it is common for multiple variant sequences to be generated for

a single targeted region; many of these variants are artifactual background "noise" induced by the reaction itself. Thus, the significance of abnormal results must be interpreted by a trained molecular pathologist using online databases and current literature to determine which variants are to be considered both non-artifact and also pathogenic (vs a SNP), a process known as "variant calling."

The final NGS report should list individual pathogenic variants detected as well as information on their relative percentage to wildtype, reported as variant allele frequency (VAF). The VAF is the percentage of variant reads detected out of all reads generated for a targeted region and is an estimate of clonal burden within a given sample. Most pathogenic variants are heterozygous and therefore occur with <50% VAF. However, if LOH or duplication of the mutation occurs, the VAF may approach 100%. Integrated Genome Viewer (IGV) is a common software platform used to visualize NGS data and contains features for identification of sequencing and analysis artifacts, while supporting viewing of large-scale structural variants detected by paired-end read technology.

A *Overview of genetic & molecular testing methodologies used in the evaluation of hematologic disorders*

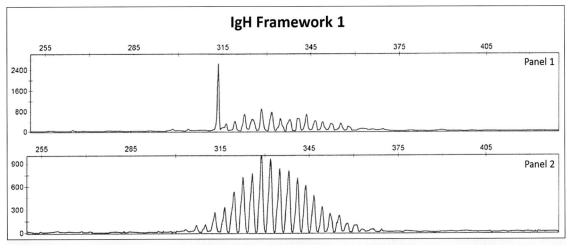

fA.9 PCR-based B-cell clonality assay using fragment length analysis. The PCR primers target the framework 1 region of the immunoglobulin heavy chain gene (IgH). Size of individual reaction products (fragments) is indicated in the top axis in base pairs, while the y axis indicates amount of each detected fragment. Panel 1 demonstrates a sample having a clonal spike within the valid size range (~310-360 bp). Panel 2 appears polyclonal with multiple peaks in a Gaussian distribution present in the appropriate size range; an appreciable clonal spike is absent, although it is possible that a tiny, obscured clonal population is present and below detection threshold

Specialized techniques for evaluating clonality in lymphoid populations

In ontogeny, each individual B and T cell physiologically undergoes its own independent immunoglobulin or T-cell receptor gene rearrangement, respectively, resulting in a robust and diverse (or polyclonal) immune repertoire. Over-proliferation of 1 lymphocyte results in a detectable predominance of 1 specific gene rearrangement (ie, a monoclonal population). The demonstration of a monoclonal immunoglobulin or T-cell receptor gene rearrangement suggests a neoplastic process and may be critical for the evaluation of lymphoid neoplasms, although clonal lymphoid populations may also be present in reactive conditions. Thus, while specialized molecular assays are highly useful for the detection of lymphocyte clonality, the results must always be interpreted within clinical and histologic context.

PCR-based fragment length analysis is currently the most widely used technique for assessment of lymphoid clonality. For T-cell receptor (TCR) assays, DNA is amplified using primers that target the conserved framework (FR) and joining (J) regions or the diversity (D) and J regions of the TCR β chain (TCRB), or the variable (V) and J regions of the TCR γ chain (TCRG). These conserved regions lie on either side of the hypervariable portion of the V-J region which is unique to each TCR in both length and sequence. A similar strategy is applied when evaluating the immunoglobulin

(Ig) receptor for B cells. When a hypervariable region is amplified using DNA primers that flank this region, a polyclonal population generates many different-sized products that form a bell-shaped curve (Gaussian distribution) around a statistically favored, average-sized rearrangement. In contrast, a clonal population of cells yields 1 or 2 prominent amplified products, or peaks, within the expected size range **fA.9**. Oligoclonal populations will produce several peaks using this method and may cause difficulties in interpretation. Generally, oligoclonal peaks are smaller in size than a single monoclonal peak; oligoclonal peaks may also be artifactual and as such will disappear upon repeat analysis. In addition, biopsies having limited material or low-level infiltrates can lead to selective amplification of a limited number of lymphocytes, yielding a false positive monoclonal or oligoclonal pattern. Guidelines have been published for interpreting peaks when using the most common primer sets. The limit of detection of typical lymphoid clonality assays is ~5 clonal cells in 100 normal cells or 5%.

For MRD detection, fragment length-based assays are not as sensitive as newer NGS-based lymphoid clonality assays, which directly sequence Ig or TCR amplicons. NGS-based clonality assays (such as clonoSEQ® from Adaptive Technologies) are currently being used in some academic centers for monitoring disease in patients having B-cell neoplasms such as lymphoma, lymphoblastic leukemia and myeloma. These assays require initial analysis of the diagnostic specimen for detection of a predominant, presumed neoplastic, sequence, which must be present at a predetermined threshold level before being designated as the clonal sequence. Subsequent follow-up samples can then be assayed for detection and quantitation of the clonal neoplastic sequence, with reported sensitivity of approximately 1 tumor cell in 10^6 normal cells.

Summary

Myeloid and lymphoid disorders are classified based on a constellation of clinical, morphologic, immunophenotypic, and cytogenetic/molecular findings. The diagnosis, prognosis, and treatment of these diseases are increasingly contingent on recurring cytogenetic and molecular abnormalities. **tA.1** summarizes the molecular and cytogenetic techniques described in this chapter as well as their appropriate specimens and expected turnaround times (TAT).

Readings

Bagg A Immunoglobulin and T-Cell Receptor Gene Rearrangements: Minding Your B's and T's in Assessing Lineage and Clonality in Neoplastic Lymphoproliferative Disorders. J Mol Diagn. 2006 Sep; 8(4):426-429.

Beck RC, Kim AS, Goswami RS, Weinberg OK, Yeung CCS, Ewalt MD. Molecular/Cytogenetic Education for Hematopathology Fellows. Am J Clin Pathol. 2020 Jul 7;154(2):149-177. **DOI: 10.1093/ajcp/aqaa038**

Buckingham L. Molecular Diagnostics, Fundamentals, Methods, and Clinical Applications. F.A.Davis Company, 2007.

Burkholder GD. The basis of chromosome banding. Appl Cytogenet.1993;19:181-186.

Evans PA, Pott Ch, Groenen PJ, et al. Significantly improved PCR-based clonality testing in B-cell malignancies by use of multiple immunoglobulin gene targets. Report of the BIOMED-2 Concerted Action BHM4-CT98-3936. Leukemia. 2007;21(2):207-214.

Hook EB. Exclusion of chromosomal mosaicism: tables of 90%, 95% and 99% confidence limits and comments on use. Am J Hum Genet. 1977;29(1):94-97.

Mardis ER. Next-generation DNA sequencing methods. Annu Rev Genomics Hum Genet. 2008;9:387-402.

McGowan-Jordan J, Simons A, Schmid M. ISCN (2016): An International System for Human Cytogenomic Nomenclature. Karger, 2016.

Mullis KB. The unusual origin of the polymerase chain reaction. Sci Am. 1990;262(4):56-65. **DOI: 10.1038/scientificamerican0490-56**

Pfeifer, JD. Molecular Genetic Testing in Surgical Pathology. Lippincott, Williams, & Wilkins, 2006.

Siebold, Alex. "Back to the Basics: Next-Generation Sequencing 101." Agilent, 7 Jan. 2017, www.agilent. com/cs/library/eseminars/public/NGS%20Data%20 Analysis%20101.pdf.

Swerdlow, S H, Campo, E, Harris, N L, Jaffe, E S, Pileri, S A, Stein, H, Thiele, J, et al. World Health Organization Classification of Tumours of Haematopoietic and Lymphoid Tissues. 4th ed. Lyon, France: IARC Press, 2017.

van Dongen JJ, Langerak AW, Brüggemann M, et al. Design and standardization of PCR primers and protocols for detection of clonal immunoglobulin and T-cell receptor gene recombinations in suspect lymphoproliferations: report of the BIOMED-2 Concerted Action BMH4-CT98-3936. Leukemia. 2003;17(12):2257-2317.

Wolff DJ, Bagg A, Cooley LD, et al. Guidance for fluorescence in situ hybridization testing in hematologic disorders. J Mol Diagn. 2007;9(2):134-143.den Dunnen JT, Dalgleish R, Maglott DR, et al. HGVS Recommendations for the Description of Sequence Variants: 2016 Update. Hum Mutat. 2016;37(6):564-569.

ISBN 978-089189-6814   ©2021 ASCP

tA.1 Summary of molecular & cytogenetic techniques used for evaluating hematologic disorders

Technique	Common applications	Tissue sources	TAT	Comments
Karyotype (chromosome analysis)	detection of quantitative & structural chromosomal abnormalities	*fresh* tissue for culture: >3 cc of marrow aspirate or 7-10 cc of leukemic blood +/− mitogenic stimulation	4-10 days	simultaneous analysis of all chromosomes at low resolution; reveals aneuploidies, rearrangements, & large gains/losses at 3-5Mb resolution
Fluorescence in situ hybridization (FISH)	detection of specific chromosomal abnormalities and recurrent translocations	fresh or fixed tissues	1-3 days	more sensitive than karyotype but only for specific abnormalities; can be performed STAT for emergent situations such as for detection of t(15;17) *PML-RARa*
Chromosomal microarray analysis	high resolution chromosome analysis for copy number changes or loss of heterozygosity	fresh or fixed tissues	5-7 days	can be used when karyotype cultures fail, to confirm hyperploidy vs hypodiploidy with endoreduplication; may not detect low level mosaicism (typically <20%)
Polymerase chain reaction (PCR)	amplification of DNA which can be evaluated directly or used as products for subsequent assays	3-5 mL of fresh whole blood or bone marrow; fresh, frozen, or fixed tissue in EDTA; ethanol fixed cytology fluids	1-3 days	highly adaptable to many different applications; PCR inhibiting agents include heparin, formalin, decalcifying agents (B5, formic acid), heavy metals (zinc, mercury), melanin, etc sensitive to contamination
Quantitative PCR (qPCR)	detection of residual disease	3-5 mL of fresh whole blood or bone marrow.	1-3 days	quantitations inferred from a standard curve; less tolerant of contamination in small DNA samples; often combined with reverse transcriptase PCR, which may require intact RNA
Reverse transcriptase PCR	detection of residual disease or specific gene fusions	similar to quantitative PCR	1-3 days	requires intact RNA; higher sensitivity than assays requiring genomic DNA; often used with qPCR
Sanger sequencing	direct, linear sequencing of a single gene or gene region	similar to PCR	2-5 days	definitive method of sequencing; with lower sensitivity than NGS sequences only 1 gene at a time
Next generation sequencing (NGS)	used for targeted multi-gene panels; allows for multiplexing multiple patient samples	similar to PCR although less initial material is required	1-2 weeks	requires specialized instruments & software; interpretation is rendered by trained molecular & bioinformatics personnel
Lymphoid clonality testing	used to evaluate clonality of B & T cells when a lymphoproliferative disorder is suspected	similar to PCR	2-5 days	interpretation of oligoclonal patterns may be difficult; clonal populations also occur in reactive states; NGS lymphoid clonality testing has some applications in residual disease detection

TAT=turnaround time.

This table is adapted from the Molecular Techniques chapter of Practical Diagnosis of Hematologic Malignancies, volume 2, 5th edition (2010) copyright by the American Society of Clinical Pathologists

Shashirekha Shetty

A Cytogenetic & molecular nomenclature

Overview

The goal in establishing cytogenetic and molecular nomenclature is to improve communication between genetic personnel by practicing a common language. In cytogenetics, the International System for Human Cytogenomic Nomenclature (ISCN) 2016 is the standard document used to describe karyotype, FISH, and MCA results and is also used in the research literature.

Karyotype nomenclature

Modal number, sex chrom, abn abbrev (first chrom; second chrom) (arm band number; arm band number)

Example 46, XX; t(9;22)(q34;q11.2) [20]

Interpretation 46 chromosomes, female (XX sex chromosomes), with a balanced translocation between chromosomes 9 and 22 with breakpoints in the long arm of chromosome 9 at band 9q34 and the long arm of chromosome 22 at band 22q11.2.

Modal number: total count of number of chromosomes in each cell of a given cell line.

Sex chromosomes: complement of X and Y chromosomes.

Band number: numerical description of the location on a chromosome arm, in order from the centromere out to the end of the chromosome. These numbers are a standard determined by ISCN 2016.

Brackets [#] - represents the number of metaphases analyzed, typically 20.

FISH nomenclature

The designation *nuc ish* ("nuclear in situ hybridization") is followed by locus designation in parenthesis with no space in between, a multiplication sign (×), and the number of signals seen. Brackets indicate the number of nuclei scored.

Examples with interpretations

nuc ish(ABL1, BCR)×2[400]
 – Normal signal pattern in 400 nuclei

nuc ish(ABL1, BCR)×2(ABL1 con BCR ×2)[400]
 – Abnormal signal pattern with *BCR-ABL1* fusion in 400 nuclei

nuc ish(ABL1, BCR)×2(ABL1 con BCR ×2)[300/400]
 – Abnormal signal pattern with *BCR-ABL1* in 300 nuclei and 100 normal nuclei

ISBN 978-089189-6814   ©2021 ASCP

Cytogenomics or microarray nomenclature

The results are expressed as follows, where *arr* refers to "array" with no space between arr and the opening parenthesis. The sex chromosomes are separated from autosomes.

Examples with interpretations

arr(1-22,X)×2
 – Normal female

arr(1-22)×2, (X,Y)×1
 – Normal male

arr(1-13)×2 mos hmz,(14)×2~3, (16-20)×2 mos hmz, (21)x2~3,(22)×2 mos hmz, (X)×1~2,(Y)×1~2
 – Abnormal, double near-haploid with a mix of normal and abnormal cells represented by *mos*. SNP array analysis shows mosaic homozygosity for chromosomes 1 to 13, 16 to 20, and 22. There is a copy number gain for chromosomes 14, 21, X, and Y.

Molecular nomenclature

Standard nomenclature recommendations of the Human Genome Variation Society (HGVS) can be found at http://varnomen.hgvs.org.

All variants detected by sequencing are compared to a *coding DNA reference sequence*, which is a cDNA-derived sequence containing the full length of all coding regions and noncoding untranslated regions [5' untranslated region (UTR) and 3'-UTR] and is designated by "NM". Individual genes often have multiple NM transcripts due to alternative splicing, etc. Nucleotide numbering is in relation to the translation initiation codon, starting with number 1 at the A of the ATG. Standard mutation nomenclature based on coding DNA reference sequences and protein-level amino acid sequences requires prefixes "c." and "p.", respectively.

Examples

NM_000222.2(KIT):c.1621A>C (p.M541L)
 – variant of *KIT* at base pair position 1621 with A changed to C, resulting in amino acid 541 changing from methionine to leucine

NM_004972.3(JAK2):c.1849G>T (c.V617F)
 – variant of *JAK2* at base pair position 1849 with G changed to T, resulting in amino acid 617 changing from valine to phenylalanine

Index

ISBN 978-089189-6814 ©2021 ASCP

ISBN 978-089189-6814 ©2021 ASCP

M

ISBN 978-089189-6814 ©2021 ASCP

ISBN 978-089189-6814   ©2021 ASCP